国学经典外译丛书（第一辑）

金匮要略英译

Essentials of the Golden Cabinet

（东汉）张仲景 ◎ 著

刘希茹 ◎ 今译　　李照国 ◎ 英译

上海三联书店

"十三五"国家重点图书出版规划项目

国家出版基金资助项目

达 于 上 下　敬 哉 有 土

——译事感怀

国学者，天人相应之积成，天人交融之精诚，天人合一之大成。盘古开天，国学与天地并生；伏羲造易，国学与六合并韵；炎黄树人，国学与三才并举；三代立本，国学与百族并融；秦汉统制，国学与万邦并荣。今日之高丽、扶桑、交趾，即其明证是也。

此非鄙人之见也，实乃历朝学人之志也、历代国人之意也。其志者，非梦也，非幻也，实乃春华秋实之景也；其意者，非妄也，非狂也，实乃天晴日明之象也。自三代以至汉唐，国学之神韵、国文之形意、国体之本末，皆悉传入中土之邻邦。其传者，非国人之意也，实异族之愿也。岁岁年年，高丽、扶桑、交趾，遣汉使，遣唐使，遣宋使，遣明使，跋山涉水，奔波神州。其行者，非劫财也，非谋利也，皆潜心研国学，习国文，求国典，由此而开辟夷人传承国学之坦途、光大国文之路径、珍储国典之金匮。

今日高丽所谓之韩医，扶桑所谓之汉方，交趾所谓之越医，皆随国学国文而传入之国医国药也。值此所谓之现代世界，国医于夷地，其形神意趣，则依然如故。其纯真，其淳朴，一如千秋万代之国学、国文与国医。自夏至清，中土虽时有改朝之举，虽偶有亡国之恨，然国学、国文与国医，则始终未因之而易，更未因之而亡。此态此势，非国人以命守之，实夷人以心继之。夷人既亡大汉之国，既立本族之邦，何以"继"大汉"往圣之绝学"？"木铎起而千里应，席珍流而万世响"，即其绝世之因由也。国学既"写天地之辉光"，既"晓生民之耳目"，自然感夷人而化夷邦，融百族而合万国。

惜哉！大明亡而大汉崩，大清衰而大汉丧！自鸦片之战，泰西列强，一如六淫七邪，借大清衰亡之际，侵入中土，劫江河，毁山川，破原野，欲攻赤县而灭神州。华夏之三才，由此而崩裂，炎黄之子孙，因此而昏聩。自此以来，反孔者，疑道者，日千千而年万万。时至今日，崇洋者，媚外者，已非千千万万，实乃举国上下。何以见之？"洋装"谓之"正装"，可谓不言自明矣。"洋装"谓之"正装"，"国装"何以谓之？"斜装"也？"邪装"也？何人可以告知？何人可以明之？

国医于高丽、扶桑，至今依然淳朴，依然纯真，此与其"国装"为"正装"之心境，自然一一而相应，时时而对应。国人以"洋装"为"正装"，其国医自然难以淳朴，难以纯真。其国学，自然难以传承，难以光大，甚或亦趋绝矣。国学之绝，何以见之？所谓"正装"者，皆系形之以形者也。而以夷人之教代之以儒道，则系神之以神者也。夷人之形，自有"直方大"之趣矣。其直形，其方形，其大形，可鉴可取，自然而然。荀子所谓之"善假于物"，即言此矣。夷人之教也，乃其祖之传，其宗之缘，国人理应知之，理应明之，此乃彼此相尊相敬是也。恰如邻人之父母，彼此知之敬之，共和同合。所谓"远亲不如近邻"，即言此举之要也。彼此虽相尊相敬，然彼之父母皆彼之父母，绝非此之父母，岂能取而代之！此理可谓人人知之，然其理之上者，其理之深者，却并非人人知之，更非人人明之。

如今中土之国医，皆遍布泰西之盗汗；神州之国药，皆洞穿西洋之涎沫。其历来之精气神韵，皆若寒冬腊月之日辉，明而无温，亮而无暖。此皆系传夷人之教、行夷人之理、遵夷人之道之故尔。国学乃国医之根，国文乃国药之本。国学绝矣，国医何以行健？国文异矣，国药何以载物？今日之神州，仰观而无吐曜，俯查而无含章。其故不辩自明矣。倘若"君子终日乾乾"，国人何以至此？"黄河之水天上来"，其水虽黄矣，必自然矣。所谓"天聪明，自我民聪明"，即言此矣。倘若"黄河之水泰西来"，其水虽清矣，然必毒矣。之所以毒矣，皆因化学元素变幻之故尔。今日闹市所售之诸水，即化学变幻之象尔，其毒矣，可谓无人不知，无人不晓。

自明晰天理以来，鄙人常告知友人学子，人人皆有两系基因，一则生理，与生俱来，无需求索。二则文化，全凭自力，仅求索而不可得，唯

达于上下 敬哉有土

修身而方可具。惜哉！此理虽可人人知之，然身处物化时代，何人甘愿自修、自取、自得？

以译事观之，则学界国之意识、民之见识、我之胆识，可谓淡而无象矣。国人之"龙"，谓之始祖。"龙之传人"，即谓此矣。然不知何人、何时、何因、何意，竟以泰西之 dragon 对译国人之"龙"。泰西所谓之 dragon，非华夏始祖之"龙"矣，实乃恶邪也，豺狼也。西人所谓之 monster，即喻 dragon 是矣。故而以 dragon 译"龙"，即以恶邪之喻神州也；以 descendants of dragon 译"龙之传人"，即以鬼魅之喻国人也。若神州为邪恶，若国人为鬼魅，岂能善乎夷人？岂能和乎异族？鄙人曾呼学界、译界、政界，明其善恶，辨其是非，除其正反。惜哉！时至今日，山依然高，水依然深。

自鸦片之战至今，泰西之言、文、学、教，一如今日之雾、霾、沙、尘，铺天盖地攻九州，山呼海啸陷神州。如今之举国上下，皆谓泰西之 Bible"圣经"，皆谓西洋之 Christmas"圣诞"，即其明证是也。某冬日时节，我为台胞授课，恰逢西洋之 Christmas，课间学子拱手谓之曰："耶诞快乐！"吾闻之不禁慨然，随问之曰："何以谓 Christmas 耶诞矣？"学子曰："吾等皆国人也。国人之'圣诞'，唯孔子之诞辰是也。"吾闻之，面红而耳赤，心酸而气滞。课后离席，魂消魄散，愧羞难已。自此以来，我以此为症痕，时常告诫学人学子。然所获者，唯子乎者也是矣。

惜哉！惜哉！

《淮南子》曰："以中制外，百事不废；中能得之，则外能收之。"此"中"若喻之"中土"，此"外"若喻之"外夷"，则国人将因之而"知所先后，则近道矣"。此乃鄙人译解《内经》、《难经》之所感也，译释《伤寒》、《金匮》之所悟也。此感此悟，非偏异之见也，实举目之望也，侧耳之闻也，扪心之问也，刻骨之切也。

李照国

丙申年五月初十于华亭康馨园

凡 例

1. 本译本以上海科学技术出版社出版的《伤寒论译释》为基础,并参考了历朝历代以及现代诸家的释本。

2. 译文每节文字包括三个部分,即"原文"、"今译"和"英译","今译"是用白话文对"原文"的释义,在此基础上将其译为英文。

3. 译文原则上以原文的文字结构和表达形式为基础,因表达需要而增加的英文单词或句子均附在方括号[ ]之中。

4. 译文中有些概念或术语出于对原文结构的传承,以直译或音译的形式予以表达,但对其实际含义则以圆括号( )的形式附录于后,作为文内注解。

5. 原文基本概念和术语原则上在译文中保持统一。但有时虽然是同一个概念和词语,但其含义则因背景的不同而有所变化,所以译文也有所调整。

6. 根据中医基本名词术语国际标准化的发展趋势,本书的所有剂量单位均采用音译,个别采用意译,基本形式和释义如下:

传统剂量单位	公制剂量单位	音译(或意译)形式
石	60 公斤	*dan*
斤	500 克	*jin*
两	31.25 克	*liang*
钱	3.125 克	*qian*
分	0.3125 克	*fen*
朱	1.3 克	*zhu*
斗	2 公升	*dou*

传统剂量单位	公制剂量单位	音译（或意译）形式
升	200 毫升	*sheng*
合	20 毫升	*ge*
钱匕	1.5—1.8 克	*qianbi*
方寸匕	5 毫升	*fangcunbi*
枚	颗、粒、片	*piece*

7. 中药和方剂名称的翻译，采用"四保险"的方式，以保证译文不出现任何差错，因为汉语同音字比较多。所谓"四保险"，即音译之后以括号形式附以中文、英文和拉丁文。如"人参"译为：Renshen（人参，ginseng，Radix Ginseng）。

8. 中文的"龙"，英文常译作 dragon，显然很不符合实际。"龙"是中华民族最具代表性的传统文化之一，而 dragon 则是西方人想象中的邪恶动物。所以西方对华友好的汉学家明确反对将"龙"译作 dragon，建议予以音译。所以本书将"龙骨"译作：Longgu（龙骨，Loong bone，Os Loong），而不译作 Longgu（龙骨，dragon bone，Os Draconis）。

目 录

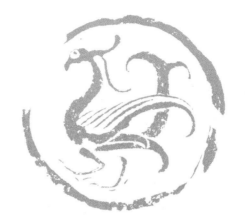

卷上

脏腑经络先后病脉证第一

【原文】

（一）

问曰：上工治未病，何也？

师曰：夫治未病者，见肝之病，知肝传脾，当先实脾。四季脾王不受邪，即勿补之。中工不晓相传，见肝之病，不解实脾，惟治肝也。

夫肝之病，补用酸，助用焦苦，益用甘味之药调之。酸入肝，焦苦入心，甘入脾。脾能伤肾，肾气微弱，则水不行；水不行，则心火气盛，则伤肺；肺被伤，则金气不行；金气不行，则肝气盛，则肝自愈。此治肝补脾之要妙也。肝虚则用此法，实则不在用之。

经曰："虚虚实实，补不足，损有余。"是其义也。余脏准此。

【今译】

问：上工治未病，是什么意思呢？

老师说：所谓治未病，举例来说，就像见到了肝病，就应该知道肝病将传到脾脏，所以应当先补脾。一年四季脾气旺盛时，就不会受邪侵袭，也就不需要补脾。一般医生不懂得这个道理，看到了肝病，就不懂得要补脾，只知道治疗肝病。

Volume 1

Volume 1

Chapter 1
Viscera, Meridians and Collaterals:
Sequence of Diseases, Pulses and Syndromes/Patterns

【英译】

Line 1. 1

Question: The great doctor only treats the disease before it has occurred. What does it mean?

The master said: To treat the disease before it has occurred [means to take measures to prevent disease from occurring]. [For example, when you have] seen the disease in the liver, [you should realize that it will] transmit from the liver to the spleen [and therefore you should take measures in advance] to strengthen the spleen. [If] in the four seasons the spleen is all strong and not attacked by pathogenic factors, there is no need to tonify the spleen. A general doctor does not know such a way [to diagnose and treat disease]. [Thus when] seeing liver disease, [he] cannot understand about how to strengthen the spleen and only treats the liver.

[To treat] liver disease, [medicinals] sour [in property should be] used to tonify [the liver], medicinals charred and bitter [in property should be used to] assist [tonification of the heart] and medicinals sweet [in property should be] used to regulate [the spleen]. Sour [flavor] enters the liver, charred and bitter [flavor]

治疗肝病,需要用酸味药来补肝,再用焦苦味的药物来补心,还要用甘味药物来调理脾脏。酸味入肝脏,焦苦味入心脏,甘味入脾脏。脾能制肾,肾气如果微弱,那么水气长久不能运行;水气不能运行,心火气就会旺盛,损伤肺脏;肺脏遭受损伤,肺气就不能运行;肺气不能运行,肝气就会旺盛,肝气旺盛则肝病就会自愈。这就是治肝补脾的妙法。肝虚就用此法治疗,肝实则不能用此法治疗。

医经上说:"虚证用泻药,虚证就更虚;实证用补药,实证就更重。补法只能用以治疗不足的病症,泻法只能用来治疗有余的病症。"说的就是这个意思,其他脏器的病变,皆可采用此法治疗。

enters the heart and sweet [flavor] enters the spleen. The spleen can control the kidney. [When] kidney qi is faint and weak, water will not move; [when] water does not move, heart fire and qi will be exuberant and the lung will be damaged. [When] the lung is damaged, lung qi cannot move. [If] lung qi cannot move, liver qi will be exuberant and liver [disease] will spontaneously heal. This is the right way to treat the liver and tonify the spleen. [If] the liver is of deficiency, this method is used; [if the spleen is of] excess, it cannot be used.

[The Medical] Canon says: "Deficiency [syndrome/pattern cannot be treated by] deficiency (purgation) and excess [syndrome/pattern cannot be treated by] excess (tonification). Insufficiency [should be] tonified and superabundance [should be] reduced. " This means what is mentioned above. [The treatment of] other viscera should follow such a way.

【原文】

(二)

夫人禀五常,因风气而生长。风气虽能生万物,亦能害万物,如水能浮舟,亦能覆舟。若五脏元真通畅,人即安和。客气邪风,中人多死。千般疢难,不越三条;一者,经络受邪,入脏腑,为内所因也;二者,四肢九窍,血脉相传,壅塞不通,为外皮肤所中也;三者,房室、金刃、虫兽所伤。以此详之,病由都尽。

若人能养慎,不令邪风干忤经络。适中经络,未流传脏腑,即医治之,四肢才觉重滞,即导引、吐纳、针灸、膏摩,勿令九窍闭塞;更能无犯王法、禽兽灾伤,房室勿令竭乏,服食节其冷热苦酸辛甘,不遗形体有衰,病则无由入其腠理。腠者,是三焦通会元真之处,为血气所注;理者,是皮肤脏腑之文理也。

【今译】

人要遵循五行的常理,其生长与自然气候息息相关。自然气候虽然能帮助万物生长,也能损害万物,就像水能浮舟也能覆舟一样。如果五脏元真之气通畅,人就能平安和合地健康生活。客气邪风严重伤害人体,就会导致死亡。疾病种类甚多,但总的来说有三类;第一类,经络遭受病邪入侵,传入脏腑,因而引起内部疾病;第二类,四肢九窍与血脉相传,壅塞不通,是外部皮肤所引起的疾病;第三类,由于房事过度、刀斧创伤、虫兽咬伤所致。按此三类情况分析,所有疾病都可以完整了解。

Volume 1

【英译】

Line 1.2

People should follow [the law of] five elements because life is integrated with natural climate. [Although] natural climate can [support] the growth of all things, [it] can also damage all things. [It is just] like water, which can float a boat, but can also capsize it. If the source qi in the five zang-organs flows freely, man will [live a] peaceful and harmonious [life]. [When] pathogenic [factors such as serious] wind attack people, death will be caused. [There are] thousands of diseases, [but] just no more than three categories. The first category is invasion of pathogenic factors into the meridians, and then entering the viscera, causing various internal [diseases]. The second category is transmission [of pathogenic factors in] the blood vessels in the four limbs and nine orifices, [causing] congestion due to attack of superficies. The third category is damage [caused by] excessive sexual intercourse, injury of metal blades and bite of insects and animals. To examine according to these [three categories], all diseases will be thoroughly understood.

If people are able to cultivate [themselves], [they will] prevent pathogenic wind from invading the meridians and collaterals. [If pathogenic factors] accidentally have invaded the meridians and collaterals, but have not transmitted to the viscera, [disease should be] treated immediately. [When] the four limbs are just felt heavy and stagnant, daoyin (a traditional way to cultivate health by guiding qi to flow naturally and smoothly all through the body), inhalation and exhalation, acupuncture and moxibustion and

如果人能注意养生，就不会令风邪侵袭经络。如果经络偶然受邪，尚未流传到脏腑，就应及时治疗。四肢刚刚感到重滞，就用导引、吐纳、针灸、膏摩等方法治疗，避免九窍闭塞不通。更不能触犯国法，要避免禽兽灾伤，房事不可过度，起居饮食要寒暖适宜，苦酸辛甘等五味要调和，不能使人体虚衰，这样病邪就不会侵入肌肤腠理。"腠"指的是三焦通会元真之处，为血气注入之处；"理"指的是皮肤与脏腑之间的纹理。

scraping with paste [should be used] to prevent blockage of the nine orifices. [Cares should be taken] to avoid violation of national laws, being injured by beasts and exhaustion due to excessive sexual intercourse. Cold and heat [should be well regulated] in wearing clothes and eating food, [and so are the tastes of] bitterness, sourness, acridness and sweetness. [Only when cares have been taken] to avoid weakening the body [can] pathogenic factors be prevented from entering the interstice and grain. Interstice refers to the site through which source [qi] and true [qi] flows, and into which blood and qi pours. Texture refers to the stripes of skin and viscera.

【原文】

(三)

问曰：病人有气色见于面部，愿闻其说。

师曰：鼻头色青，腹中痛，苦冷者死；鼻头色微黑色，有水气；色黄者，胸上有寒；色白者，亡血也。设微赤，非时者死；其目正圆者痉，不治。又色青为痛，色黑为劳，色赤为风，色黄者便难，色鲜明者有留饮。

【今译】

问：病人面部气色是怎样的，想听听您的解说。

老师说：鼻头色青的，主腹中疼痛，如果还怕冷，就可能导致死亡；鼻头色微黑的，说明内部有水气；面色黄的，说明胸上有寒气；面色白的，说明有失血。如果鼻头微赤，不该出现的时候出现，患者就可能死亡；眼睛正视转动不灵的，是痉病，不易治疗。另外面色青的，为疼痛；面色黑的，为劳损；面色红的，为风热；面色黄的，为便秘；面色鲜明的，体内有留饮。

Volume 1

【英译】

Line 1.3

Question: There are various complexions in patients. I'd like to listen to your explanation.

The master said: [If] the tip of nose is blue in color, [there is] pain in the abdomen, [and if there is] aversion to cold, [the patient will] die; [if] the tip of nose is slightly black in color, there is water qi (edema); [if] the face is yellow in color, there is cold in the chest; [if the face is] white in color, [there is] collapse of blood. If [the tip of nose is] slightly red in the time [when it should] not be so, [the patient will] die; [if] the eyes are straight and round, [it] is tetany, difficult to treat. Besides, blue color also means pain, black color means overstrain, red color means wind, yellow color means constipation and bright color means fluid retention.

【原文】

(四)

师曰：病人语声寂然喜惊呼者,骨节间病;语声喑喑然不彻者,心膈间病;语声啾啾然细而长者,头中病。

【今译】

老师说：平静的病人突然惊呼,是骨节间有病;病人声音低微不清楚,是心膈间有病;病人声音微小而长,是头中有病。

【原文】

(五)

师曰：息摇肩者,心中坚;息引胸中上气者咳;息张口短气者,肺痿唾沫。

【今译】

老师说：病人呼吸时肩膀摇动的,说明心中有实邪阻滞;病人呼吸引起胸中之气上冲,说明有咳嗽病症;病人呼吸时张口短气,说明有肺痿唾沫之症。

Volume 1

【英译】

Line 1.4

The master said: [If] a quiet patient suddenly cries, [it indicates that] the disease is in the joints; [if] the voice [of a patient] is dull and unclear, [it indicates that] the disease [is located] between the heart and diaphragm; [if] the voice [of a patient] is faint and long, [it indicates that] the disease [is located] in the head.

【英译】

Line 1.5

The master said: [The patient's] shoulders are shaking when breathing, [indicating] hardness in the heart; qi surging up from the chest [when the patient is] breathing [indicates disease with] cough; shortness of breath [when the patient] opens the mouth to breathe [indicates] lung wilting with spitting of drool.

【原文】

（六）

师曰：吸而微数，其病在中焦，实也，当下之即愈，虚者不治；在上焦者，其吸促；在下焦者，其吸远，此皆难治。呼吸动摇振振者，不治。

【今译】

老师说：病人呼吸微数，说明病在中焦，为实证，应当用下法治愈，如果病人身体虚弱，就不易治疗。病在上焦的，呼吸急促；病在下焦的，呼吸深长，都很难治。呼吸时全身动摇震颤的，更难治疗。

【原文】

（七）

师曰：寸口脉动者，因其王时而动，假令肝王色青，四时各随其色。肝色青而反色白，非其时色脉，皆当病。

【今译】

老师说：寸口脉搏动，是因其随季节而变动，如果肝旺季节色青的，四时所表现的颜色都与此相关。肝旺的季节其色应为青，但反而为白的，就不是该季节应有的颜色和脉象，都属于疾病的表现。

Volume 1

【英译】

Line 1.6

The master said: Faint and rapid breath [indicates that] the disease is in the middle energizer, [it is an] excess [syndrome/ pattern] and can be cured by purgation. [If the patient is] weak, [it is] difficult to treat. [If the disease is] in the upper energizer, while the breath is hasty; [if the disease is] in the lower energizer, while the breath is deep and long, [they are] difficult to treat; [if the body is] shaking [when the patient is] breathing, [it is] very difficult to treat.

【英译】

Line 1.7

The master said: [When] cunkou pulse is moving, [it is] the result of [its adaptation to] the movement [in the season when the liver] is effulgent. If it is blue [in the season when] the liver is effulgent, all [the viscera] will follow such [a change of] color. [When] the effulgent liver should be blue in color but actually is white in color, [it is] not the normal color and pulse [condition], all indicating disease.

【原文】

（八）

问：有未至而至，有至而不至，有至而不去，有至而太过，何谓也？

师曰：冬至之后，甲子夜半少阳起，少阳之时阳始生，天得温和。以未得甲子，天因温和，此为未至而至也；以得甲子，而天未温和，此为至而不至也；以得甲子，而天大寒不解，此为至而不去也；以得甲子，而天温和如盛夏五六月时，此为至而太过也。

【今译】

问：典籍上说，有未至而至，有至而不至，有至而不去，有至而太过。这是什么意思呢？

老师说：冬至节之后，甲子日夜半少阳起始，少阳起始之时阳气开始产生，天气逐步变得温和。如果冬至后甲子之日未到，但天气却变得温和了，这就是"未至而至"的意思；甲子之日已经到了，但天气并未变得温和，这就是"至而不至"的意思；甲子之日已经到了，但天气却大寒不解，这就是"至而不去"的意思；甲子之日已经到了，但天气却温热得像盛夏五六月份的时候，这就是"为至而太过"的意思。

Volume 1

【英译】

Line 1.8

Question: [Medical Canon says:] There are [problems that] the one has not arrived but the other has arrived, the one has arrived but the other has not arrived, the one has arrived but the other has not left, the one has arrived but it is too hyperactive. What does it mean?

The master said: After winter solstice, at the midnight of the jiazi day (60 days after winter solstice), shaoyang begins to rise. The time [when] shaoyang [begins to rise], yang [qi] starts to grow and the weather becomes warm. [If] the weather is warm [but] the jiazi day has not arrived yet, this is what "the one has not arrived but the other has arrived" means; [if] the jiazi day has already arrived, but the weather is not warm, this is what "the one has arrived but the other has not arrived" means; [if] the jiazi day has already arrived but the weather is very cold and difficult to resolve, this is what "the one has arrived but the other has not left" means; [if] the jiazi day has arrived, but the weather is as hot as that in May and June in summer, this is what "the one has arrived but it is too hyperactive" means.

【原文】

(九)

师曰：病人脉浮者在前，其病在表；浮者在后，其病在里，腰痛背强不能行，必短气而极也。

【今译】

老师说：病人脉浮见于关前的寸部，说明病在表；病人脉浮见于关后的尺部，说明病在里，所以腰痛背强不能行动，必然引起气短困倦。

【原文】

(十)

问曰：经云厥阳独行，何谓也？师曰：此为有阳无阴，故称厥阳。

【今译】

问：医经上说，"厥阳独行"。这是什么意思呢？

老师说：意思是说，只有阳没有阴，所以称为厥阳。

Volume 1

【英译】

Line 1.9

The master said: Floating pulse in patients that appears before [the guan region and in the cun region] indicates the disease [located] in the external; floating [pulse] that appears after [the guan region and in the chi region] indicates the disease [located] in the internal. [The manifestations include] pain of the waist, stiffness of the back, inability to move, shortness of breath and extreme [fatigue].

【英译】

Line 1.10

Question: [The Medical Canon says:] "Reversal yang moves alone". What does it mean?

The master said: That means that there is only yang without yin. That is why it is called reversal yang.

【原文】

(十一)

问曰：寸脉沉大而滑，沉则为实，滑则为气，实气相搏，血气入脏即死，入腑即愈，此为卒厥。何谓也？

师曰：唇口青，身冷，为入脏，即死；如身和，汗自出，为入腑，即愈。

【今译】

问：寸口脉象沉大而滑，脉象沉为血实，脉象滑为气实，血实和气实相搏，血气就会入脏，造成死亡，血气入腑就会治愈，这就叫卒厥。这是什么意思呢？

老师说：口唇为青，身体寒冷，这就是血气入脏的表现，就会导致死亡；如果全身温和，有汗自出，这就是血气入腑，就易于治愈。

Volume 1

【英译】

Line 1. 11

[Question]: Cunkou pulse is sunken, large and slippery. Sunken [pulse] indicates [blood] excess and slippery [pulse] indicates qi [excess]. [When blood] excess and qi [excess] contend with each other, blood and qi will enter the zang-organs and [cause] death. [When blood and qi] have entered the fu-organs, [the disease is easy to be] cured. This is called fainting suddenly. What is the reason?

The master said: Blue lips and cold body indicate [that blood and qi] have entered the zang-organs and [will cause] death. If the body is warm and there is spontaneous sweating, [it] indicates [that blood and qi] have entered the fu-organs and [the disease is easy to be] cured.

【原文】

（十二）

问曰：脉脱入脏即死，入腑即愈，何谓也？

师曰：非为一病，百病皆然。譬如浸淫疮，从口起流向四肢者，可治，从四肢流来入口者，不可治。病在外者可治，入里者即死。

【今译】

问：脉脱而邪入脏，即会导致死，邪入腑则易于治愈，这是什么原因呢？

老师说：这并不是脉脱这一种病，百病皆是如此。比如浸淫疮，从口发生蔓延到四肢，就可以治愈，但从四肢蔓延入口，就不可治愈。病在外的可以治愈，病入里的就会死亡。

【英译】

Line 1. 12

Question: [When] the pulse [is] undetectable, [pathogenic factors will] enter the zang-organs and [cause] death. [When pathogenic factors] have entered the fu-organs, [the disease is easy to be] cured. What is the reason?

The master said: This is not [the case of just] one disease, [in fact] all diseases are the same. Take spreading sore for example. [When] spreading from the mouth to the four limbs, [it is] curable. [But when] spreading from the four limbs to the mouth, [it is] incurable. Disease in the external is curable while [disease] in the internal is incurable.

【原文】

(十三)

问曰：阳病十八,何谓也?

师曰：头痛,项、腰、脊、臂、脚掣痛。

阴病十八,何谓也?

师曰：咳、上气、喘、哕、咽、肠鸣、胀满、心痛、拘急。五脏病各有十八,合为九十病。人又有六微,微有十八病,合为一百八病。五劳、七伤、六极、妇人三十六病,不在其中。

清邪居上,浊邪居下,大邪中表,小邪中里,檠饪之邪,从口入者,宿食也。五邪中人,各有法度,风中于前,寒中于暮,湿伤于下,雾伤于上,风令脉浮,寒令脉急,雾伤皮腠,湿流关节,食伤脾胃,极寒伤经,极热伤络。

【今译】

问：阳病有十八种,指的是什么呢?

老师说：头痛,项、腰、脊、臂、脚掣痛。

问：阴病有十八种,指的是什么呢?

老师说：咳、上气、喘、哕、咽、肠鸣、胀满、心痛、拘急。五脏的病各有十八,合起来为九十种。人又有六微,又各有十八病,合起来共有一百零八种。五劳、七伤、六极、妇女三十六种病,不在其中。

雾霾这样的清邪居于上,水湿这样的浊邪居于下,风邪这样的大邪多伤于表,寒邪这样的小邪多伤于里,饮食失节所造成的病邪,从口而入,即宿食。风、寒、湿、雾、饮食这样的五种病邪伤人,各有规律,风邪侵袭主要在上午,寒邪侵袭主要在下午,湿邪伤人体于下部,雾邪伤人体于上部,风邪使脉象浮,寒邪使脉象急,雾邪伤皮腠,湿邪则流入关节,食邪则损伤脾胃,寒邪盛则伤经,热邪盛则伤络。

Volume 1

【英译】

Line 1. 13

Question: There are 18 kinds of yang diseases. What are they?

The master answered: They include headache and pulling pain in the neck, waist, spine, arm and foot.

[Question]: There are 18 kinds of yin diseases. What are they?

The master answered: They include cough, asthma, panting, belching, dysphagia, borborygmus, abdominal fullness, heart pain and spasm. In the five zang-organs, each [of them] has 18 kinds of diseases, altogether there are 90. [Usually] people have six mild [pathological conditions], each [of which] has 18 kinds of diseases, altogether there are 108 diseases. [But] five kinds of overstrain, seven kinds of damage, six kinds of extreme [exhaustions] and thirty-six woman diseases are not involved in these diseases.

Clear pathogenic factors (fog and haze) are in the upper and turbid pathogenic factors (water and dampness) are in the lower. Major pathogenic factors attack the external while minor pathogenic factors attack the internal. Cereal pathogenic factor that has entered [the internal] from the mouth [causes] retention of undigested food. The five kinds of pathogenic factors attack human beings in their own way. [Pathogenic] wind attacks [human beings] in the morning, [pathogenic] cold attacks [human beings] in the afternoon, [pathogenic] dampness damages the lower part [of human body] and [pathogenic] fog damages the upper part [of human body]. [Pathogenic] wind makes the pulse floating, [pathogenic] cold makes the pulse tense, [pathogenic] fog damages the skin and interstices, [pathogenic] dampness flows into the joints, [pathogenic] food damages the spleen and stomach, extreme cold damages the meridians and extreme heat damages the collaterals.

【原文】

（十四）

问曰：病有急当救里救表者，何谓也？

师曰：病，医下之，续得下利清谷不止，身体疼痛者，急当救里；后身体疼痛，清便自调者，急当救表也。

【今译】

问：有的病先要急救其里，然后再救治其表。这是为什么呢？

老师说：如果医生误用攻下法治疗在表之病，就会造成持续不断的下利清谷，虽然身体疼痛，但还是应当急救其里。治疗后如果病人依然身体疼痛，但大便已经恢复正常，就应急救其表。

【原文】

（十五）

夫病痼疾，加以卒病，当先治其卒病，后乃治其痼疾也。

【今译】

平素有痼疾的病人，新病旧病均有，应当先治其新病，后治其痼疾。

【英译】

Line 1.14

Question: [In treating] diseases, [doctors] sometimes quickly rescue the internal, then quickly rescue the external. What is the reason?

The master answered: [In treating] diseases, [if] doctors [have wrongly used] purgation, there will be incessant diarrhea with undigested food. [Even if there is] generalized pain, [measures should be taken] to quickly rescue the internal. [If there is] still generalized pain [after application of purgation] and defecation is spontaneously normalized, [measures should be taken] to quickly rescue the external.

【英译】

Line 1.15

[In a patient, some times] the old disease [is not cured yet], [but] a new disease has occurred. [Doctor] should first treat the new disease and then treat the old disease.

【原文】

(十六)

师曰：五脏病各有所得者愈，五脏病各有所恶，各随其所不喜者为病。病者素不应食，而反暴思之，必发热也。

【今译】

老师说：五脏疾病，各有其所适应的饮食。能得到所适应的饮食，就能逐步治愈。五脏疾病，也各有其所不适应的饮食。如果食用了不适应的饮食，病情就会加重。如果病人突然想吃自己平素不喜欢的饮食，就会提升病气，必然引起发热。

【原文】

(十七)

夫诸病在脏，欲攻之，当随其所得而攻之，如渴者，与猪苓汤。余皆仿此。

【今译】

凡在内脏的病，如果治疗时想采用攻下法，应当根据其所得的病邪而攻下。如有口渴，可用猪苓汤治疗。其他疾病的治疗均可按此方法进行。

【英译】

Line 1. 16

[In] five zang-organs diseases, each of them needs [certain food appropriate for it]. [When they] have obtained [what are appropriate for them], [the diseases will be eventually] cured. [In] the five zang-organs diseases, each of them dislikes [certain food inappropriate for it]. [When they] have obtained [what is inappropriate for them], [the diseases will be] worsened. [If] the patient suddenly wants to eat what he usually dislikes to eat, [pathogenic qi will] immediately increase and inevitably cause heat.

【英译】

Line 1. 17

[In treating] visceral diseases, attacking and purging [therapies] can be used according to the pathogenic factors that have attacked it. If there is thirst, Zhuling Decoction (猪苓汤, polyporus decoction) [can be used] to treat it. [Treatment of] the other [diseases] also can follow such a way.

痉湿暍病脉证治第二

【原文】

（一）

太阳病，发热无汗，反恶寒者，名曰刚痉。

【今译】

太阳病患者，身体发热而无汗，反而有恶寒症状的，称为刚痉。

【原文】

（二）

太阳病，发热汗出，而不恶寒，名曰柔痉。

【今译】

太阳病患者，身体发热而汗出，但却不恶寒的，称为柔痉。

Volume 1

Chapter 2
Tetany, Dampness and Summer Disease:
Pulses, Syndrome/Patterns and Treatment

【英译】

Line 2. 1

Taiyang disease, [characterized by] fever, no sweating and aversion to cold, is called hard tetany.

【英译】

Line 2.2

Taiyang disease, [characterized by] fever, sweating and no aversion to cold, is called soft tetany.

【原文】

（三）

太阳病，发热，脉沉而细者，名曰痉，为难治。

【今译】

太阳病患者，身体发热，脉象沉而细的，称为痉，很难治疗。

【原文】

（四）

太阳病，发汗太多，因致痉。

【今译】

太阳病患者，发汗太多，因而导致痉的发作。

【原文】

（五）

夫风病，下之则痉，复发汗，必拘急。

【今译】

外感风邪为病，误用下法则可导致痉病，再度发汗后，必然引起筋脉拘急。

【英译】

Line 2.3

Taiyang disease, [characterized by] fever, sunken and thin pulse, is called tetany, very difficult to treat.

【英译】

Line 2.4

[In] taiyang disease, excessive sweating causes tetany.

【英译】

Line 2.5

In wind disease, purgation will cause tetany and repeated [application of] diaphoresis will cause spasm.

【原文】

（六）

疮家虽身疼痛，不可发汗，汗出则痓。

【今译】

身患疮疡的病人虽然身体疼痛，但不可用发汗法治疗，汗出后就会引发痓病。

【原文】

（七）

病者身热足寒，颈项强急，恶寒，时头热，面赤目赤，独头动摇，卒口噤，背反张者，痓病也。若发其汗者，寒湿相得，其表益虚，即恶寒甚。发其汗已，其脉如蛇。

【今译】

病人身体发热，足部寒冷，颈项部强直拘急，恶寒，时时感到头部发热，面红目赤，唯有头部摇动，牙关突然紧闭，背部反张，这就是痓病。如果用发汗之法治疗，寒湿就会搏结，卫表就会更虚，恶寒因此更甚。发汗以后，其脉就屈曲如蛇一样。

【英译】

Line 2.6

Although the patient with sores suffers from generalized pain, diaphoresis cannot be used [because] sweating causes tetany.

【英译】

Line 2.7

The disease, [characterized by] generalized fever, cold feet, stiffness of the neck and nape, aversion to cold, occasionally heat in the head, red face and eyes, shaking of the head only, sudden lockjaw and rigidity of the back, is tetany disease. If sweating is promoted, cold and dampness will be worsened, and the external will be even more weakened, indicating that aversion to cold is severe. After promoting sweating, the pulse will move like a snake.

【原文】

(八)

暴腹胀大者,为欲解,脉如故,反伏弦者,痉。

【今译】

患者突然腹部胀大,这是病情好转的征兆,脉象如果不变,反而伏弦,说明是痉病。

【原文】

(九)

夫痉脉,按之紧如弦,直上下行。

【今译】

痉病的脉象,按时寸关尺三部之脉象均紧而弦。

【原文】

(十)

痉病有灸疮,难治。

【今译】

有灸疮的人患痉病,就很难治。

【英译】

Line 2.8

Sudden distension and enlargement of the abdomen indicates [that the disease is] about to resolve. [If] the pulse remains the same as before or becomes hidden and taut，it is tetany.

【英译】

Line 2.9

The pulse in tetany [disease] is tight and taut when pressed，moving upwards and downwards (from the cun region to the chi region).

【英译】

Line 2. 10

Tetany disease with sores [caused by] moxibustion is difficult to treat.

【原文】

（十一）

太阳病，其证备，身体强，几几然，脉反沉迟，此为痉，栝蒌桂枝汤主之。

栝蒌桂枝汤方

栝蒌根（二两）　桂枝（三两）　芍药（三两）　甘草（二两）　生姜（三两）　大枣（十二枚）

右六味，以水九升，煮取三升。分温三服，取微汗。汗不出，食顷，啜热粥发之。

【今译】

太阳病患者，具有太阳病的症状，但身体强直，不能侧转，脉象反而沉迟，这就是痉病，用栝蒌桂枝汤主治。

【英译】

Line 2. 11

[In] taiyang disease，all the symptoms and signs are present，[the patient's] body is rigid and in vain to move，and the pulse is sunken and slow. Such [a pathological condition is called] tetany. Gualou Guizhi Decoction（栝蒌桂枝汤，trichosanthes and cinnamon twig decoction）[can be used] to treat it.

Gualou Guizhi Decoction（栝蒌桂枝汤，trichosanthes and cinnamon twig decoction）[is composed of] 2 *liang* of Gualougen（栝蒌根，trichosanthes root，Radix Trichosanthis），3 *liang* of Guizhi（桂枝，cinnamon twig，Ramulus Cinnamomi），3 *liang* of Shaoyao（芍药，peony，Radix Paeoniae），2 *liang* of Gancao（甘草，licorice，Radix Glycyrrhizae Praeparata），3 *liang* of Shengjiang（生姜，fresh ginger，Rhizoma Zingiberis Recens）and 12 pieces of Dazao（大枣，jujube，Fructus Ziziphus Jujubae）.

These six ingredients are decocted in 9 *sheng* of water to get 3 *sheng* [after] boiling. [The decoction is] divided into three [doses] and taken warm to induce slight sweating. [If there is] no sweating, after a little while，[the patient can] sip hot porridge to promote sweating.

【原文】

(十二)

太阳病,无汗而小便反少,气上冲胸,口噤不得语,欲作刚痉,葛根汤主之。

葛根汤方

葛根(四两)　麻黄(三两,去节)　桂枝(三两,去皮)　芍药(二两)甘草(二两,炙)　生姜(三两)　大枣(十二枚)

右七味,咬咀,以水七升,先煮麻黄、葛根,减二升,去沫,内诸药,煮取三升,去滓。温服一升,覆取微似汗,不须啜粥,余如桂枝汤法将息及禁忌。

【今译】

太阳病患者,无汗但小便反而少,气上冲胸,牙关紧闭,不能言语,这是将要发作刚痉病的征兆,用葛根汤主治。

【英译】

Line 2. 12

[In] taiyang disease, [there is] no sweating, urine is scanty, qi surges upwards to the chest, [the patient is] unable to speak [due to] lockjaw and hard tetany is about to occur. Gegen Decoction (葛根汤, pueraria decoction) [can be used] to treat it.

Gegen Decoction (葛根汤, pueraria decoction) [is composed of] 4 *liang* of Gegen (葛根, pueraria, Radix Puerariae), 3 *liang* of Mahuang (麻黄, ephedra, Herba Ephedrae)(remove nodes), 3 *liang* of Guizhi (桂枝, cinnamon twig, Ramulus Cinnamomi)(remove the bark), 2 *liang* of Shaoyao (芍药, peony, Radix Paeoniae), 2 *liang* of Gancao (甘草, licorice, Radix Glycyrrhizae Praeparata)(broil), 3 *liang* of Shengjiang (生姜, fresh ginger, Rhizoma Zingiberis Recens) and 12 pieces of Dazao (大枣, jujube, Fructus Ziziphus Jujubae).

These seven ingredients are pounded [into small pieces] and decocted in 7 *sheng* of water. Mahuang (麻黄, ephedra, Herba Ephedrae) and Gegen (葛根, pueraria, Radix Puerariae) are boiled first to reduce 2 *sheng* [of water]. [After] removal of foam, all the other ingredients are put into [it] to boil and get 3 *sheng*. The dregs are removed and [the decoction is] taken warm 1 *sheng* [each time]. [The patient should be] covered with quilt [so as] to induce slight sweating, [and there is] no need to sip hot porridge. Methods, rest and contraindications are the same as that for Guizhi Decoction (桂枝汤, cinnamon twig decoction).

【原文】

（十三）

痉为病，胸满口噤，卧不着席，脚挛急，必齘齿，可与大承气汤。

大承气汤方

大黄（四两，酒洗）　厚朴（半斤，炙，去皮）　枳实（五枚，炙）　芒硝
（三合）

右四味，以水一斗，先煮二物，取五升，去滓，内大黄，煮取二升，去
滓，内芒硝，更上火微一二沸。分温再服，得下止服。

【今译】

痉病发作时，胸部胀满，牙关紧闭，卧睡时脊背无法接触床席，脚部
挛急，上下牙齿紧咬，可用大承气汤主治。

【英译】

Line 2. 13

［When］tetany develops into disease，［it is characterized by］chest fullness，lockjaw，lying but unable to lie on the mat，spasm of the feet and grinding of the teeth. ［It］can be treated by Da Chengqi Decoction（大承气汤，major decoction for harmonizing qi）.

Da Chengqi Decoction（大承气汤，major decoction for harmonizing qi）［is composed of］4 *liang* of Dahuang（大黄，rhubarb，Radix et Rhizoma Rhei）（wash in wine），0. 5 *jin* of Houpo（厚朴，magnolia bark，Cortex Magnoliae Officinalis）（broil and remove the bark），5 pieces of Zhishi（枳实，processed unripe bitter orange，Fructus Aurantii Imma-turus）（broil）and 3 *ge* of Mangxiao（芒硝，mirabilite，Mirabilitum）.

These four ingredients are decocted in 1 *dou* of water. Two ingredients are boiled first to get 5 *sheng* of water. ［When］the dregs are removed，Dahuang（大黄，rhubarb，Radix et Rhizoma Rhei）is added and boiled to get 2 *sheng* of water. ［When］the dregs are removed，Mangxiao（芒硝，mirabilite，Mirabilitum）is added and boiled once or twice with mild fire. ［The decoction is］divided into two［doses］and taken warm. ［When there is］defecation，stop taking［the decoction］.

【原文】

(十四)

太阳病,关节疼痛而烦,脉沉而细者,此名湿痹。湿痹之候,小便不利,大便反快,但当利其小便。

【今译】

太阳病患者,关节疼痛,烦躁不安,脉象沉而细,此证称为湿痹。湿痹的症候,主要是小便不利,大便反而畅快,但治疗应当以利其小便为先。

【原文】

(十五)

湿家之为病,一身尽疼,发热,身色如熏黄也。

【今译】

患湿病的人,周身疼痛,发热,皮肤如烟熏一样的发黄。

【英译】

Line 2. 14

Taiyang disease，[characterized by] joint pain with vexation and sunken and thin pulse，is called dampness impediment. [The symptoms and signs of] dampness impediment are inhibited urination and free defecation. But [in such a case,] urination should be made free first.

【英译】

Line 2. 15

Patients with dampness disease [usually suffer from] generalized pain，fever and yellow body as if being fumigated.

【原文】

（十六）

湿家，其人但头汗出，背强，欲得被覆向火。若下之早则哕，或胸满，小便不利，舌上如胎者，以丹田有热，胸上有寒，渴欲得饮而不能饮，则口燥烦也。

【今译】

患湿病的人，头部汗出，背部强直，只想近火取暖。如果攻下法使用得早，则会出现呃逆，或胸中胀满，小便不利，舌上湿润如胎一样，这是由于丹田有热，胸上有寒所致，虽然渴得想饮水但却不能饮水，使得口腔干燥更甚。

【原文】

（十七）

湿家下之，额上汗出，微喘，小便利者死，若下利不止者亦死。

【今译】

患湿病的人，若用下法治疗，额上就会出汗，微有气喘，小便清长频数的，病情危险。若腹泻不止的，预后也不良。

Volume 1

【英译】

Line 2. 16

Patients with dampness disease suffer from sweating over the head, rigidity of the back and desire to be covered with quilt and meet fire. If purgation is used earlier, [it will] cause hiccup, or chest fullness, inhibited urination and thick tongue fur because there is heat in dantian (cinnabar region) and cold in the chest. [If the patient feels] thirsty and wants to drink water but is unable to drink, dryness and vexation [will be caused].

【英译】

Line 2. 17

[When] the patient with dampness [disease is treated by] purgation, [there will be] sweating on the forehead with slight panting. [If] urination is disinhibited, [the patient will] die. If [there is] incessant diarrhea, [the patient will] also die.

【原文】

(十八)

风湿相搏,一身尽疼痛,法当汗出而解,值天阴雨不止,医云此可发汗,汗之病不愈者,何也? 盖发其汗,汗大出者,但风气去,湿气在,是故不愈也。若治风湿者,发其汗,但微微似欲出汗者,风湿俱去也。

【今译】

风邪与湿邪相搏,会使患者全身疼痛,治疗应用汗法解除病邪。正值天阴下雨不止,医生认为可用汗法治疗,但发汗后病却没有痊愈,这是什么原因呢? 主要是因为发汗不当,致使汗出太急太多,使得风邪虽然除去,但湿邪依然存在,所以病就无法治愈。如果治疗风湿证用发汗法,即使全身有微微的湿润之感,而不要大汗淋漓,这样才能使风湿逐步消解。

【原文】

(十九)

湿家病,身疼发热,面黄而喘,头痛,鼻塞而烦,其脉大,自能饮食,腹中和无病,病在头中寒湿,故鼻塞,内药鼻中则愈。

【今译】

湿病患者,身体疼痛,浑身发热,面黄气喘,头痛,鼻塞,烦闷,脉象大,但饮食正常,腹中调和,内脏无病,只是头中有寒湿之邪,所以鼻塞。将药纳入鼻中,病就能痊愈。

【英译】

Line 2. 18

[When] wind and dampness contend with each other, [there will appear] generalized pain [which] can be resolved only by perspiration. [If] it is cloudy and incessantly rainy, doctors say that it can [be treated by] perspiration. [But] the disease is not always cured after perspiration. What is the reason? Because diaphoresis has promoted great sweating, and although wind qi is removed, dampness qi is still present. That is why [the disease is] not cured. If wind-dampness is treated [by diaphoresis to promote sweating], sweating should be mild as if going to perspire. [In such a way of treatment,] both wind and dampness will disappear.

【英译】

Line 2. 19

Patients with dampness disease suffer from generalized pain, fever, yellow complexion, panting, headache, nasal congestion and vexation. [Besides,] the pulse is large, [the patient is] able to drink and eat, [there is] harmony in the abdomen without any disease, [indicating that there is] cold-dampness disease in the head. That is why [there is] nasal congestion. To insert medicine into the nose will cure [the disease].

【原文】

(二十)

湿家身烦疼,可与麻黄加术汤发其汗为宜,慎不可以火攻之。

麻黄加术汤方

麻黄(三两,去节) 桂枝(二两,去皮) 甘草(一两,炙) 杏仁(七十个,去皮尖) 白术(四两)

右五味,以水九升,先煮麻黄,减二升,去上沫,内诸药,煮取二升半,去滓。温服八合,覆取微似汗。

【今译】

湿病患者,烦闷,疼痛,可用麻黄加术汤发汗治疗,不可以用火攻法治疗。

【英译】

Line 2.20

［When there is］ vexation and pain in the patient with dampness ［disease］，Mahuang Decoction（麻黄汤，ephedra decoction）added with Baizhu（白术，rhizome of largehead atractylodes，Rhizoma Atractylodis Macrocephalae）［is］ the appropriate ［formula used］ to treat it. Cares should be taken to avoid using fire attack therapy.

Mahuang Decoction（麻黄汤，ephedra decoction）added with Baizhu（白术，rhizome of largehead atractyloes，Rhizoma Atractylodis Macrocephalae）［is composed of］3 *liang* of Mahuang（麻黄，ephedra，Herba Ephedrae）（remove nodes），2 *liang* of Guizhi（桂枝，cinnamon twig，Ramulus Cinnamomi）（remove the bark），1 *liang* of Gancao（甘草，licorice，Radix Glycyrrhizae Praeparata）（broil），70 pieces of Xingren（杏仁，apricot kernel，Semen Armeniacae Amarum）（remove the peel and tips）and 4 *liang* of Baizhu（白术，rhizome of largehead atractylodes，Rhizoma Atractylodis Macrocephalae）.

These five ingredients are decocted in 9 *sheng* of water. Mahuang（麻黄，ephedra，Herba Ephedrae）is boiled first to reduce 2 *sheng* of water. ［After］ removal of foam，all the other ingredients are put into it to boil and get 2.5 *sheng*. The dregs are removed and ［the decoction is］ taken warm 8 *ge* ［each time］. ［After taking the decoction, the patient is］ covered with quilt to induce slight sweating.

【原文】

(二十一)

病者一身尽疼,发热,日晡所剧者,名风湿。此病伤于汗出当风,或久伤取冷所致也。可与麻黄杏仁薏苡甘草汤。

麻黄杏仁薏苡甘草汤方

麻黄(去节,半两,汤泡) 甘草(一两,炙) 薏苡仁(半两) 杏仁(十个,去皮尖,炒)

右剉麻豆大,每服四钱匕,水盏半,煮八分,去滓。温服,有微汗,避风。

【今译】

病人全身疼痛,浑身发热,下午 3 时至 5 时病情加剧,此病情称为风湿。此病是因汗出受风所致,或因长期贪恋冷气所致。可用麻黄杏仁薏苡甘草汤主治。

【英译】

Line 2.21

[In] the patient, [the disease marked by symptoms and signs of] generalized pain all through the body with fever [that is] more serious in the late afternoon is called wind-dampness. This disease is caused by exposure to wind [when] sweating or enduring injury resulting from cold. Mahuang Xingren Yiyi Gancao Decoction (麻黄杏仁薏苡甘草汤, ephedra, apricot kernel, coix and licorice decoction) [can be used] to treat it.

Mahuang Xingren Yiyi Gancao Decoction (麻黄杏仁薏苡甘草汤, ephedra, apricot kernel, coix and licorice decoction) [is composed of] 0.5 *liang* of Mahuang (麻黄, ephedra, Herba Ephedrae) (remove the nodes and soak in boiled water), 1 *liang* of Gancao (甘草, licorice, Radix Glycyrrhizae Praeparata) (broil), 0.5 *liang* of Yiyiren (薏苡仁, coix, Semen Coicis) and 10 pieces of Xingren (杏仁, apricot kernel, Semen Armeniacae Amarum) (remove the peel and tips, and stir-fry).

These four ingredients are grated to the size of hemp seeds. [In] each dose, 4 *qianbi* [of the grated elements] is added. [These grated ingredients are] boiled in one and a half cups of water to get 8 *fen*. The dregs are removed and [the decoction is] taken warm. There is slight sweating [after taking the decoction, and therefore] wind [must be] avoided.

【原文】

(二十二)

风湿,脉浮,身重,汗出,恶风者,防己黄芪汤主之。

防己黄芪汤方

防己(一两) 甘草(半两,炒) 白术(七钱半) 黄芪(一两一分,去芦)

右剉麻豆大,每抄五钱匕,生姜四片,大枣一枚,水盏半,煎八分,去滓。温服,良久再服。喘者,加麻黄半两;胃中不和者,加芍药三分;气上冲者,加桂枝三分;下有陈寒者,加细辛三分。服后当如虫行皮中,从腰下如冰,后坐被上,又以一被绕腰以下,温,令微汗,差。

【今译】

风湿病患者,脉象浮,身体沉重,汗出,恶风,可用防己黄芪汤主治。

【英译】

Line 2.22

[Disease, characterized by] wind-dampness, floating pulse, heaviness of the body, sweating and aversion to cold, [can be] treated by Fangji Huangqi Decoction (防己黄芪汤, the root of stephania tetrandra and astragalus decoction).

Fangji Huangqi Decoction (防己黄芪汤, the root of stephania tetrandra and astragalus decoction) [is composed of] 1 *liang* of Fangji (防己, the root of stephania tetrandra, Radix Stephaniae Tetrandrae), 0.5 *liang* of Gancao (甘草, licorice, Radix Glycyrrhizae Praeparata) (fry), 7.5 *qian* of Baizhu (白术, rhizome of largehead atractylodes, Rhizoma Atractylodis Macrocephalae) and 1 *liang* and 1 *fen* of Huangqi (黄芪, astragalus, Radix Astragali) (remove the tips).

These ingredients are grated to the size of hemp seeds, each dose is scooped up 5 *qianbi*, [added with] 4 slices of Shengjiang (生姜, fresh ginger, Rhizoma Zingiberis Recens) and 1 piece of Dazao (大枣, jujube, Fructus Ziziphus Jujubae), boiling in one and a half cup of water to get 8 *fen*. The dregs are removed and [the decoction is] taken warm. To take it again, [one must] wait for a certain period of time. For panting, 0.5 *liang* of Mahuang (麻黄, ephedra, Herba Ephedrae) is added; for disharmony of the stomach, 3 *fen* of Shaoyao (芍药, peony, Radix Paeoniae) is added; for qi surging upwards, 3 *fen* of Guizhi (桂枝, cinnamon twig, Ramulus Cinnamomi) is added; for old cold in the lower part of the body, 3 *fen* of Xixin (细辛, asarum, Herba Asari) is added. After taking [the decoction, the patient will feel] as if there were worms beneath the skin and there was icy coldness from the waist downwards. [For effective treatment, the patient should] sit on the quilt and wrap the waist with another quilt to warm the body and induce slight sweating, [eventually the disease will be] cured.

【原文】

(二十三)

伤寒八九日，风湿相搏，身体疼烦，不能自转侧，不呕不渴，脉浮虚而涩者，桂枝附子汤主之。若大便坚，小便自利者，去桂加白术汤主之。

桂枝附子汤方

桂枝（四两，去皮）　生姜（三两，切）　附子（三枚，炮，去皮，破八片）　甘草（二两，炙）　大枣（十二枚，擘）

右五味，以水六升，煮取二升，去滓，分温三服。

白术附子汤方

白术（二两）　附子（一枚半，炮，去皮）　甘草（一两，炙）　生姜（一两半，切）　大枣（六枚）

右五味，以水三升，煮取一升，去滓，分温三服。一服觉身痹，半日许再服，三服都尽，其人如冒状，勿怪，即是术、附并走皮中逐水气，未得除故耳。

【今译】

伤寒发作八九日后，风邪与湿邪相搏，身体疼痛，烦躁，不能转侧，不呕吐，也不口渴，脉象浮虚而涩，宜用桂枝附子汤主治。如果大便坚硬，小便自利，可用去桂枝加白术汤主治。

Volume 1

【英译】

Line 2.23

Eight or nine days [after occurrence of] cold damage [disease], wind and dampness contend with each other, [causing] generalized pain with vexation, inability to turn [the body], no retching and thirst, floating, weak and rough pulse. Guizhi Fuzi Decoction (桂枝附子汤, cinnamon twig and aconite decoction) [can be used] to treat it. If stool is hard and urination is disinhibited, Guizhi (桂枝, cinnamon twig, Ramulus Cinnamomi) is removed and Baizhu Decoction (白术汤, largehead atractylodes rhizome decoction) is added.

Guizhi Fuzi Decoction (桂枝附子汤, cinnamon twig and aconite decoction) [is composed of] 4 *liang* of Guizhi (桂枝, cinnamon twig, Ramulus Cinnamomi)(remove the bark), 3 *liang* of Shengjiang (生姜, fresh ginger, Rhizoma Zingiberis Recens)(cut), 3 pieces of Fuzi (附子, aconite, Radix Aconiti Lateralis Preparata)(broil heavily, remove the bark and pound into eight small pieces), 2 *liang* of Gancao (甘草, licorice, Radix Glycyrrhizae Praeparata)(broil) and 12 pieces of Dazao (大枣, jujube, Fructus Ziziphus Jujubae)(break).

These five ingredients are decocted in 6 *sheng* of water to get 2 *sheng* [after] boiling. The dregs are removed and [the decoction is] divided into three [doses] and taken warm.

Baizhu Fuzi Decoction (白术附子汤, largehead atractylodes rhizome and aconite decoction) [is composed of] 2 *liang* of Baizhu (白术, rhizome of largehead atractylodes, Rhizoma Atractylodis Macrocephalae), 1.5 piece of Fuzi (附子, aconite, Radix Aconiti Lateralis Preparata) (fry heavily and remove the bark), 1 *liang* of Gancao (甘草, licorice, Radix Glycyrrhizae Praeparata) (broil), 1.5 *liang* of Shengjiang (生姜, fresh ginger, Rhizoma Zingiberis Recens)(cut) and 6 pieces of Dazao (大枣, jujube, Fructus Ziziphus Jujubae).

These five ingredients are decocted in 3 *sheng* of water to get 1 *sheng* [after] boiling. The dregs are removed and [the decoction is] divided into three [doses] and taken warm. [If the patient] feels generalized pain [after] taking the first [dose], the second [dose] is taken half a day later. [After] taking the three [doses], if the patient feels vexing, it is not strange. The reason is that Baizhu (白术, rhizome of largehead atractyloes, Rhizoma Atractylodis Macrocephalae) and Fuzi (附子, aconite, Radix Aconiti Lateralis Preparata) have penetrated into the skin to remove water qi but have failed to eliminate it.

【原文】

(二十四)

风湿相搏,骨节烦,掣痛不得屈伸,近之则痛剧,汗出短气,小便不利,恶风不欲去衣,或身微肿者,甘草附子汤主之。

甘草附子汤方

甘草(二两,炙)　附子(二枚,炮,去皮)　白术(二两)　桂枝(四两,去皮)

右四味,以水六升,煮取三升,去滓。温服一升,日三服。初服得微汗则解。能食,汗出复烦者,服五合。恐一升多者,服六七合为妙。

【今译】

风邪与湿邪相搏,骨节疼,屈伸不利,触按则疼痛加剧,汗出短气,小便不利,恶风,但却不敢脱去衣服,有的身体微肿,宜用甘草附子汤主治。

Volume 1

【英译】

Line 2.24

[When] wind and dampness contend with each other, [there will be symptoms and signs of] pain of joints with vexation, inability to stretch [the joints due to] spasmatic pain, acute pain when touched, sweating, shortness of breath, disinhibited urination, aversion to cold, no desire to remove clothes, or slight swelling of the body. Gancao Fuzi Decoction (甘草附子汤, licorice and aconite decoction) [can be used] to treat it.

Gancao Fuzi Decoction (甘草附子汤, licorice and aconite decoction) [is composed of] 2 *liang* of Gancao (甘草, licorice, Radix Glycyrrhizae Praeparata)(broil), 2 pieces of Fuzi (附子, aconite, Radix Aconiti Lateralis Preparata)(fry heavily and remove the bark), 2 *liang* of Baizhu (白术, rhizome of largehead atractylodes, Rhizoma Atractylodis Macrocephalae) and 4 *liang* of Guizhi (桂枝, cinnamon twig, Ramulus Cinnamomi)(remove the bark).

These four ingredients are decocted in 6 *sheng* of water to get 3 *sheng* [after] boiling. The dregs are removed and [the decoction is] taken warm 1 *sheng* [each time] and three times a day. [If there is] slight sweating [after] taking [the decoction for] the first [time], [the disease will be] resolved. [If the patient] can eat, [but there is] sweating and vexation again, 5 *ge* [of the decoction should be] taken. [If one] feels that 1 *sheng* is too much, it is better to take 6 or 7 *ge*.

【原文】

(二十五)

太阳中暍,发热恶寒,身重而疼痛,其脉弦细芤迟。小便已,洒洒然毛耸,手足逆冷,小有劳,身即热,口开,前板齿燥。若发其汗,则其恶寒甚;加温针,则发热甚;数下之,则淋甚。

【今译】

太阳病中暑,发热恶寒,身体沉重而疼痛,脉象弦细芤迟。小便时,有洒洒寒栗之感,毫毛耸起,手足逆冷,稍有体劳便身热,张口喘气,门牙干燥。如果用发汗法治疗,恶寒就会加重;如果食用温针治疗,则发热更甚;如果反复使用攻下法,则会引起淋病。

Volume 1

【英译】

Line 2.25

Summer-heat in taiyang ［disease is characterized by］ fever, aversion to cold, heaviness and pain of the body, taut, thin, hollow and slow pulse. After urination, ［the patient feels］ shivering and body hair ［seems］ to erect. ［Other symptoms and signs include］ reversal cold of hands and feet, slight overstrain, generalized fever, open-mouth and panting, and dryness of the front teeth. If diaphoresis is used, aversion to cold will be severe. ［If acupuncture with］ warmed needle is applied, fever will be severe. ［If］ purgation ［is used］ repeatedly, stranguria will be severe.

【原文】

（二十六）

太阳中热者,暍是也。汗出恶寒,身热而渴,白虎加人参汤主之。

白虎加人参汤方

知母（六两）　石膏（一斤,碎）　甘草（二两）　粳米（六合）　人参
（三两）

右五味,以水一斗,煮米熟汤成,去滓。温服一升,日三服。

【今译】

太阳病中有热者,即为暍病。症见汗出,恶寒,身热,口渴,用白虎
加人参汤主治。

Volume 1

【英译】

Line 2. 26

Heat attack in taiyang ［disease］ is caused by summer-heat. ［If there are symptoms and signs of］ sweating, aversion to cold, generalized fever and thirst, Baihu Decoction（白虎汤, white tiger decoction）added with Renshen（人参, ginseng, Radix Ginseng）［can be used］ to treat it.

Baihu Decoction（白虎汤, white tiger decoction）added with Renshen （人参, ginseng, Radix Ginseng）［is composed of］ 6 *liang* of Zhimu（知母, rhizome of common anemarrhena, Rhizoma Anemarrhenae）, 1 *jin* of Shigao（石膏, gypsum, Gypsum Fibrosum）(pound), 2 *liang* of Gancao（甘草, licorice, Radix Glycyrrhizae Praeparata）, 6 *ge* of Jingmi（粳米, polished round-grained rice, Semen Oryzae Nonglutinosae） and 3 *liang* of Renshen（人参, ginseng, Radix Ginseng）.

These five ingredients are decocted in 1 *dou* of water and the rice is well cooked. The dregs are removed and ［the decoction is］ taken warm 1 *sheng* ［each time］ and three times a day.

【原文】

(二十七)

太阳中暍,身热疼重,而脉微弱,此以夏月伤冷水,水行皮中所致也,一物瓜蒂汤主之。

一物瓜蒂汤方

瓜蒂(二七个)

右剉,以水一升,煮取五合,去滓,顿服。

【今译】

太阳病中暑,身热疼重,脉象微弱,这是由于夏季过度饮用冷水,以致水湿侵袭皮肤所致,宜用一物瓜蒂汤主治。

【英译】

Line 2.27

Heat attack in taiyang [disease is marked by] generalized fever, pain and heaviness of the body, faint and weak pulse, caused by damage from cold water that moves beneath the skin in summer. Yiwu Guadi Decoction (一物瓜蒂汤, one single melon stalk decoction) [can be used] to treat it.

Yiwu Guadi Decoction (一物瓜蒂汤, one single melon stalk decoction [is composed of] 27 pieces of Guadi (瓜蒂, melon stalk, Pedicellus Melo).

This ingredient is grated and decocted in 1 *sheng* of water to get 5 *ge* [after] boiling. The dregs are removed and [the decoction is] taken in a single [dose].

百合狐惑阴阳毒病脉证治第三

【原文】

(一)

论曰：百合病者，百脉一宗，悉致其病也。意欲食，复不能食，常默默，欲卧不能卧，欲行不能行，饮食或有美时，或有不用闻食臭时，如寒无寒，如热无热，口苦，小便赤，诸药不能治，得药则剧吐利，如有神灵者，身形如和，其脉微数。

每溺时头痛者，六十日乃愈；若溺时头不痛，淅然者，四十日愈；若溺快然，但头眩者，二十日愈。

其证或未病而预见，或病四五日而出，或病二十日、或一月微见者，各随证治之。

【今译】

据说，百合病，是百脉同出一源，皆源自心肺，心肺病则百脉皆病。百合病的表现为，想吃饭却不能吃，经常默默不语，想躺卧也不能卧，想行走也不能走，有时想饮食而且感觉也鲜美，但有时连食物的味道都不想闻，似乎像寒证但却没有寒象，似乎像热证但却没有热象，唯独口苦，

Volume 1

Chapter 3
Lily Disease, Huhuo (erosion of throat, anus and genitalia) and Yin Yang Toxin: Pulses, Syndromes/Patterns and Treatment

【英译】

Line 3. 1

It is said that lily disease [results from] the source of all vessels (heart and lung), [the disorder of which] causes all diseases. [The manifestations of lily disease is marked by] desire to eat but being unable to eat, frequent silence, desire to lie down but being unable to do so, desire to walk but being unable to walk, desire to drink and eat with delicious feeling, unwilling even to smell food, [signs] similar to cold but without cold, [signs] similar to heat but without heat, bitterness in the mouth and red urine. No medicine can treat [it]. Taking medicine will cause vomiting and diarrhea, like being haunted by spirit and ghost. [But] the body seems to be normal, only the pulse is slightly rapid.

[If there is] headache in urination, [it will be] cured in sixty days; if [there is] no headache [but only] chilliness in urination, [it will be] cured in forty days; if urination is smooth and [there is only] dizziness, [it will be] cured in twenty days.

[The symptoms and signs of lily disease are quite different.]

小便赤,一般的药物都不能治,服药后呕吐下利剧烈,就像有神灵作祟一样,但身体似乎没有任何变异,唯脉象有些微数。

如果小便时头痛,六十天左右就能治愈;如果小便时头不痛,只有寒栗之感,四十天左右就能治愈;如果小便畅快,但头目眩晕,二十天左右就能治愈。

百合病的症状各有不同,有的提前出现,有的发病四五天后才出现,有的发病二十天或一个月左右才略有出现,应各随其证治疗。

Sometimes they appear before occurrence, sometimes appear four or five days after occurrence, sometimes appear twenty days or one month after occurrence. [Each case is] treated according to the manifestations.

【原文】

(二)

百合病,发汗后者,百合知母汤主之。

百合知母汤方

百合(七枚,擘) 知母(三两,切)

右先以水洗百合,渍一宿,当白沫出,去其水,更以泉水二升,煎取一升,去滓;别以泉水二升煎知母,取一升,去滓;后合和煎,取一升五合。分温再服。

【今译】

百合病误用发汗法后,用百合知母汤主治。

Volume 1

【英译】

Line 3.2

Lily disease，after ［application of］ perspiratioin，［can be］ treated by Baihe Zhimu Decoction（百合知母汤，lily bulb and common anemarrhena rhizome decoction）.

Baihe Zhimu Decoction（百合知母汤，lily bulb and common anemarrhena rhizome decoction）［is composed of］7 pieces of Baihe （百合，lily bulb，Bulbus Lilii）(break)and 3 *liang* of Zhimu（知母，rhizome of common anemarrhena，Rhizoma Anemarrhenae）(cut).

In these ingredients，Baihe（百合，lily bulb，Bulbus Lilii）is washed first in water and soaked for one night. The white foam is removed and ［soaking］ water is eliminated. ［It is then］ decocted in 2 *sheng* of spring water to get 1 *sheng* ［after］ boiling. The dregs are removed. Another 2 *sheng* of spring water is used to boil Zhimu（知母，rhizome of common anemarrhena，Rhizoma Anemarrhenae）and get 1 *sheng* ［after］ boiling. The dregs are removed. Finally ［these two decoctions are］ mixed to boil and get 1. 5 *sheng*. ［The final decoction is］ divided ［into two doses］ and taken warm.

【原文】

(三)

百合病,下之后者,滑石代赭汤主之。

滑石代赭汤方

百合(七枚,擘) 滑石(三两,碎,绵裹) 代赭石(如弹丸大一枚,碎,绵裹)

右先以水洗百合,渍一宿,当白沫出,去其水,更以泉水二升,煎取一升,去滓;别以泉水二升煎滑石、代赭,取一升,去滓;后合和重煎,取一升五合,分温服。

【今译】

百合病误用下法治疗后,用滑石代赭汤主治。

Volume 1

【英译】

Line 3.3

Lily disease, after [application of] purgation, [can be] treated by Huashi Daizhe Decoction（滑石代赭汤，talcum and hematite decoction）.

Huashi Daizhe Decoction（滑石代赭汤，talcum and hematite decoction）[is composed of] 7 pieces of Baihe（百合，lily bulb, Bulbus Lilii）(break), 3 *liang* of Huashi（滑石，talcum，Talcum）(pound and wrap in the gauze)and 1 piece of Daizheshi（代赭石，hematite，Haematitum）(as large as a pellet，pound and wrap in the gauze).

In these ingredients，Baihe（百合，lily bulb, Bulbus Lilii）is washed first in water and soaked for one night. The white foam is removed and [soaking] water is eliminated. [It is then] decocted in 2 *sheng* of spring water to get 1 *sheng* [after] boiling. The dregs are removed. Another 2 *sheng* of spring water is used to boil Huashi（滑石，talcum，Talcum）and get 1 *sheng* [after] boiling. The dregs are removed. Finally [these two decoctions are] mixed to boil and get 1.5 *sheng*. [The final decoction is] divided [into two doses] and taken warm.

【原文】

(四)

百合病,吐之后者,百合鸡子汤主之。

百合鸡子汤方

百合(七枚,擘)　鸡子黄(一枚)

右先以水洗百合,渍一宿,当白沫出,去其水,更以泉水二升,煎取一升,去滓,内鸡子黄,搅匀,煎五分,温服。

【今译】

百合病误用吐法治疗后,用百合鸡子汤主治。

【英译】

Line 3.4

Lily disease，after ［application of］ vomiting ［therapy］，［can be］ treated by Baihe Jizi Decoction（百合鸡子汤方，lily bulb and chicken egg decoction）.

Baihe Jizi Decoction（百合鸡子汤方，lily bulb and chicken egg decoction）［is composed of］7 pieces of Baihe（百合，lily bulb，Bulbus Lilii）(break) and 1 piece of Jizihuang（鸡子黄，egg yolk，Galli Vitellus）.

In these ingredients，Baihe（百合，lily bulb，Bulbus Lilii）is washed first in water and soaked for one night. The white foam is removed and ［soaking］ water is eliminated. ［It is then］ decocted in 2 *sheng* of spring water to get 1 *sheng* ［after］ boiling. The dregs are removed and Jizihuang（鸡子黄，egg yolk，Galli Vitellus）is put into ［it］ to mix with it. ［Finally it is］ boiled into 5 *fen* and taken warm.

【原文】

(五)

百合病,不经吐、下、发汗,病形如初者,百合地黄汤主之。

百合地黄汤方

百合(七枚,擘) 生地黄汁(一升)

右以水洗百合,渍一宿,当白沫出,出其水,更以泉水二升,煎取一升,去滓,内地黄汁,煎取一升五合,分温再服。中病,勿更服,大便当如漆。

【今译】

百合病没有经过吐法、下法、汗法治疗,病情仍如初发时一样,用百合地黄汤主治。

【英译】

Line 3.5

Lily disease which, without ［application of］ vomiting, purgation and diaphoresis ［therapies］, still appears the same as ［it manifests］ at the beginning, ［can be］ treated by Baihe Dihuang Decoction （百合地黄汤方, lily bulb and rehmannia decoction）.

Baihe Dihuang Diecoction （百合地黄汤方, lily bulb and rehmannia decoction）［is composed of］7 pieces of Baihe （百合, lily bulb, Bulbus Lilii）（break）and 1 *sheng* of Shengdihuang （生地黄, fresh rehmannia, Radix Rehmanniae）（juice）.

In these ingredients, Baihe （百合, lily bulb, Bulbus Lilii) is washed first in water and soaked for one night. The white foam is removed and ［soaking］ water is eliminated. ［It is then］ decocted in 2 *sheng* of spring water to get 1 *sheng* ［after］ boiling. The dregs are removed and Shengdihuang （生地黄, fresh rehmannia, Radix Rehmanniae）is put into ［it］ to get 1 *sheng* and 5 *ge* ［after］ boiling. ［Finally it is］ divided ［into two doses］ and taken warm. ［When］ the disease is attacked, ［the patient should］ not take ［the decoction］ any more and the stool will appear like lacquer.

【原文】

（六）

百合病一月不解，变成渴者，百合洗方主之。

百合洗方

右以百合一升，以水一斗，渍之一宿，以洗身。洗已，食煮饼，勿以盐豉也。

【今译】

百合病发作一月后不解，出现口渴之症，用百合洗方主治。

【原文】

（七）

百合病，渴不差者，栝蒌牡蛎散主之。

栝蒌根　牡蛎（熬，等分）

右为细末，饮服方寸匕，日三服。

【今译】

百合病患者有口渴症状，尚未治愈的，用栝蒌牡蛎散主治。

Volume 1

【英译】

Line 3.6

[When] lily disease is not resolved in one month and changes into thirst，[it should be] treated by Baihe Xi Decoction（百合洗方，lily bulb washing decoction）.

Baihe Xi Decoction（百合洗方，lily bulb washing decoction）[is just composed of] 1 *sheng* of Baihe（百合，lily bulb, Bulbus Lilii）. It is decocted in 1 *dou* of water and soaked for one night. [It is used] to wash the body. After washing [the body，the patient can] eat boiled cake，but not salty [food made of] fermented beans.

【英译】

Line 3.7

[When] lily disease with thirst is not improved，Gualou Muli Powder（栝蒌牡蛎散方，trichosanthes root and oyster shell powder）[can be used] to treat it.

Gualou Muli Powder（栝蒌牡蛎散方，trichosanthes root and oyster shell powder）[is composed of] Gualougen（栝蒌根，Radix Trichosanthis）and Muli（牡蛎，oyster shell，Concha Ostreae）（simmer and of the same amount）.

These ingredients are pounded into fine powder. [The powder is] taken 1 *fangcunbi* [each time] and three times a day.

【原文】

（八）

百合病,变发热者,百合滑石散主之。

百合滑石散方

百合(一两,炙)　滑石(三两)

右为散,饮服方寸匕,日三服。当微利者,止服,热则除。

【今译】

百合病患者,有发热症状的,用百合滑石散主治。

【原文】

（九）

百合病见于阴者,以阳法救之;见于阳者,以阴法救之。见阳攻阴,复发其汗,此为逆;见阴攻阳,乃复下之,此亦为逆。

【今译】

百合病见到属于阴的症候,以阳法救治;见到属于阳的症候,以阴法救治。见到属于阳的症候,反而攻阴,再用发汗之法,这属于误治;见到属于阴的症候反而攻阳,继而使用下法,这也属于误治。

【英译】

Line 3.8

［When］ lily disease has transformed into heat，Baihe Huashi Powder（百合滑石散，lily bulb and talcum powder）［can be used］to treat it.

Baihe Huashi Powder（百合滑石散，lily bulb and talcum powder）［is composed of］1 *liang* of Baihe（百合，lily bulb，Bulbus Lilii)(broil) and 3 *liang* of Huashi（滑石，talcum，Talcum）.

This powder is taken 1 *fangcunbi* ［each time］and three times a day. When there is slight diarrhea，［the patient should］stop taking ［the powder］. ［In this way，］heat will be eliminated.

【英译】

Line 3.9

［When the manifestation of］lily disease is seen in yin，［it can be］rescued by yang method；［when the manifestation of lily disease］is seen in yang，［it can be］rescued by yin method. ［When］seen in yang but attacking yin with promotion of sweating，it is an adverse ［treatment］. ［When］seen in yin but attacking yang with ［application of］purgation，it is also an adverse ［treatment］.

【原文】

（十）

狐惑之为病,状如伤寒,默默欲眠,目不得闭,卧起不安,蚀于喉为惑,蚀于阴为狐,不欲饮食,恶闻食臭,其面目乍赤、乍黑、乍白。蚀于上部则声喝,甘草泻心汤主之。

甘草泻心汤方

甘草（四两）、黄芩、人参、干姜（各三两） 黄连一两 大枣（十二枚） 半夏（半斤）

右七味,水一斗,煮取六升,去滓,再煎。温服一升,日三服。

【今译】

狐惑病的症候,一般的表现类似于伤寒,常见症状为默默欲眠,但却不能闭目,卧起不宁,喉咙溃烂称为惑,阴部溃烂称为狐,不思饮食,不愿闻饮食之味,面目突然发红、发黑或发白。喉咙上部溃烂则声音嘶哑,宜用甘草泻心汤主之治。

Volume 1

【英译】

Line 3. 10

As a disease, huhuo（erosion of throat, anus and genitalia）manifests as cold damage ［disease］, ［usually characterized by］silence with desire to sleep, inability to close the eyes and disquietude either in lying or in getting up. ［When］eroding the throat, ［the patient is］in confusion; ［when］eroding yin（anus and genitals）, ［the patient is］unwilling to drink and eat and dislikes odor of food. ［As a result, the face of the patient］suddenly ［turns］red, or black or white. ［When］eroding the upper ［part of the body］, the voice ［of the patient will sound］husky, Gancao Xiexin Decoction（甘草泻心汤, licorice decoction for draining the heart）［can be used］to treat it.

Gancao Xiexin Decoction（甘草泻心汤, licorice decoction for draining the heart）［is composed of］4 *liang* of Gancao（甘草, licorice, Radix Glycyrrhizae Praeparata）, 3 *liang* of Huangqin（黄芩, scutellaria, Radix Scutellariae）, 3 *liang* of Renshen（人参, ginseng, Radix Ginseng）, 3 *liang* of Ganjiang（干姜, dried ginger, Rhizoma Zingiberis）, 1 *liang* of Huanglian（黄连, coptis, Rhizoma Coptidis）, 12 pieces of Dazao（大枣, jujube, Fructus Ziziphus Jujubae）and 0.5 *jin* of Banxia（半夏, pinellia, Rhizoma Pinelliae）.

These seven ingredients are decocted in 1 *dou* of water to get 6 *sheng* ［after］boiling. The dregs are removed and ［these ingredients are］boiled again. ［The decoction is］taken warm 1 *sheng* ［each time］and three times a day.

【原文】

(十一)

蚀于下部则咽干,苦参汤洗之。

苦参汤方

苦参(一升)

以水一斗,煎取七升,去滓,熏洗,日三服。

【今译】

阴部溃烂,咽干,用苦参汤洗之。

【原文】

(十二)

蚀于肛者,雄黄熏之。

雄黄

右一味为末,筒瓦二枚合之,烧,向肛熏之。

【今译】

肛部溃烂的,宜用雄黄熏治。

【英译】

Line 3. 11

［When the disease］erodes the anus and genitals，the throat will become dry，and Kushen Decoction（苦参汤，flavescent sophora decoction）［can be used to treat it through］washing.

Kushen Decoction（苦参汤，flavescent sophora decoction）［is composed of］1 *sheng* of Kushen（苦参，flavescent sophora，Radix Sophorae Flavescentis）.

This ingredient is decocted in 1 *dou* of water to get 7 *sheng* ［after］boiling. The dregs are removed and［the decoction is used］to fumigate and wash，three times a day.

【英译】

Line 3. 12

［When the disease］erodes the anus，［it can be treated by］fumigation with Xionghuang（雄黄，realgar，Realgar）.

Xionghuang（雄黄，realgar，Realgar）is the only ingredient. ［It is］put between two concave tiles［that form a tube in which the ingredient is］burning to fumigate the anus.

【原文】

（十三）

病者脉数，无热，微烦，默默但欲卧，汗出，初得之三四日，目赤如鸠眼；七八日，目四眦黑。若能食者，脓已成也，赤豆当归散主之。

赤豆当归散方

赤小豆（三升，浸令芽出，曝干） 当归（三两）

右二味，杵为散，浆水服方寸匕，日三服。

【今译】

病人脉数，无发热症状，微有烦躁，沉默欲卧，汗出。病发初期的三四天，病人眼睛红赤得像斑鸠的眼一样；发作七八天后，两眼的内外眦均变黑。如果能饮食，说明热度已经蕴结成脓，宜用赤豆当归散主治。

【英译】

Line 3. 13

The patient ［suffers from］ rapid pulse，no fever，slight vexation，silence with desire to sleep，and sweating. Three or four days ［after］ occurrence ［of the disease］，［the patient's］ eyes are as red as that of the turtledove. Seven or eight days ［after］ occurrence ［of the disease］，［the patient's］ outer and inner corners of two eyes become black. If ［the patient］ is able to eat，［it indicates that］ pus is formed and Chidou Danggui Powder （赤豆当归散方，Chinese angelica and rice bean powder） ［can be used］ to treat it.

Chidou Danggui Powder （赤豆当归散方，Chinese angelica and rice bean powder） ［is composed of］ 3 *sheng* of Chixiaodou （赤小豆，rice bean，Semen Phaseoli）（soak to sprout and dry thoroughly）and 3 *liang* of Danggui （当归，Chinese angelica，Radix Angelicae Sinensis）.

These two ingredients are pounded into powder and mixed in water. ［It is］ taken 1 *fangcunbi* ［each time］ and three times a day.

【原文】

（十四）

阳毒之为病，面赤斑斑如锦文，咽喉痛，唾脓血。五日可治，七日不可治。升麻鳖甲汤主之。

升麻鳖甲汤方

升麻（二两）　当归（一两）　蜀椒（炒去汗，一两）　甘草（二两）鳖甲（手指大一片，炙）　雄黄（半两，研）

右六味，以水四升，煮取一升，顿服之。老少再服，取汗。

【今译】

阳毒病的症状表现，一般为面部有赤斑，犹如花纹一样，咽喉痛，唾脓血。发作五日之内可治，超过七天则病情危重，难以治疗。用升麻鳖甲汤主治。

【英译】

Line 3. 14

The disease caused by yang toxin ［is characterized by］ red complexion like silk, sore-throat and vomiting pus and blood. Five days ［after its occurrence, it is］ curable, seven days ［after occurrence, it is］ incurable. Shengma Biejia Decoction (升麻鳖甲汤, cimicifuga and turtle shell decoction) ［can be used］ to treat it.

Shengma Biejia Decoction (升麻鳖甲汤, cimicifuga and turtle shell decoction) ［is composed of］ 2 *liang* of Shengma (升麻, cimicifuga, Rhizoma Cimicifuga), 1 *liang* of Danggui (当归, Chinese angelica, Radix Angelicae Sinensis), 1 *liang* of Shujiao (蜀椒, zanthoxylum, Pericarpium Zanthoxyli) (fry to remove sweating), 2 *liang* of Gancao (甘草, licorice, Radix Glycyrrhizae Praeparata), 1 piece of Biejia (鳖甲, turtle shell, Carapax Trionycis Praeparata)(as big as a thumb, broil)and 0.5 *liang* of Xionghuang (雄黄, realgar, Realgar)(brush).

These six ingredients are decocted in 4 *sheng* of water to get 1 *sheng* ［after］ boiling and take once the whole. Both old and young ［patients need］ to take ［two doses of this decoction］ to promote sweating.

【原文】

(十五)

阴毒之为病，面目青，身痛如被杖，咽喉痛。五日可治，七日不可治。升麻鳖甲汤去雄黄、蜀椒主之。

【今译】

阴毒病的症状表现，一般为面目发青，身体疼痛，就像被拷打了一样，咽喉疼痛。发作五日之内可治，超过七日的便不可治。用升麻鳖甲汤去雄黄、蜀椒主治。

【英译】

Line 3. 15

The disease caused by yin toxin [is characterized by] bluish face and eyes, generalized pain like [being beaten by] a stick and sore-throat. Five days [after its occurrence, it is] curable, seven days [after occurrence, it is] incurable. Shengma Biejia Decoction (升麻鳖甲汤, cimicifuga and turtle shell decoction) with removal of Xionghuang (雄黄, realgar, Realgar) and Shujiao (蜀椒, zanthoxylum, Pericarpium Zanthoxyli) [can be used] to treat it.

疟病脉证并治第四

【原文】

（一）

师曰：疟，脉自弦，弦数者多热，弦迟者多寒。弦小紧者下之差，弦迟者可温之，弦紧者可发汗，针灸也。浮大者可吐之，弦数者风发也，以饮食消息止之。

【今译】

老师说：疟病之脉象多为自弦。如果脉象弦而数，则多有热；如果脉象弦而迟，则多有寒。如果脉象又弦又小又紧，可以用攻下法治愈；如果脉象弦而迟的，可用温法治疗；如果脉象弦而紧的，可用发汗法或针灸法治疗；如果脉象浮而大的，可用吐法治疗；如果脉象弦而数的，因风邪所致，可以饮食调理斟酌治疗。

Chapter 4
Malaria: Pulses, Syndromes/Patterns and Treatment

【英译】

Line 4. 1

The master said: [In] malaria, the pulse is spontaneously taut. [If] the pulse is taut and rapid, [there is] excessive heat; [if] the pulse is taut and slow, [there is] excessive cold. [When the pulse is] small and tight, [it can be] resolved by purgation. [When the pulse is] taut and slow, [it can be] resolved by warming [therapy]. [If the pulse is] taut and tight, [it can be resolved through] sweating by acupuncture and moxibustion. [When the pulse is] floating and large, [it can be resolved by] vomiting [therapy]; [when the pulse is] taut and rapid, [it is] caused by [pathogenic] wind and can be resolved by regulation of drinking water and taking food.

【原文】

(二)

病疟,以月一日发,当以十五日愈;设不差,当月尽解。如其不差,当云何?师曰:此结为症瘕,名曰疟母,急治之,宜鳖甲煎丸。

鳖甲煎丸方

鳖甲(十二分,炙)　乌扇(三分,烧)　黄芩(三分)　柴胡(六分)鼠妇(三分,熬)　干姜(三分)　大黄(三分)　芍药(五分)　桂枝(三分)　葶苈(一分,熬)　石苇(三分,去毛)　厚朴(三分)　牡丹(五分,去心)　瞿麦(二分)　紫威(三分)　半夏(一分)　人参(一分)　䗪虫(五分,熬)　阿胶(三分,炙)　蜂窠(四分,熬)　赤硝(十二分)　蜣螂(六分,熬)　桃仁(二分)

右二十三味为末,取锻灶下灰一斗,清酒一斛五斗,浸灰,候酒尽一半,着鳖甲于中,煮令泛烂如胶漆,绞取汁,内诸药,煎为丸,如梧子大。空心服七丸,日三服。

【今译】

疟病如果每月初一发作,一般应当在十五日内治愈;如果十五天内没有治愈,一个月内应当治愈。如果一个月内也没有治愈,该

【英译】

Line 4.2

Malaria which occurs in the first day of each month will be cured in fifteen days. If [it is] not cured [in fifteen days], [it will be] cured at the end of this month. If it is not cured, how to explain it?

The master said: This is binding into lump syndrome/pattern, known as source of malaria. Biejiajian Pill (鳖甲煎丸, turtle shell pill) is the appropriate [formula for treating it].

Biejiajian Pill (鳖甲煎丸, turtle shell pill) [is composed of] 12 *fen* of Biejia (鳖甲, turtle shell, Carapax Trionycis Praeparata) (broil), 3 *fen* of Wushan (乌扇, belamcanda, Rhizoma Belamcandae)) (burn), 3 *fen* of Huangqin (黄芩, scutellaria, Radix Scutellariae), 6 *fen* of Chaihu (柴胡, bupleurum, Radix Bupleuri), 3 *fen* of Shufu (鼠妇, wood louse, Armadillidium) (simmer), 3 *fen* of Ganjiang (干姜, dried ginger, Rhizoma Zingiberis), 3 *fen* of Dahuang (大黄, rhubarb, Radix et Rhizoma Rhei), 5 *fen* of Shaoyao (芍药, peony, Radix Paeoniae), 3 *fen* of Guizhi (桂枝, cinnamon twig, Ramulus Cinnamomi), 1 *fen* of Tingli (葶苈, tingli, Semen Lepidii seu Descurainiae) (simmer), 3 *fen* of Shiwei (石苇, pyrrosia, Folium Pyrrosiae) (remove the hair), 5 *fen* of Houpo (厚朴, magnolia bark, Cortex Magnoliae Officinalis), 5 *fen* of Mudan (牡丹, moutan, Cortex Moutan Radicis) (remove center), 2 *fen* of Qumai (瞿麦, dianthus, Herba Dianthi), 3 *fen* of Ziwei (紫威, campsis flower, Flos Campsis), 1 *fen* of Banxia (半夏, pinellia, Rhizoma Pinelliae), 1 *fen* of Renshen (人参, ginseng, Radix Ginseng), 5 *fen* of Zhechong (蟅虫, ground beetle, Eupolyphaga seu Steleophaga) (simmer), 3 *fen* of Ejiao (阿胶,

怎么办呢?

老师说：这是疟邪结于胁下成为症瘕，称为疟母，应紧急治疗，用鳖甲煎丸主治。

ass-hide glue, Colla Corii Asini)（broil）, 4 *fen* of Fengke（蜂窠, hornet's rest, Nidus Vespae Praeparata）（boil）, 12 *fen* of Chixiao（赤硝, red niter, Nitrum Rubrum）, 6 *fen* of Qianglang（蜣螂, dung beetle, Catharsius）（simmer）and 2 *fen* of Taoren（桃仁, peach kernel, Semen Persicae）.

These twenty-three ingredients are pounded into powder to produce 1 *dou* of ashes ［after being］ burnt and fried. ［It is］ soaked in 5 *dou* of clear wine till half of the wine has disappeared. ［Then］ Biejia（鳖甲, turtle shell, Carapax Trionycis Praeparata）is put into ［it］, boiling like glue lacquer to obtain juice. All the ingredients in it are boiled to produce pills the size of firmiana seeds. ［The patient］ takes 7 pills ［each time when］ the stomach is empty and three times a day.

【原文】

（三）

师曰：阴气孤绝，阳气独发，则热而少气烦冤，手足热而欲呕，名曰瘅疟。若但热不寒者，邪气内脏于心，外舍分肉之间，令人消铄脱肉。

【今译】

老师说：如果阴气衰绝，阳气独盛，则患者热盛而少气，烦躁，郁闷，手足发热，时时想吐，称为瘅疟。如果只有热而没有寒，则邪气内藏于心，外伏于分肉之间，令人肌肉消损。

【原文】

（四）

温疟者，其脉如平，身无寒但热，骨节疼烦，时呕，白虎加桂枝汤主之。

白虎加桂枝汤方

知母（六两）　甘草（二两，炙）　石膏（一斤）　粳米（二合）　桂枝（三两，去皮）

右剉，每五钱，水一盏半，煎至八分，去滓。温服，汗出愈。

【今译】

温疟病患者，脉象像正常一样，身上无寒但有热，骨节疼痛剧烈，时时呕吐，宜用白虎加桂枝汤主治。

Volume 1

【英译】

Line 4.3

The master said: [When] yin qi is exhausted and yang qi is exuberant, [there will be] heat, shortness of breath, vexation, feverish hands and feet and nausea. It is called heat malaria. If [there is] just heat but no cold, [it indicates that] pathogenic factors are [internally] hidden in the heart and externally penetrating in the interstices, [consequently] causing wasting of fleshes.

【英译】

Line 4.4

[In] warm malaria, the pulse is normal, there is no generalized cold but heat, the joints are painful and vexing, and there is occasional nausea. Baihu Decoction (白虎汤, white tiger decoction) added with Guizhi (桂枝, cinnamon twig, Ramulus Cinnamomi) [can be used] to treat it.

Baihu Decoction (白虎汤, white tiger decoction) added with Guizhi (桂枝, cinnamon twig, Ramulus Cinnamomi) [is composed of] 6 *liang* of Zhimu (知母, rhizome of common anemarrhena, Rhizoma Anemarrhenae), 2 *liang* of Gancao (甘草, licorice, Radix Glycyrrhizae Praeparata) (broil), 1 *jin* of Shigao (石膏, gypsum, Gypsum Fibrosum), 2 *ge* of Jingmi (粳米, polished round-grained rice, Semen Oryzae Nonglutinosae) and 3 *liang* of Guizhi (桂枝, cinnamon twig, Ramulus Cinnamomi) (remove the bark).

These ingredients are grated and each [dose] is 5 *qian*, put into one and a half cup of water to boil and get 8 *fen*. The dregs are removed and [the decoction is] taken warm. [When there is] sweating, [the disease is about] to heal.

【原文】

（五）

疟多寒者，名曰牝疟，蜀漆散主之。

蜀漆散方

蜀漆（烧去腥）　云母（烧二日夜）　龙骨（等分）

右三味，杵为散，未发前，以浆水服半钱。温疟加蜀漆半分，临发时，服一钱匕。

【今译】

疟病多寒的，称为牝疟，宜用蜀漆散主治。

【原文】

附《外台秘要》方

牡蛎汤　治牝疟

牡蛎（四两，熬）　麻黄（四两，去节）　甘草（二两）　蜀漆（三两）

右四味，以水八升，先煮蜀漆、麻黄，去上沫，得六升，内诸药，煮取二升，温服一升。若吐，则勿更服。

【今译】

附方：选自《外台秘要》的牡蛎汤方，用以治疗牝疟。

Volume 1

【英译】

Line 4.5

Malaria with excessive cold is called female malaria, Shuqi Powder（蜀漆散, dichroa powder）[can be used] to treat it.

Shuqi Powder（蜀漆散, dichroa powder）[is composed of] Shuqi（蜀漆, dichroa, Ramulus et Folium Dichroae）(burn to remove fishy smell), Yunmu（云母, muscovite, Muscovitum）(burn two days and nights)and Longgu（龙骨, Loong bone, Os Loong）, of the same amount.

These three ingredients are grated into powder. Before [it] attacks, [the powder is] taken 0.5 *qian* with thin porridge. For warm malaria, 0.5 *fen* of Shuqi（蜀漆, dichroa, Ramulus et Folium Dichroae）is added. [When it is] attacking, 1 *qianbi* [of the powder is] taken.

【英译】

Line 4.6

Appendix: Formula [from the book entitled] *Waitai Miyao*（《外台秘要》, *The Medical Secrets of an Official Named Wang Tao*）.

Muli Decoction（牡蛎汤, oyster shell decoction）[is used] to treat female malaria.

Muli Decoction（牡蛎汤, oyster shell decoction）[is composed of] 4 *liang* of Muli（牡蛎, oyster shell, Concha Ostreae）(simmer), 4 *liang* of Mahuang（麻黄, ephedra, Herba Ephedrae）(remove the nodes), 2 *liang* of Gancao（甘草, licorice, Radix Glycyrrhizae Praeparata）and 3 *liang* of Shuqi（蜀漆, dichroa, Ramulus et Folium Dichroae）.

These four ingredients are decocted in 8 *sheng* of water. Shuqi（蜀漆, dichroa, Ramulus et Folium Dichroae）and Mahuang（麻黄, ephedra, Herba Ephedrae）are boiled first. Remove the foam and get 6 *sheng* [after] boiling. The rest ingredients are put into it and boiled to get 2 *sheng*. [The decoction is] taken warm 1 *sheng* [each time]. If [there is] vomiting, [it is] forbidden to take [the decoction] any more.

【原文】

《外台》柴胡去半夏加栝蒌汤治疟病发渴者,亦治劳疟。

柴胡(八两)　人参、黄芩、甘草(各三两)　栝蒌根(四两)　生姜(二两)　大枣(十二枚)

右七味,以水一斗二升,煮取六升,去滓,再煎取三升。温服一升,日二服。

【今译】

源自《外台秘要》的柴胡去半夏加栝蒌汤,用以治疗疟病有口渴症状的,可以治疗劳疟。

【原文】

柴胡桂姜汤治疟寒多,微有热,或但寒不热。

柴胡(半斤)　桂枝(三两,去皮)　干姜(二两)　栝蒌根(四两)　黄芩(三两)　牡蛎(三两,熬)　甘草(二两,炙)

右七味,以水一斗二升,煮取六升,去滓,再煎取三升。温服一升,日三服。初服微烦,复服汗出便愈。

【今译】

柴胡桂姜汤用以治疗疟病寒多,有微热,或者只有寒而没有热。

Volume 1

【英译】
　　Chaihu Decoction (柴胡汤, bupleurum decoction) with removal of Banxia (半夏, pinellia, Rhizoma Pinelliae) and addition of Gualou (栝蒌, trichosanthes root, Radix Trichosanthis) [can be used] to treat malaria with thirst and also consumptive malaria.

　　Chaihu Decoction (柴胡汤, bupleurum decoction) with removal of Banxia (半夏, pinellia, Rhizoma Pinelliae) and addition of Gualou (栝蒌, trichosanthes root, Radix Trichosanthis) [is composed of] 8 *liang* of Chaihu (柴胡, bupleurum, Radix Bupleuri), 3 *liang* of Renshen (人参, ginseng, Radix Ginseng), 3 *liang* of Huangqin (黄芩, scutellaria, Radix Scutellariae), 3 *liang* of Gancao (甘草, licorice, Radix Glycyrrhizae Praeparata), 4 *liang* of Gualougen (栝蒌根, trichosanthes root, Radix Trichosanthis), 2 *liang* of Shengjiang (生姜, fresh ginger, Rhizoma Zingiberis Recens) and 12 pieces of Dazao (大枣, jujube, Fructus Ziziphus Jujubae).

　　These seven ingredients are decocted in 1 *dou* and 2 *sheng* of water to get 6 *sheng* [after] boiling. The dregs are removed [and it is] boiled again to get 3 *sheng*. [The decoction is] taken warm 1 *sheng* [each time] and twice a day.

【英译】
　　Chaihu Guijiang Decoction (柴胡桂姜汤, bupleurum, cinnamon twig and ginger decoction) [can be used] to treat malaria with excessive cold and slight heat, or only cold and no heat.

　　Chaihu Guijiang Decoction (柴胡桂姜汤, bupleurum, cinnamon twig and ginger decoction) [is composed of] 0.5 *jin* of Chaihu (柴胡, bupleurum, Radix Bupleuri), 3 *liang* of Guizhi (桂枝, cinnamon twig, Ramulus Cinnamomi)(remove the bark), 2 *liang* of Ganjiang (干姜, dried ginger, Rhizoma Zingiberis), 4 *liang* of Gualougen (栝蒌根, trichosanthes root, Radix Trichosanthis), 3 *liang* of Huangqin (黄芩, scutellaria, Radix Scutellariae), 3 *liang* of Muli (牡蛎, oyster shell, Concha Ostreae)(simmer)and 2 *liang* of Gancao (甘草, licorice, Radix Glycyrrhizae Praeparata)(broil).

　　These seven ingredients are decocted in 1 *dou* and 2 *sheng* of water to get 6 *sheng* [after] boiling. The dregs are removed and [it is] boiled again to get 3 *sheng*. [The decoction is] taken warm 1 *sheng* [each time] and three times a day. [If the patient feels] slightly vexed [when] taking the first [dose], [there will be] sweating [after] taking the second [dose] and [the disease is] about to heal.

中风历节病脉证并治第五

【原文】

（一）

夫风之为病，当半身不遂，或但臂不遂者，此为痹。脉微而数，中风使然。

【今译】

因风引发的病，其症状应当是半身不遂，或者只有手臂不遂，这是痹证。脉象微而数的，就是中风的征兆。

Volume 1

Chapter 5
Wind Stroke and Joint Disease:
Pulses, Syndromes/Patterns and Treatment

【英译】

Line 5. 1

The disease caused by wind [is characterized by] hemplegia or paralysis of the arm only. This is called impediment. Faint and rapid pulse is due to wind stroke.

【原文】

(二)

寸口脉浮而紧,紧则为寒,浮则为虚,寒虚相搏,邪在皮肤。浮者血虚,络脉空虚,贼邪不泻,或左或右,邪气反缓,正气即急,正气引邪,喎僻不遂。

邪在于络,肌肤不仁;邪在于经,即重不胜;邪入于腑,即不识人;邪入于脏,舌即难言,口吐涎。

【今译】

寸口脉象浮而紧,脉象紧则为寒,脉象浮则为虚,寒虚相搏,邪首先留滞于皮肤。脉象浮的表示血虚,如果络脉空虚,则邪气无法外泻,或者滞留在左侧,或者滞留在右侧。总之邪气侵犯的一侧表现为弛缓状态,未受邪气侵袭的一方则显得拘急,由于健侧牵引患侧,使得口眼歪斜向健侧,无法随意运动。

如果邪气侵犯了络脉,则表现为肌肤麻木不仁;邪气如果侵入经脉,脉体则沉重无力;邪气侵入于腑,则导致患者神昏;邪气侵入于脏,则导致舌强难言,口吐痰涎。

【原文】

侯氏黑散治大风,四肢烦重,心中恶寒不足者。

菊花(四十分) 白术(十分) 细辛(三分) 茯苓(三分) 牡蛎

Volume 1

【英译】

Line 5.2

[There are cases where] the pulse in the cunkou [region] is floating and tight. Tight [pulse] indicates cold while floating [pulse] indicates deficiency. Contention between cold and deficiency [indicates that] pathogenic [factors] are in the skin. Floating [pulse indicates] blood deficiency. [As a result,] the collaterals and vessels are void and deficient, thief-like pathogenic [factors] are not drained and hidden either in the left or in the right. [When] pathogenic qi is slack, healthy qi is tense. [When] healthy qi draws pathogenic factors, it [will cause] distorsion and deviation of the mouth and eyes. [When] pathogenic factors are in the collaterals, the skin is numb; [when] pathogenic factors are in the meridians, [the body] is heavy and hampered; [when] pathogenic factors are in the fu-organs, [the patient is] unable to recognize others; [when] pathogenic factors are in the zang-organs, the tongue is difficult in speaking and the mouth is vomiting and drooling.

【英译】

Houshi Heisan Powder（侯氏黑散，Hou's black powder）[is used] to treat severe wind [stroke characterized by] vexing heaviness of the four limbs and insufficient aversion to cold in the heart.

Houshi Heisan（侯氏黑散，Hou's black powder）[is composed of] 40 *fen* of Juhua（菊花，chrysanthemum，Flos Chrysanthemi），10 *fen* of Baizhu（白术，rhizome of largehead atractylodes，Rhizoma

（三分）　桔梗（八分）　防风（十分）　人参（三分）　矾石（三分）　黄芩
（五分）　当归（三分）　干姜（三分）　芎䓖（三分）　桂枝（三分）

　　右十四味，杵为散，酒服方寸匕，日一服。初服二十日，温酒调服。禁一切鱼肉大蒜，常宜冷食，六十日止，即药积在腹中不下也，热食即下矣，冷食自能助药力。

【今译】

　　侯氏黑散可用以治疗大风病症，表现为四肢烦重，心中恶寒，阳气不足。

Volume 1

Atractylodis Macrocephalae), 3 *fen* of Xixin (细辛，asarum，Herba Asari)，3 *fen* of Fuling (茯苓，poria，Poria)，3 *fen* of Muli (牡蛎，oyster shell，Concha Ostreae)，8 *fen* of Jiegeng (桔梗，platycodon grandiflorum，Radix Platycodi)，10 *fen* of Fangfeng (防风，saposhnikovia，Radix Saposhnikoviae)，3 *fen* of Renshen (人参，ginseng，Radix Ginseng)，3 *fen* of Fanshi (矾石，alum，Alumen)，5 *fen* of Huangqin (黄芩，scutellaria，Radix Scutellariae)，3 *fen* of Danggui (当归，Chinese angelica，Radix Angelicae Sinensis)，3 *fen* of Ganjiang (干姜，dried ginger，Rhizoma Zingiberis)，3 *fen* of Xiongqiong (芎䓖，xiongqiong，Rhizoma Chuanxiong) and 3 *fen* of Guizhi (桂枝，cinnamon twig，Ramulus Cinnamomi).

These fourteen ingredients are pounded into powder. Take 1 *fangcunbi* of wine and 1 [dose] each time. Initially [the powder is] taken for 20 days with warm wine. It is forbidden to take any fish and garlic. [The patient] usually takes cold food，[but it should] stop after sixty days because medicine accumulates in the abdomen and cannot descend. Hot food will enable it to descend. [But] cold food can strengthen the effect of medicine.

【原文】

(三)

寸口脉迟而缓,迟则为寒,缓则为虚,荣缓则为亡血,卫缓则为中风。邪气中经,则身痒而瘾疹。心气不足,邪气入中,则胸满而短气。

【今译】

寸口脉象迟而缓,脉象迟则为寒,脉象缓则为虚。脉象沉而缓的,是营气不足,导致亡血;脉象浮而缓的,是卫气不足,引起中风。邪气侵袭了经脉,则出现身痒和瘾疹。如果心气不足,邪气入侵,则导致胸满和短气等症。

【原文】

风引汤　除热瘫痫。

大黄、干姜、龙骨(各四两)　桂枝(三两)　甘草、牡蛎(各二两)寒水石、滑石、赤石脂、白石脂、紫石英、石膏(各六两)

右十二味,杵,粗筛,以韦囊盛之,取三指撮,井花水三升,煮三沸,温服一升。

【今译】

风引汤主治热性风瘫及癫痫。

【英译】

Line 5.3

[There are cases where]the pulse in the cunkou [region] is slow and moderate. Slow [pulse] means cold and moderate [pulse] means deficiency. Moderate [pulse] in the nutrient [aspect] indicates blood collapse while in the defense [aspect] indicates wind stroke. [When] pathogenic qi invades the meridians, [it] will cause generalized itching and dormant papules. [When] heart qi is insufficient, pathogenic qi will enter the center and cause chest fullness and shortness of breath.

【英译】

Fengyin Decoction (风引汤, wind pulling decoction) eliminates heat, paralysis and epilepsy.

Fengyin Decoction (风引汤, wind pulling decoction) [is composed of] 4 *liang* of Dahuang (大黄, rhubarb, Radix et Rhizoma Rhei), 4 *liang* of Ganjiang (干姜, dried ginger, Rhizoma Zingiberis), 4 *liang* of Longgu (龙骨,Loong bone, Os Loong), 3 *liang* of Guizhi (桂枝, cinnamon twig, Ramulus Cinnamomi), 2 *liang* of Gancao (甘草, licorice, Radix Glycyrrhizae Praeparata), 2 *liang* of Muli (牡蛎, oyster shell, Concha Ostreae), 6 *liang* of Hanshuishi (寒水石, glauberite, Gypsum seu Calcitum), 6 *liang* of Huashi (滑石, talcum, Talcum), 6 *liang* of Chishizhi (赤石脂, halloysite, Halloysitum Rubrum), 6 *liang* of Baishizhi (白石脂, kaolin, Kaolin), 6 *liang* of Zishiying (紫石英, fluorite, Fluoritum) and 6 *liang* of Shigao (石膏, gypsum, Gypsum Fibrosum).

These twelve ingredients are pounded and sieved into powder, kept in a leather bag. A three-finger pinch is taken out and 3 *sheng* of clear water is added to boil for three times. [The decoction is] taken warm 1 *sheng* [each time].

【原文】

防己地黄汤治病如狂状,妄行,独语不休,无寒热,其脉浮。

防己(一分)　桂枝(三分)　防风(三分)　甘草(二分)

右四味,以酒一杯,浸之一宿,绞取汁,生地黄二斤,咬咀,蒸之如斗米饭久,以铜器盛其汁,更绞地黄汁,和分再服。

【今译】

防己地黄汤主治的疾病症状为狂躁不宁,行为反常,自言自语不休,无寒无热,脉象浮。

【原文】

头风摩散方

大附子(一枚,炮)　盐(等分)

右二味为散,沐了,以方寸匕,已摩疢上,令药力行。

【今译】

头风摩散方由一枚大附子和适量的盐所构成。融合后服用。

【英译】

Fangji Dihuang Decoction（防己地黄汤，stephania tetrandra root and fresh rehmannia decoction）treats the disease ［with the manifestations］like mania，abnormal behavior，incessant soliloquy，no cold and heat，and floating pulse.

Fangji Dihuang Decoction（防己地黄汤，stephania tetrandra root and fresh rehmannia decoction）［is composed of］1 *fen* of Fangji（防己，the root of stephania tetrandra，Radix Stephaniae Tetrandrae），3 *fen* of Guizhi（桂枝，cinnamon twig，Ramulus Cinnamomi），3 *fen* of Fangfeng（防风，saposhnikovia，Radix Saposhnikoviae）and 2 *fen* of Gancao（甘草，licorice，Radix Glycyrrhizae Praeparata）.

These four ingredients are soaked in a cup of wine for one night and wringed out the juice. 2 *jin* of Shengdihuang（生地黄，fresh rehmannia，Radix Rehmanniae）is steamed like cooking 1 *dou* of rice and the juice is poured into a copper vessel. Shengdihuang（生地黄，fresh rehmannia，Radix Rehmanniae）is wringed out to produce more juice. ［These two juices are］mixed and divided into two ［doses］before being taking.

【英译】

Toufeng Mosan Powder（头风摩散方，head wind rubbing powder）.

This formula ［is composed of］1 piece of big Fuzi（附子，aconite，Radix Aconiti Lateralis Preparata）（fry heavily）and salt，of the same amount.

These two ingredients are pounded into powder. Wash ［the head］with 1 *fangcunbi* and rub the affected area to strengthen the effect of medicine.

【原文】

（四）

寸口脉沉而弱，沉即主骨，弱即主筋，沉即为肾，弱即为肝。汗出入水中，如水伤心，历节黄汗出，故曰历节。

【今译】

寸口脉象沉而弱，脉象沉主骨病，脉象弱主筋病，脉象沉表现的是肾的状况，脉象弱表现的是肝的状况。出汗后入冷水沐浴，水湿从汗孔入内，伤及心脏，关节肿胀，有黄汗溢出，称为历节。

【译文】

（五）

跌阳脉浮而滑，滑则谷气实，浮则汗自出。

【今译】

跌阳脉象浮而滑，脉象滑则说明谷气实，脉象浮则说明汗自出。

【英译】

Line 5.4

[There are cases where] the pulse in the cunkou [region] is sunken and weak. Sunken [pulse] indicates [a symptom of] bones while weak [pulse] indicates [a symptom of] sinews. Sunken [pulse] is [a manifestation of] the kidney while weak [pulse] is [a manifestation of] the liver. [When a person] enters into water [when] sweating and if water injures the heart, the joints [will be affected] with yellow sweating [all over the body]. That is why it is called [pain of] joints.

【英译】

Line 5.5

[There are cases where] the pulse at fuyang (the pulsation on the dorsum of the foot) is floating and slippery. Slippery [pulse] indicates excess of cereal qi while floating [pulse] indicates spontaneous sweating.

【原文】

（六）

少阴脉浮而弱，弱则血不足，浮则为风，风血相搏，即疼痛如掣。

【今译】

少阴脉象浮而弱，脉象弱则表示阴血不足，脉象浮则表示外受风邪，风血相搏，导致疼痛如同抽掣。

【原文】

（七）

盛人脉涩小，短气，自汗出，历节疼，不可屈伸，此皆饮酒汗出当风所致。

【今译】

肥胖之人脉象涩而小，气短，自汗，关节疼，不可屈伸，这都是由于饮酒汗出而遭受风邪侵袭所致。

【英译】

Line 5.6

[In this disease,] the shaoyin pulse is floating and weak. Weak [pulse] indicates insufficient blood while floating [pulse] indicates [pathogenic] wind. [When] wind and blood are contending with each other, there will be pain as if being pulled.

【英译】

Line 5.7

[When] the pulse of an obese person is rough and small, [there will be] shortness of breath, spontaneous sweating, pain of joints and inability to bend and stretch [joints]. All these [symptoms and signs] are caused by drinking wine, sweating and exposure to wind.

【原文】

(八)

诸肢节疼痛,身体魁羸,脚肿如脱,头眩短气,温温欲吐,桂枝芍药知母汤主之。

桂枝芍药知母汤方

桂枝(四两) 芍药(三两) 甘草(二两) 麻黄(二两) 生姜(五两) 白术(五两) 知母(四两) 防风(四两) 附子(二枚,炮)

右九味,以水七升,煮取二升,温服七合,日三服。

【今译】

各关节疼痛,身体消瘦,双脚肿大,头眩短气,心中闷闷不乐,时常想吐,用桂枝芍药知母汤主治。

【英译】

Line 5.8

[The patient with] pain of all joints, emaciation and weakness, swollen feet as if falling off [the legs], dizziness, shortness of breath, seething and nausea [can be] treated by Guizhi Shaoyao Zhimu Decoction (桂枝芍药知母汤, cinnamon twig, peony and common anemarrhena rhizome decoction).

Guizhi Shaoyao Zhimu Decoction (桂枝芍药知母汤, cinnamon twig, peony and common anemarrhena rhizome decoction) [is composed of] 4 *liang* of Guizhi (桂枝, cinnamon twig, Ramulus Cinnamomi), 3 *liang* of Shaoyao (芍药, peony, Radix Paeoniae), 2 *liang* of Gancao (甘草, licorice, Radix Glycyrrhizae Praeparata), 2 *liang* of Mahuang (麻黄, ephedra, Herba Ephedrae), 5 *liang* of Shengjiang (生姜, fresh ginger, Rhizoma Zingiberis Recens), 5 *liang* of Baizhu (白术, rhizome of largehead atractylodes, Rhizoma Atractylodis Macrocephalae), 4 *liang* of Zhimu (知母, rhizome of common anemarrhena, Rhizoma Anemarrhenae), 4 *liang* of Fangfeng (防风, saposhnikovia, Radix Saposhnikoviae) and 2 pieces of Fuzi (附子, aconite, Radix Aconiti Lateralis Preparata) (fry heavily).

These nine ingredients are decocted in 7 *sheng* of water to get 2 *sheng* [after] boiling. [The decoction is] taken warm 7 *ge* [each time] and three times a day.

【原文】

(九)

味酸则伤筋,筋伤则缓,名曰泄;咸则伤骨,骨伤则痿,名曰枯。枯泄相搏,名曰断泄。荣气不通,卫不独行,荣卫俱微,三焦无所御,四属断绝,身体羸瘦,独足肿大,黄汗出,胫冷。假令发热,便为历节也。

【今译】

偏食酸味则伤筋,筋伤则驰缓不用,称为泄。偏食咸味则伤骨,骨伤则痿软无力,称为枯。筋骨弛缓痿软,称为断泄。营气虚濡而不通,卫气虚弱而行,营气和卫气俱衰微,三焦就失去了正常功能,肢体四部(即皮、肉、脂、髓)即失去充养,身体消瘦,足部肿大,黄汗溢出,两胫发冷。如果两胫发热,则为历节。

【英译】

Line 5.9

Sour flavor damages the sinews. [When] damaged, the sinews become slack, known as looseness. Salty [flavor] damages the bones. [When] damaged, the bones become wilted, known as desiccation. [When] looseness and desiccation are contending with each other, it is called breaking looseness. [When] nutrient qi fails to flow freely and defense qi cannot flow normally, nutrient [qi] and defense [qi] all become faint, [resulting in] inability to control the triple energizer, fracture (deprival of nourishment) of the four portions (skin, flesh, fat and marrow), marked emaciation, swollen feet, yellow sweating and coldness of lower legs. If there is fever, it is the case of joint acuteness.

【原文】

(十)

病历节,不可屈伸,疼痛,乌头汤主之。

乌头汤方治脚气疼痛,不可屈伸。

麻黄、芍药、黄芪(各三两) 甘草(三两,炙) 川乌(五枚,哎咀,以蜜二升,煎取一升,即出乌头)

右五味,哎咀四味,以水三升,煮取一升,去滓,内蜜煎中,更煎之。服七合,不知,尽服之。

【今译】

历节病,关节疼痛,不可屈伸,宜用乌头汤主治。

【英译】

Line 5. 10

Joint acuteness disease with inability to bend and stretch and pain [can be] treated by Wutou Decoction (乌头汤，aconite decoction).

Wutou Decoction (乌头汤，aconite decoction) can treat pain of foot and inability to bend and stretch.

Wutou Decoction (乌头汤，aconite decoction) [is composed of] 3 *liang* of Mahuang (麻黄，ephedra，Herba Ephedrae)，3 *liang* of Shaoyao (芍药，peony，Radix Paeoniae)，3 *liang* of Huangqi (黄芪，astragalus，Radix Astragali)，3 *liang* of Gancao (甘草，licorice，Radix Glycyrrhizae Praeparata) (broil) and 5 pieces of Chuanwu (川乌，aconite main root，Radix Aconiti)(chew，boil in 2 *sheng* of honey to get 1 *sheng*，and remove aconite).

These five ingredients，[among which] four are chewed，are decocted in 3 *sheng* of water to get 1 *sheng* [after] boiling. The dregs are removed，honey is put into [it] to boil again. [The decoction is] taken 7 *ge* [each time]. [If there is] no effect，all the decoction should be taken.

【原文】

(十一)

矾石汤治脚气冲心。

矾石(二两)

右一味,以浆水一斗五升,煎三五沸,浸脚良。

【今译】

矾石汤主治脚气冲心,这是一种外治法。

附方

【原文】

《古今录验》续命汤治中风痱,身体不能自收,口不能言,冒昧不知痛处,或拘急不得转侧。

麻黄、桂枝、当归、人参、石膏、干姜、甘草(各三两) 芎䓖(一两) 杏仁(四十枚) 右九味,以水一斗,煮取四升,温服一升,当小汗,薄覆脊,凭几坐,汗出则愈。不汗更服,无所禁,勿当风。并治但伏不得卧,咳逆上气,面目浮肿。

【今译】

续命汤源自《古今录验》,主治中风所致的痱病,症状为身体弛缓,不能自收,口不能说话,昏冒不知疼痛,或者肢体拘急不能转侧。

【英译】

Line 5. 11

Fanshi Decoction（矾石汤，alum decoction）treats beriberi that strikes the heart.

Fanshi Decoction（矾石汤，alum decoction）[is composed of] 2 *liang* of Fanshi（矾石，alum，Alumen）.

This single ingredient is boiled in 1 *dou* and 5 *sheng* of cereal water for three or five times. It is good to soak the feet [with such a decoction].

Appendded formulas

【英译】

Xuming Decoction（续命汤，decoction for prolonging life）[from the book entitled] *Gujin Luyan*（《古今录验》，*Ancient and Present Records of Experiences*）[is used to treat] wind stroke [with difficulty to move the body and inability to feel pain and itching]. [This disease is characterized by] inability of the body to control itself, aphasia, mental confusion without knowing the location of pain, or spasm and inability to turn the body.

Xuming Decoction（续命汤，decoction for prolonging life）[is composed of] 3 *liang* of Mahuang（麻黄，ephedra，Herba Ephedrae），3 *liang* of Guizhi（桂枝，cinnamon twig，Ramulus Cinnamomi），3 *liang* of Danggui（当归，Chinese angelica，Radix Angelicae Sinensis），3 *liang* of Renshen（人参，ginseng，Radix Ginseng），3 *liang* of Shigao（石膏，gypsum，Gypsum Fibrosum），3 *liang* of Ganjiang（干姜，dried ginger，Rhizoma Zingiberis），3 *liang* of Gancao（甘草，licorice，Radix Glycyrrhizae Praeparata），1 *liang* of Xiongqiong（芎䓖，xiongqiong，Rhizoma Chuanxiong）and 40 pieces of Xingren（杏仁，apricot kernel，Semen Armeniacae Amarum）.

These nine ingredients are decocted in 1 *dou* of water to get 4 *sheng*. [The decoction is] taken warm 1 *sheng* [each time] to induce slight sweating. [The patient should] cover his back with thin [clothes or quilt] and leans on a chair. [When] there is sweating, [the disease will] heal. [If there is] no sweating, more [decoction should be] taken. [There is] no contraindication, [but cares must be taken] to avoid exposure to wind. [This decoction also can be used] to treat [the patients who] curl up [in bed] but cannot lie down [with the symptoms and signs of] cough, retching, dyspnea and dropsy of face and eyes.

【原文】

《千金》三黄汤治中风手足拘急，百节疼痛，烦热心乱，恶寒，经日不欲饮食。

麻黄(五分)　独活(四分)　细辛(二分)　黄芪(二分)　黄芩(三分)

右五味，以水六升，煮取二升。分温三服，一服小汗，二服大汗。心热加大黄二分，腹满加枳实一枚，气逆加人参三分，悸加牡蛎三分，渴加栝蒌根三分，先有寒加附子一枚。

【今译】

三黄汤源自《千金方》，主治中风后手足拘急，所有关节疼痛不已，烦躁不安，身体发热，心情烦乱，恶寒，数日不想饮食。

Volume 1

【英译】

Sanhuang Decoction（三黄汤，three yellow decoction）［from the book entitled］ *Qianjin* ［*fang*］（《千金方》，*Thousand Golden Formulas*）［is used］ to treat wind storke ［with the symptoms and signs of］ spasm of hands and feet, pain of all joints, vexing heat, dysphoria, aversion to cold and no desire to drink water and eat food for several days.

Sanhuang Decoction （三黄汤，three yellow decoction）［is composed of］ 5 *fen* of Mahuang（麻黄，ephedra, Herba Ephedrae）, 4 *fen* of Duhuo （独活，pubescent angelica, Radix Angelicae Pubescentis）, 2 *fen* of Xixin（细辛，asarum, Herba Asari）, 2 *fen* of Huangqi（黄芪，astragalus, Radix Astragali） and 3 *fen* of Huangqin （黄芩，scutellaria, Radix Scutellariae）.

These five ingredients are decocted in 6 *sheng* of water to get 2 *sheng* ［after］ boiling. ［The decoction is］ divided into three ［doses］ and taken warm. ［After］ taking the first ［dose］, ［there will be］ slight sweating. ［After］ taking the second ［dose］, ［there will be］ profuse sweating. For heart heat, 2 *fen* of Dahuang （大黄，rhubarb, Radix et Rhizoma Rhei） is added; for abdominal fullness, 1 piece of Zhishi （枳实，processed unripe bitter orange, Fructus Aurantii Immaturus） is added; for conuterflow of qi, 3 *fen* of Renshen（人参，ginseng, Radix Ginseng） is added; for palpitation, 3 *fen* of Muli（牡蛎，oyster shell, Concha Ostreae） is added; for thirst, 3 *fen* of Gualougen （栝蒌根，trichosanthes root, Radix Trichosanthis） is added; for initial cold, 1 piece of Fuzi（附子，aconite, Radix Aconiti Lateralis Preparata） is added.

【原文】

《近效方》术附汤治风虚头重眩,苦极,不知食味,暖肌补中,益精气。

白术(二两)　附子(一枚半,炮,去皮)　甘草(一两,炙)

右三味,剉,每五钱匕,姜五片,枣一枚,水盏半,煎七分,去滓,温服。

【今译】

术附汤源自《近效方》,主治正气虚而外感风寒,头重目眩,非常难受,饮食乏味。治宜暖肌补中,补益精气。

【英译】

Shufu Decoction（术附汤，rhizome of largehead atractylodes and aconite decoction）[from the book entitled] *Jinxiao Formulas* (《近效方》，*Significant Effective Formulas*) [is used] to treat wind-deficiency，heaviness of the head，dizziness，extreme bitterness and inability to taste food [by means of] warming the fleshes，tonifying the middle and replenishing essential qi.

Shufu Decoction（术附汤，rhizome of largehead atractylodes and aconite decoction）[is composed of] 2 *liang* of Baizhu（白术，rhizome of largehead atractylodes，Rhizoma Atractylodis Macrocephalae），1 piece of Fuzi（附子，aconite，Radix Aconiti Lateralis Preparata）(fry heavily and remove the bark) and 1 *liang* of Gancao（甘草，licorice，Radix Glycyrrhizae Praeparata)(broil).

These three ingredients are pounded [into powder]. 5 *qianbi* [of each ingredient]，5 slices of ginger and 1 piece of Dazao（大枣，jujube，Fructus Ziziphus Jujubae）are boiled in half a cup of water to get 7 *fen* [after] boiling. The dregs are removed and [the decoction is] taken warm.

【原文】

崔氏八味丸治脚气上入,少腹不仁。

干地黄(八两) 山茱萸、薯蓣(各四两) 泽泻、茯苓、牡丹皮(各三两) 桂枝、附子(炮,各一两)

右八味,末之,炼蜜和丸梧子大。酒下十五丸,日再服。

【今译】

崔氏八味丸用以治疗脚气入腹,导致少腹麻木不仁,拘急不适。

【原文】

《千金方》越婢加术汤治肉极,热则身体津脱,腠理开,汗大泄,厉风气,下焦脚弱。

麻黄(六两) 石膏(半斤) 生姜(三两) 甘草(二两) 白术(四两) 大枣(十五枚)

右六味,以水六升,先煮麻黄,去上沫,内诸药,煮取三升,分温三服。恶风加附子一枚,炮。

【今译】

越婢加术汤源自《千金方》,用以治疗肌肉极,热则身体津液虚脱,腠理开泄,大汗淋漓,形成厉风气,导致下肢软弱无力。

【英译】

Cuishi Bawei Pill（崔氏八味丸，Cui's Eight Ingredients Pill）[is used] to treat beriberi entering the upper [part of the body] and numbness of the lower abdomen.

Cuishi Bawei Pill（崔氏八味丸，Cui's Eight Ingredients Pill）[is composed of] 8 *liang* of Gandihuang（干地黄，dried rehmannia，Radix Rehmanniae），4 *liang* of Shanzhuyu（山茱萸，cornus，Fructus Corni），4 *liang* of Shuyu（薯蓣，dioscorea，Rhizoma Dioscoreae），3 *liang* of Zexie（泽泻，alisma，Rhizoma Alismatis），3 *liang* of Fuling（茯苓，poria，Poria），3 *liang* of Mudanpi（牡丹皮，moutan，Cortex Moutan Radicis），1 *liang* of Guizhi（桂枝，cinnamon twig，Ramulus Cinnamomi）and 1 *liang* of Fuzi（附子，aconite，Radix Aconiti Lateralis Preparata）(fry heavily).

These eight ingredients are ground [into powder] and blended with Lianmi（炼蜜，processed honey，Mel Praeparatum）to form pills the size of firmiana seeds. [Each time] 15 pills are swallowed in wine and twice a day.

【英译】

Yuebi Decoction（越婢汤，decoction for effusing the spleen）added with Baizhu Decoction（白术汤，rhizome of largehead atractylodes decoction）[is used] to treat extreme heat in fleshes [that causes] exhaustion of fluid and humor，opening of interstices，great discharge of sweating，pestilent wind qi and weakness of the triple energizer and feet.

Yuebi Decoction（越婢汤，decoction for effusing the spleen）[is composed of] 6 *liang* of Mahuang（麻黄，ephedra，Herba Ephedrae），0.5 *jin* of Shigao（石膏，gypsum，Gypsum Fibrosum），3 *liang* of Shengjiang（生姜，fresh ginger，Rhizoma Zingiberis Recens），2 *liang* of Gancao（甘草，licorice，Radix Glycyrrhizae Praeparata），4 *liang* of Baizhu（白术，rhizome of largehead atractylodes，Rhizoma Atractylodis Macrocephalae）and 15 pieces of Dazao（大枣，jujube，Fructus Ziziphus Jujubae）.

These six ingredients are decocted in 6 *sheng* of water. Mahuang（麻黄，ephedra，Herba Ephedrae）is boiled first. The dregs are removed and the rest ingredients are put into [it] to boil and get 3 *sheng*. [The decoction is] divided into three [doses] and taken warm. For aversion to cold, 1 piece of Fuzi（附子，aconite，Radix Aconiti Lateralis Preparata）is added [after being heavily fried].

血痹虚劳病脉证并治第六

【原文】

(一)

问曰：血痹病从何得之？师曰：夫尊荣人，骨弱肌肤盛，重因疲劳汗出，卧不时动摇，加被微风，遂得之。但以脉自微涩，在寸口、关上小紧，宜针引阳气，令脉和紧去则愈。

【今译】

问：血痹病是怎么引起的呢？

老师说：那些尊养处优的人，筋骨脆弱，肌肤丰满，由于疲劳汗出，卧床时辗转反侧，受风遇寒，因此就得了病。但是如果脉象微而涩，寸口、关部的脉象微小而紧，宜用针刺引动阳气，使脉和不紧，疾病就会痊愈。

Chapter 6
Blood Impediment and Consumptive Disease: Pulses, Syndrome/Patterns and Treatment

【英译】

Line 6. 1

Question: How is blood impediment disease caused?

The master said: Those living a comfortable life [often suffer from] weakness of bones and exuberant fleshes, [accompanied by] heaviness [of the body] and sweating [after] fatigue, restlessness [when] lying [on bed] and invasion of mild wind. [That is why such a disease] is caused. But if the pulse is faint and rough, [especially the pulse] in the cunkou [region] and guan [region] is small and tight, [it is] appropriate [to use] acupuncture [to conduct] yang qi. [When] the pulse becomes harmonious and not tight, [the disease will be] cured.

【原文】

（二）

血痹阴阳俱微，寸口关上微，尺中小紧，外证身体不仁，如风痹状，黄芪桂枝五物汤主之。

黄芪桂枝五物汤方

黄芪（三两）　芍药（三两）　桂枝（三两）　生姜（六两）　大枣（十二枚）

右五味，以水六升，煮取二升。温服七合，日三服。

【今译】

血痹病因阴阳俱微，所以寸口脉象和关部脉象微，尺部脉象小而紧，症见身体不仁，症状如风痹一样，宜用黄芪桂枝五物汤主治。

【原文】

（三）

夫男子平人，脉大为劳，极虚，亦为劳。

【今译】

男子外形上看身体是正常的，但脉象大而无力，或者极度虚弱，也属于虚劳病。

【英译】

Line 6. 2

[In] blood impediment [disease], both yin and yang are weak，[the pulse on] the upper of cunkou [region] is faint，[the pulse on] the middle of chi [area] is small and tight, the body is numb in external syndrome/pattern like wind impediment. [It should be] treated by Huangqi Guizhi Wuwu Decoction（黄芪桂枝五物汤，astragalus and cinnamon twig decoction with five medicinals）.

Huangqi Guizhi Wuwu Decoction（黄芪桂枝五物汤，astragalus and cinnamon twig decoction with five medicinals）[is composed of] 3 *liang* of Huangqi（黄芪，astragalus, Radix Astragali），3 *liang* of Shaoyao（芍药，peony, Radix Paeoniae），3 *liang* of Guizhi（桂枝，cinnamon twig, Ramulus Cinnamomi），6 *liang* of Shengjiang（生姜，fresh ginger, Rhizoma Zingiberis Recens）and 12 pieces of Dazao（大枣，jujube, Fructus Ziziphus Jujubae）.

These five ingredients are decocted in 6 *sheng* of water to get 2 *sheng* [after] boiling. [The decoction is] taken warm 7 *ge* [each time] and three times a day.

【英译】

Line 6. 3

Man [who looks] healthy [but has a large pulse is actually ill]. The large pulse indicates consumptive [disease] and extremely weak [pulse] also indicates consumptive [disease].

【原文】

(四)

男子面色薄者,主渴及亡血,卒喘悸,脉浮者,里虚也。

【今译】

男子面色淡白的,表现为口渴,失血,稍动则气喘心悸,脉象浮弱的,是里虚。

【原文】

(五)

男子脉虚沉弦,无寒热,短气里急,小便不利,面色白,时目瞑,兼衄,少腹满,此为劳使之然。

【今译】

男子脉象虚沉而弦,无寒无热,短气,里急,小便不利,面色苍白,时有视物不清,兼有衄血,少腹胀满,这是虚劳病的表现。

【英译】

Line 6.4

Men with a thin [pale] complexion are mainly [characterized by] thirst, blood collapse, sudden panting, palpitation, floating pulse and internal deficiency.

【英译】

Line 6.5

Men [with] weak, sunken and taut pulse, no cold and heat, shortness of breath, tenesmus, inhibited urination, pale complexion, occasional dim vision, accompanied by nosebleed and fullness of lower abdomen [actually suffer from consumptive disease]. Such [symptoms and signs are in] fact the manifestations of consumptive [disease].

【原文】

（六）

劳之为病，其脉浮大，手足烦，春夏剧，秋冬瘥，阴寒精自出，酸削不能行。

【今译】

虚劳病者，其脉象浮而大，手足烦热，春夏加剧，秋冬减轻，阴部寒冷，有精液滑出，双腿酸痛无力而行。

【原文】

（七）

男子脉浮弱而涩，为无子，精气清冷。

【今译】

男子脉象浮弱而涩，是没有生育能力的表现，这是由于精液清稀而冷所致。

【英译】

Line 6.6

The disease caused by consumption [is characterized by] floating and large pulse, vexing feeling of hands and feet, aggravation in spring and summer, remission in autumn and winter, genital cold with spontaneous seminal emission, weak and emaciated [legs] and inability to walk.

【英译】

Line 6.7

Men with floating, weak and rough pulse are sterile because the essential qi is cold.

【原文】

（八）

夫失精家,少腹弦急,阴头寒,目眩,发落,脉极虚芤迟,为清谷,亡血,失精。脉得诸芤动微紧,男子失精,女子梦交,桂枝龙骨牡蛎汤主之。

桂枝加龙骨牡蛎汤方

桂枝、芍药、生姜（各三两）　甘草（二两）　大枣（十二枚）　龙骨、牡蛎（各三两）

右七味,以水七升,煮取三升,分温三服。

天雄散方

天雄（三两,炮）　白术（八两）　桂枝（六两）　龙骨（三两）

右四味,杵为散,酒服半钱匕,日三服,不知,稍增之。

【今译】

经常梦遗或失精的男子,少腹弦急,阴部寒冷,双目眩晕,头发脱落,脉象极虚,又空又迟,为下利清谷,失血失精。此种患者还会有各种空动微紧的脉象。男子失精,女子梦交,均可用桂枝龙骨牡蛎汤主治。

【英译】

Line 6.8

The patients with seminal emission [suffer from] taut tension in the lower abdomen, coldness of glans penis, dizziness of eyes, loss of hair and extreme weak, hollow and slow pulse indicating diarrhea with undigested food, blood collapse and seminal emission. [When] the pulse is hollow, stirring, faint and tight, [it indicates] seminal emission in men and sexual intercourse in dream in women. [This disease can be] treated by Guizhi Longgu Muli Decoction (桂枝龙骨牡蛎汤, cinnamon twig, Loong bone and oyster shell decoction).

Guizhi Longgu Muli Decoction (桂枝龙骨牡蛎汤, cinnamon twig, Loong bone and oyster shell decoction) [is composed of] 3 *liang* of Guizhi (桂枝, cinnamon twig, Ramulus Cinnamomi), 3 *liang* of Shaoyao (芍药, peony, Radix Paeoniae), 3 *liang* of Shengjiang (生姜, fresh ginger, Rhizoma Zingiberis Recens), 2 *liang* of Gancao (甘草, licorice, Radix Glycyrrhizae Praeparata), 12 pieces of Dazao (大枣, jujube, Fructus Ziziphus Jujubae), 3 *liang* of Longgu (龙骨, Loong bone, Os Loong) and 3 liang of Muli (牡蛎, oyster shell, Concha Ostreae).

These seven ingredients are decocted in 7 *sheng* of water to get 3 *sheng* [after] boiling. [The decoction is] divided into three [doses] and taken warm.

Tianxiong Powder (天雄散, tianxiong conite decoction)[is composed of] 3 *liang* of Tianxiong (天雄, tianxiong conite, Aconiti Radix Lateralis Tianxiong)(fry heavily), 8 *liang* of Baizhu (白术, rhizome of largehead atractylodes, Rhizoma Atractylodis Macrocephalae), 6 *liang* of Guizhi (桂枝, cinnamon twig, Ramulus Cinnamomi) and 3 *liang* of Longgu (龙骨,Loong bone, Os Loong).

These four ingredients are pounded into powder. Half a *qianbi* is taken in wine [each time] and three times a day. [If there is] no effect, slightly increase the dose.

【原文】

（九）

男子平人，脉虚弱细微者，善盗汗也。

【今译】

男子形体无明显症状，但脉象却虚弱细微，经常盗汗。

【原文】

（十）

人年五六十，其病脉大者，痹侠背行，若肠鸣，马刀侠瘿者，皆为劳得之。

【今译】

患者年龄到了五六十岁的时候，脉象大，脊柱两边麻木僵硬，如果伴有肠鸣，或腋下颈旁有瘰疬的，都属于劳病症状。

【原文】

（十一）

脉沉小迟，名脱气，其人疾行则喘喝，手足逆寒，腹满，甚则溏泄，食不消化也。

【今译】

脉象沉小而迟，称为脱气，患者行走略快，就会出现气喘促，手足逆寒，腹部胀满，甚至出现大便溏泄，饮食不能消化等症状。

【英译】

Line 6.9

[If] a man [who appears] healthy [but whose] pulse is deficient, weak, thin and faint, a tendency to sweat at night [is indicated].

【英译】

Line 6.10

[In] a person of fifty or sixty years of age, [if] the pathological pulse is large, [there is] impediment along the spine. If [there are symptoms and signs of] borborygmus and [cervical scrofula looking like] saber, consumption is the cause.

【英译】

Line 6.11

The sunken, small and slow pulse [of a patient] is called exhaustion of qi. Such a patient [suffers from] panting when walking quickly, reversal cold of hands and feet, abdominal fullness, or even sloppy diarrhea and indigestion.

【原文】

(十二)

脉弦而大,弦则为减,大则为芤,减则为寒,芤则为虚,虚寒相搏,此名为革。妇人则半产漏下,男子则亡血失精。

【今译】

脉象弦而大,脉象弦则无力,脉象大则空弱,脉象无力则为寒象的表现,脉象空弱则为虚的表现,虚寒并见,则为革脉。妇女出现革脉,则多见于半产漏下,男子出现革脉,则多见于失血失精。

【原文】

(十三)

虚劳里急,悸,衄,腹中痛,梦失精,四肢酸疼,手足烦热,咽干口燥,小建中汤主之。

小建中汤方

桂枝(三两,去皮) 甘草(三两,炙) 大枣(十二枚) 芍药(六两)

生姜(二两) 胶饴(一升)

右六味,以水七升,煮取三升,去滓,内胶饴,更上微火消解。温服一升,日三服。

【今译】

虚劳病的症状为,腹中拘急,心悸,衄血,腹中疼痛,梦中失精,四肢酸疼,手足烦热,咽干口燥,用小建中汤主治。

【英译】

Line 6. 12

[There are cases where] the pulse [of a patient] is taut and large. Taut [pulse] indicates reduction while large [pulse] indicates hollowness. Reduction means cold while hollowness means deficiency. [When] deficiency and cold contend with each other, it is called tympanic [pulse]. [In] women, [such a pulse] indicates premature delivery and vaginal discharge of blood; [in] men, [such a pulse] indicates blood collapse and seminal emission.

【英译】

Line 6. 13

[The disease, characterized by] deficiency-consumption, abdominal urgency, palpitation, nosebleed, abdominal pain, seminal emission in dream, aching pain of the four limbs, vexing heat in the hands and feet, dryness of the throat and mouth, [can be] treated by Xiao Jianzhong Decoction (小建中汤, minor decoction for strengthening the middle).

Xiao Jianzhong Decoction (小建中汤, minor decoction for strengthening the middle) [is composed of] 3 *liang* of Guizhi (桂枝, cinnamon twig, Ramulus Cinnamomi) (remove the bark), 3 *liang* of Gancao (甘草, licorice, Radix Glycyrrhizae Praeparata) (broil), 12 pieces of Dazao (大枣, jujube, Fructus Ziziphus Jujubae), 6 *liang* of Shaoyao (芍药, peony, Radix Paeoniae), 2 *liang* of Shengjiang (生姜, fresh ginger, Rhizoma Zingiberis Recens) and 1 *sheng* of Jiaoyi (胶饴, malt, Maltosum).

These six ingredients are decocted in 7 *sheng* of water to get 3 *sheng* [after] boiling. The dregs are removed and Jiaoyi (胶饴, malt, Maltosum) is put into it to melt with mild fire. [The decoction is] taken warm 1 *sheng* [each time] and three times a day.

【原文】

(十四)

虚劳里急,诸不足,黄芪建中汤主之。

【今译】

虚劳病有腹中里急,阴阳气血均不足等症状的,用黄芪建中汤主治。

【原文】

(十五)

虚劳腰痛,少腹拘急,小便不利者,八味肾气丸主之。

干地黄(八两) 山药、山茱萸(各四两) 泽泻(三两) 茯苓(三两) 牡丹皮(三两) 桂枝、附子(炮)(各一两)

右八味,末之,炼蜜和丸梧子大,酒下十五丸,加二十五丸,日再服。

【今译】

虚劳病有腰痛,少腹拘急,小便不利等症状的,宜用八味肾气丸主治。

【英译】

Line 6. 14

［In］ deficiency-consumption with abdominal urgency and insufficiency of all ［other aspects］, Huangqi Jianzhong Decoction （黄芪建中汤，astragalus decoction for strengthening the middle） ［can be used］ to treat it.

【英译】

Line 6. 15

［In］ deficiency-consumption with lumbago, abdominal hypertonicity and inhibited urination，Bawei Shenqi Pill （八味肾气丸，eight ingredients pill for strengthening kidney qi） ［can be used］ to treat it.

Bawei Shenqi Pill （八味肾气丸，eight ingredients pill for strengthening kidney qi） ［is composed of］ 8 *liang* of Gandihuang （干地黄，dried rehmannia，Radix Rehmanniae），4 *liang* of Shanyao （山药，dioscorea，Rhizoma Dioscoreae），4 *liang* of Shanzhuyu （山茱萸，cornus，Fructus Corni），3 *liang* of Zexie （泽泻，alisma，Rhizoma Alismatis），3 *liang* of Fuling （茯苓，poria，Poria），3 *liang* of Mudanpi （牡丹皮，moutan，Cortex Moutan），1 *liang* of Guizhi （桂枝，cinnamon twig，Ramulus Cinnamomi） and 1 *liang* of Fuzi （附子，aconite，Radix Aconiti Lateralis Preparata） （fry heavily）.

These eight ingredients are pounded into powder and blended with Lianmi （炼蜜，processed honey，Mel Praeparatum） to produce pills the size of firmiana seeds. ［Usually］ 15 pills，or increasing to 25 pills，are swallowed in wine ［each time］ and twice a day.

【原文】

(十六)

虚劳诸不足,风气百疾,薯蓣丸主之。

薯蓣丸方

薯蓣(三十分)　当归　桂枝　曲　干地黄　豆黄卷(各十分)　甘草(二十八分)　人参(七分)　芎䓖　芍药　白术　麦门冬　杏仁(各六分)　柴胡　桔梗　茯苓(各五分)　阿胶(七分)　干姜(三分)　白敛(二分)　防风(六分)　大枣(百枚,为膏)

右二十一味,末之,炼蜜和丸,如弹子大。空腹酒服一丸,一百丸为剂。

【今译】

虚劳病中有阴阳气血均不足,又有风邪所致的多种疾病,用薯蓣丸主治。

Volume 1

【英译】

Line 6. 16

Deficiency-consumption with insufficiency of all ［aspects］ and various diseases ［caused by］ pathogenic wind ［can be］ treated by Shuyu Pill（薯蓣丸，dioscorea pill）.

Shuyu Pill（薯蓣丸，dioscorea pill）［is composed of］ 30 *fen* of Shuyu（薯蓣，dioscorea，Rhizoma Dioscoreae），10 *fen* of Danggui（当归，Chinese angelica，Radix Angelicae Sinensis），10 *fen* of Guizhi（桂枝，cinnamon twig，Ramulus Cinnamomi），10 *fen* of Qu（曲，medicated leaven，Massa Medicata Fermentata），10 *fen* of Gandihuang（干地黄，dried rehmannia，Radix Rehmanniae），10 *fen* of Douhuangjuan（豆黄卷，dried soybean sprout，Sojae Semen Sojae Germinatum），28 *fen* of Gancao（甘草，licorice，Radix Glycyrrhizae Praeparata），7 *fen* of Renshen（人参，ginseng，Radix Ginseng），6 *fen* of Xiongqiong（芎䓖，xiongqiong，Rhizoma Chuanxiong），6 *fen* of Shaoyao（芍药，peony，Radix Paeoniae），6 *fen* of Baizhu（白术，rhizome of largehead atractylodes，Rhizoma Atractylodis Macrocephalae），6 *fen* of Maimendong（麦门冬，ophiopogon，Radix Ophiopogonis），6 *fen* of Xingren（杏仁，apricot kernel，Semen Armeniacae Amarum），5 *fen* of Chaihu（柴胡，bupleurum，Radix Bupleuri），5 *fen* of Jiegeng（桔梗，platycodon grandiflorum，Radix Platycodi），5 *fen* of Fuling（茯苓，poria，Poria），7 *fen* of Ejiao（阿胶，ass-hide glue，Colla Corii Asini），3 *fen* of Ganjiang（干姜，dried ginger，Rhizoma Zingiberis），2 *fen* of Bailian（白敛，ampelopsis，Radix Ampelopsis），6 *fen* of Fangfeng（防风，saposhnikovia，Radix Saposhnikoviae）and 100 pieces of Dazao（大枣，jujube，Fructus Ziziphus Jujubae）（make into paste）.

These twenty-one ingredients are pounded into powder and blended with Lianmi（炼蜜，processed honey，Mel Praeparatum）to produce pills the size of pellets. One pill is taken in wine ［each time］ when the stomach is empty. This formula ［is composed of］ one hundred pills.

【原文】

（十七）

虚劳虚烦不得眠，酸枣汤主之。

酸枣汤方

酸枣仁（二升）　甘草（一两）　知母（二两）　茯苓（二两）　芎䓖（二两）

右五味，以水八升，煮酸枣仁，得六升，内诸药，煮取三升，分温三服。

【今译】

虚劳病中有虚烦不能安眠等症状的，用酸枣汤主治。

Volume 1

【英译】

Line 6. 17

Deficiency-consumption with deficiency-vexation and inability to sleep [can be] treated by Suanzao Decoction (酸枣汤, spiny jujube decoction).

Suanzao Decoction (酸枣汤, spiny jujube decoction) [is composed of] 2 *sheng* of Suanzaoren (酸枣仁, spiny jujube, Semen Ziziphi Spinosi), 1 *liang* of Gancao (甘草, licorice, Radix Glycyrrhizae Praeparata), 2 *liang* of Zhimu (知母, rhizome of common anemarrhena, Rhizoma Anemarrhenae), 2 *liang* of Fuling (茯苓, poria, Poria) and 2 *liang* of Xiongqiong (芎藭, xiongqiong, Rhizoma Chuanxiong).

These five ingredients are decocted in 8 *sheng* of water. Suanzaoren (酸枣仁, spiny jujube, Semen Ziziphi Spinosi) is boiled [first] to get 6 *sheng* [of water]. [Then] the rest ingredients are put into [it] to boil and get 3 *sheng*. [The decoction is] divided into three [doses] and taken warm.

【原文】

（十八）

五劳虚极羸瘦，腹满，不能饮食，食伤、忧伤、饮伤、房室伤、饥伤、劳伤、经络营卫气伤，内有干血，肌肤甲错，两目黯黑。缓中补虚，大黄蟅虫丸主之。

大黄蟅虫丸方

大黄（十分，蒸）　黄芩（二两）　甘草（三两）　桃仁（一升）　杏仁（一升）　芍药（四两）　干地黄（十两）　干漆（一两）　虻虫（一升）　水蛭（百枚）　蛴螬（一升）　蟅虫（半升）　右十二味，末之，炼蜜和丸小豆大。酒饮服五丸，日三服。

【今译】

五劳过度则导致身体消瘦，腹部胀满，不能饮食。这是由于饮食不节、忧虑不尽、饮酒过量、房事太过、饥饱不均、劳累太过，损伤经络营卫气血，导致体内瘀血，肌肤甲错，两眼黯黑。治疗应以缓中补虚为主，宜用大黄蟅虫丸主治。

附方

【原文】

《千金翼方》炙甘草汤治虚劳不足，汗出而闷，脉结悸，行动如常，不出百日，危急者，十一日死。

甘草（四两，炙）　桂枝、生姜（各三两）　麦门冬（半升）　麻仁（半

【英译】

Line 6. 18

[In the disease of] five consumptions with extreme deficiency and emaciation, [there are symptoms and signs of] abdominal fullness, inability to drink and eat, damage caused by food, anxiety, drinking, sexual intercourse, hunger, overexertion, damage of meridians, collaterals, nutrient qi and defense qi, dry blood in the body, squamous and dry skin and dark eyes. [To resolve such symptoms and signs, measures should be taken] to harmonize the middle and improve deficiency. Dahuang Zhechong Pill (大黄蟅虫丸, rhubarb and ground beetle pill) [can be used] to treat it.

Dahuang Zhechong Pill (大黄蟅虫丸, rhubarb and ground beetle pill) [is composed of] 10 *fen* of Dahuang (大黄, rhubarb, Radix et Rhizoma Rhei)(steam), 2 *liang* of Huangqin (黄芩, scutellaria, Radix Scutellariae), 3 *liang* of Gancao (甘草, licorice, Radix Glycyrrhizae Praeparata), 1 *sheng* of Taoren (桃仁, peach kernel, Semen Persicae), 1 *sheng* of Xingren (杏仁, apricot kernel, Semen Armeniacae Amarum), 4 *liang* of Shaoyao (芍药, peony, Radix Paeoniae), 10 *liang* of Gandihuang (干地黄, dried rehmannia, Radix Rehmanniae), 1 *liang* of Ganqi (干漆, lacquer, Toxicodendri Resina), 1 *sheng* of Mengchong (虻虫, tabanus, Tabanus), 100 pieces of Shuizhi (水蛭, leech, Hirudo), 1 *sheng* of Qicao (蛴螬, june beetle grub, Holotrichiae Vermiculus) and 0. 5 *sheng* of Zhechong (蟅虫, ground beetle, Eupolyphaga seu Steleophaga).

These twelve ingredients are pounded into powder and blended with Lianmi (炼蜜, processed honey, Mel Praeparatum) [to produce] pills the size of small beans. [Usually] five pills are taken in wine [each time] and three times a day.

Appended formulas

【英译】

Zhi Gancao Decoction (炙甘草汤, moxa licorice decoction) [from the book entitled] *Qianjin Yifang* (《千金翼方》, *Supplemented Thousand Golden Formulas*).

升） 人参、阿胶（各二两） 大枣（三十枚） 生地黄（一斤）

右九味，以酒七升，水八升，先煮八味，取三升，去滓，内胶消尽。温服一升，日三服。

【今译】

炙甘草汤源自《千金翼方》，用以治疗虚劳不足，汗出胸闷，脉结心悸。患者虽然行动如常，但由于阴阳气血皆虚，不出百日就会导致死亡。病情危急者，延续十一日就会死亡。

【原文】

《肘后》獭肝散治冷劳，又主鬼疰一门相染。

獭肝一具，炙干，末之。水服方寸匕，日三服。

【今译】

獭肝散源自《肘后备急方》，用以治疗寒性虚劳证，也主治鬼疰病。

[This formula is used] to treat deficiency-consmuption with insufficiency [and other symptoms and signs of] sweating, oppression, bound pulse and palpitation. [Although the patient] behaves normally, [he will] die in eleven days [because the disease becomes] urgent within one hundred days.

Zhi Gancao Decoction (炙甘草汤, moxa licorice decoction) [is composed of] 4 *liang* of Gancao (甘草, licorice, Radix Glycyrrhizae Praeparata) (broil), 3 *liang* of Guizhi (桂枝, cinnamon twig, Ramulus Cinnamomi), 3 *liang* of Shengjiang (生姜, fresh ginger, Rhizoma Zingiberis Recens), 0.5 *sheng* of Maimendong (麦门冬, ophiopogon, Radix Ophiopogonis), 0.5 *sheng* of Maren (麻仁, cannabis seed, Semen Cannabis), 2 *liang* of Renshen (人参, ginseng, Radix Ginseng), 2 *liang* of Ejiao (阿胶, ass-hide glue, Colla Corii Asini), 30 pieces of Dazao (大枣, jujube, Fructus Ziziphi Jujubae) and 1 *jin* of Shengdihuang (生地黄, fresh rehmannia, Radix Rehmanniae).

[Among] these nine ingredients, eight are boiled first in 7 *sheng* of wine and 7 *sheng* of water to get 3 *sheng* [after] boiling. The dregs are removed and put Ejiao (阿胶, ass-hide glue, Colla Corii Asini) into [it] to melt completely. [The decoction is] taken warm 1 *sheng* [each time] and three times a day.

【英译】

Tagan Powder (獭肝散, otter's liver powder) [from the book entitled] *Zhouhou Beiji Formulas* (《肘后备急方》, *A Handbook of Formulas For Emergencies*)

[Tagan Powder (獭肝散, otter's liver powder) is used] to treat cold consumptive [disease] and an infectious disease of the same nature.

[Tagan Powder (獭肝散, otter's liver powder) is composed of] one otter's liver [which is] broiled dry and pounded into powder. [The powder is] taken one *fangcunbi* in water [each time] and three times a day.

肺痿肺痈咳嗽上气病脉证治第七

【原文】

(一)

问曰：热在上焦者，因咳为肺痿。肺痿之病何从得之？师曰：或从汗出，或从呕吐，或从消渴，小便利数，或从便难，又被快药下利，重亡津液，故得之。

【今译】

问：热在上焦的人，因为咳嗽而发展成肺痿病。肺痿病是怎么造成的呢？

老师说：造成肺痿病的原因，或是因为发汗，或是因为呕吐，或是从消渴多尿之证转化而来，或是因为大便困难而用峻烈药物通利大便，因而损伤津液所致。

【原文】

曰：寸口脉数，其人咳，口中反有浊唾涎沫者何？师曰：为肺痿之病。若口中辟辟燥，咳即胸中隐隐痛，脉反滑数，此为肺痈，咳唾脓血。脉数虚者为肺痿，数实者为肺痈。

【今译】

问：患者寸口脉数，咳嗽，口中为什么反而有浊唾涎沫呢？

老师说：因为这是肺痿之病。如果患者口中干燥，咳嗽时感到胸中隐隐作痛，脉象反而滑数，这就是肺痈病，所以就咳吐脓血。

脉象数虚的为肺痿，脉象数实的为肺痈。

Volume 1

Chapter 7
Lung Wilting, Lung Abscess, Cough and Ascending Qi
Disease: Pulses, Syndromes/Patterns and Treatment

【英译】

Line 7. 1

Question: [In patients with] heat in the upper energizer, cough will cause lung wilting. How does the disease of lung wilting occur?

The master said: [It is] either caused by sweating, or by vomiting, or by wasting-thirst with frequent urination, or by difficulty in defecation that is heavily purged and causes heavy collapse of fluid and humor.

【英译】

Question: The patient with rapid pulse in the cunkou [region] coughs, but there is sputum and foamy drool in the mouth. What is the reason?

The master said: [This] is lung wilting disease. If the mouth is dry, there is dull pain in the chest and the pulse is slippery and rapid. This is lung abscess [marked by] cough with pus and blood.

Rapid and weak pulse indicates lung wilting while rapid and strong [pulse] indicates lung abscess.

【原文】

（二）

问曰：病咳逆，脉之，何以知此为肺痈？当有脓血，吐之则死，其脉何类？师曰：寸口脉微而数，微则为风，数则为热；微则汗出，数则恶寒。风中于卫，呼气不入；热过于荣，吸而不出。风伤皮毛，热伤血脉。风舍于肺，其人则咳，口干喘满，咽燥不渴，时唾浊沫，时时振寒。热之所过，血为之凝滞，畜结痈脓，吐如米粥。始萌可救，脓成则死。

【今译】

问题：患咳嗽气逆病的人，通过脉诊怎么知道患的是肺痈呢？一定会有脓血，呕吐时就会死亡，其脉象属于哪一类的呢？

老师说：这种患者的寸口脉象应该是微而数，微脉为风邪，数脉为热邪；脉微则有汗出，脉数则有恶寒。风邪中于卫，邪气随着呼气而排出；热象进入荣血，则随吸气而更加深入其中，不会排出。风邪损伤皮毛，热邪损伤血脉。风邪停滞于肺，患者就会咳嗽、口干、气喘、胸满、咽喉干燥但口不渴、呕唾浊沫，时时振寒。热邪侵犯之后，血就会凝滞。热邪与血液畜结，酿成痈脓，患者因此呕吐米粥样的浓痰。此病初期无脓时可救，脓形成后就会危及生命。

Volume 1

【英译】

Line 7.2

Question: [In] disease with cough and counterflow [of qi], why taking pulse can diagnose it lung abscess? When there is pus and blood, [the patient will] die when vomiting. What kind of pulse does the patient have?

The master said: The pulse in the cunkou [region] is faint and rapid. Faint [pulse] indicates [pathogenic] wind while rapid [pulse] indicates [pathogenic] heat. [When the pulse is] faint, [there will be] sweating; [when the pulse is] rapid, [there will be] aversion to cold. [When] wind attacks the defense [aspect], exhalation will prevent it from entering [into the internal]. [When pathogenic] heat penetrates through the blood, inhalation makes it enter [into the internal]. [Pathogenic] wind damages the skin and hair, [pathogenic] heat damages the blood and vessels. [When pathogenic] wind has entered the lung, the patient will [suffer from] cough, dry mouth, panting, chest fullness, dry throat without thirst, frequent spitting of saliva and foam and occasional quivering. [When pathogenic] heat has penetrated through [the blood], the blood will be stagnated, [consequently] amassing and binding into abscess and pus, and [causing] vomiting [of sputum with blood and pus] like porridge. At the initial stage, [the patient] can be rescued [because there is no pus in vomiting]. [When] there is pus [in vomiting], [the patient] will die.

【原文】

(三)

上气,面浮肿,肩息,其脉浮大,不治。又加利,尤甚。

【今译】

喘急气逆,面部浮肿,抬肩呼吸,脉象浮大,为不治之症。如果又有下利,病情则更为危重。

【原文】

(四)

上气,喘而躁者,属肺胀,欲作风水,发汗则愈。

【今译】

喘急气逆,喘息而烦躁的,属于肺胀,有欲作风水之势,发汗则可治愈。

Volume 1

【英译】

Line 7.3

[The disease, characterized by] rapid breath [with counterflow of qi], puffy swollen face and floating and large pulse, is incurable. If there is diarrhea, it is more severe.

【英译】

Line 7.4

[The disease, characterized by] rapid breath [with counterflow of qi], panting and vexation, is lung distension, consequently developing into wind-water [disease]. [It can be] cured by diaphoresis.

【原文】

（五）

肺痿吐涎沫而不咳者，其人不渴，必遗尿，小便数。所以然者，以上虚不能制下故也。此为肺中冷，必眩，多涎唾，甘草干姜汤以温之。若服汤已渴者，属消渴。

甘草干姜汤方

甘草（四两，炙）　干姜（二两，炮）

右㕮咀，以水三升，煮取一升五合，去滓，分温再服。

【今译】

肺痿患者吐涎沫但却不咳嗽，是因为患者不渴，但必然会遗尿，小便频数。之所以如此，是因为上虚不能制下的缘故。这是因为肺中虚寒，必然产生头眩，多唾涎沫，宜用甘草干姜汤温补。如果服用汤药后出现口渴的，属于消渴。

【英译】

Line 7.5

[The patient suffering from] lung wilting spits with foamy drool, but does not cough [because] he is not thirsty. [However] there must be enuresis and frequent urination. The reason is that the upper [part of the body is] deficient and therefore cannot control the lower [part of the body]. This is caused by cold in the lung [which] inevitably [leads to] dizziness and increased drool and spittle. Gancao Ganjiang Decoction (甘草干姜汤, licorice and dried ginger decoction) [can be used to treat it] by warming. If [the patient feels] thirsty after taking the decoction, it belongs to wasting-thirst.

Gancao Ganjiang Decoction (甘草干姜汤, licorice and dried ginger decoction) [is composed of] 4 *liang* of Gancao (甘草, licorice, Radix Glycyrrhizae Praeparata)(broil) and 2 *liang* of Ganjiang (干姜, dried ginger, Rhizoma Zingiberis)(fry heavily).

These two ingredients are chewed and decocted in 3 *sheng* of water to get 1.5 *sheng* [after] boiling. The dregs are removed and [the decoction is] divided into two [doses] and taken warm.

【原文】

(六)

咳而上气,喉中水鸡声,射干麻黄汤主之。

射干麻黄汤方

射干(十三枚。一法三两) 麻黄(四两) 生姜(四两) 细辛 紫菀、款冬花(各三两) 五味子(半升) 大枣(七枚) 半夏(大者洗,八枚。一法半升)

右九味,以水一斗二升,先煮麻黄两沸,去上沫,内诸药,煮取三升,分温三服。

【今译】

咳嗽气喘的患者,喉中痰鸣如水鸡声,用射干麻黄汤主治。

【原文】

(七)

咳逆上气,时时吐浊,但坐不得眠,皂荚丸主之。

皂荚丸方

皂荚(八两,刮去皮,用酥炙)

一味,末之,蜜丸梧子大。以枣膏和汤服三丸,日三、夜一服。

【今译】

患者咳嗽、喘逆、气急,时时呕吐浊痰,只能坐而不得睡眠,用皂荚丸主治。

【英译】

Line 7.6

[The patient with] cough, panting and rale in the throat [sounding like] crow of rooster in water [can be] treated by Shegan Mahuang Decoction (射干麻黄汤, belamcanda and ephedra decoction).

Shegan Mahuang Decoction (射干麻黄汤, belamcanda and ephedra decoction) [is composed of] 13 pieces of Shegan (射干, belamcanda, Rhizoma Belamcandae) (or 3 *liang*), 4 *liang* of Mahuang (麻黄, ephedra, Herba Ephedrae), 4 *liang* of Shengjiang (生姜, fresh ginger, Rhizoma Zingiberis Recens), 3 *liang* of Xixin (细辛, asarum, Herba Asari), 3 *liang* of Ziwan (紫菀, aster, Radix Asteris), 3 *liang* of Kuandonghua (款冬花, coltsfoot, Flos Farfarae), 0.5 *sheng* of Wuweizi (五味子, schisandra, Fructus Schisandrae), 7 pieces of Dazao (大枣, jujube, Fructus Ziziphus Jujubae) and 8 pieces of Banxia (半夏, pinellia, Rhizoma Pinelliae) (big, wash; or 0.5 *sheng*).

These nine ingredients are decocted in 1 *dou* and 2 *sheng* of water. Mahuang (麻黄, ephedra, Herba Ephedrae) is boiled first for twice. [After] removal of the foam, the rest ingredients are put into [it] to boil and get 3 *sheng*. [The decoction is] divided into three [doses] and taken warm.

【英译】

Line 7.7

[The patient suffering from] cough, panting, rapid breath, frequent vomiting of turbid sputum and can only sit but inability to sleep [can be] treated by Zaojia Pill (皂荚丸, gelditsia Pill).

Zaojia Pill (皂荚丸, gelditsia Pill) [is composed of] 8 *liang* of Zaojia (皂荚, gelditsia, Fructus Gleditsiae) (remove the bark and broil in butter).

This ingredient is pounded into powder and made into honey pills the size of firminana seeds. Mixed with jujube paste and hot water, the pills are taken three [each time], thrice a day and once at night.

【原文】

（八）

咳而脉浮者，厚朴麻黄汤主之。

厚朴麻黄汤方

厚朴（五两）　麻黄（四两）　石膏（如鸡子大）　杏仁（半升）　半夏（半升）　干姜（二两）　细辛（二两）　小麦（一升）　五味子（半升）

右九味，以水一斗二升，先煮小麦熟，去滓，内诸药，煮取三升。温服一升，日三服。

【今译】

咳嗽而脉象浮，用厚朴麻黄汤主治。

【原文】

（九）

脉沉者，泽漆汤主之。

泽漆汤方

半夏（半升）　紫参（五两。一作紫菀）　泽漆（三斤，以东流水五斗，煮取一斗五升）　生姜（五两）　白前（五两）　甘草　黄芩　人参　桂枝（各三两）

右九味，㕮咀，内泽漆汁中，煮取五升。温服五合，至夜尽。

【今译】

患者脉象沉的，用泽漆汤主治。

【英译】

Line 7.8

[The disease marked by] cough and floating pulse [can be] treated by Houpo Mahuang Decoction (厚朴麻黄汤，magnolia bark and ephedra decoction).

Houpo Mahuang Decoction (厚朴麻黄汤，magnolia bark and ephedra decoction) [is composed of] 5 *liang* of Houpo (厚朴，magnolia bark，Cortex Magnoliae Officinalis), 4 *liang* of Mahuang (麻黄，ephedra，Herba Ephedrae), Shigao (石膏，gypsum，Gypsum Fibrosum) (as big as a chichen egg), 0.5 *sheng* of Xingren (杏仁，apricot kernel，Semen Armeniacae Amarum), 0.5 *sheng* of Banxia (半夏，pinellia，Rhizoma Pinelliae), 2 *liang* of Ganjiang (干姜，dried ginger，Rhizoma Zingiberis), 2 *liang* of Xixin (细辛，asarum，Herba Asari), 1 *sheng* of Xiaomai (小麦，wheat，Semen Tritici) and 0.5 *sheng* of Wuweizi (五味子，schisandra，Fructus Schisandrae).

These nine ingredients are decocted in 1 *dou* and 2 *sheng* of water. Xiaomai (小麦，wheat，Semen Tritici) is cooked first. The dregs are removed and all other ingredients are put into it to boil and get 3 *sheng*. [The decoction is] taken warm 1 *sheng* [each time] and three times a day.

【英译】

Line 7.9

[The patient with] sunken pulse [can be] treated by Zeqi Decoction (泽漆汤，sun spurge decoction).

Zeqi Decoction (泽漆汤，sun spurge decoction) [is composed of] 0.5 *sheng* of Banxia (半夏，pinellia，Rhizoma Pinelliae), 5 *liang* of Zishen (紫参) [or Ziwan (紫菀，aster，Radix Asteris)], 3 *jin* of Zeqi (泽漆，sun spurge，Herba Euphorbiae Helioscopiae) (get 1 *dou* and 5 *sheng* after boiling in 5 *dou* of water running toward the east), 5 *liang* of Shengjiang (生姜，fresh ginger，Rhizoma Zingiberis Recens), 5 *liang* of Baiqian (白前，willowleaf wallowwort，Rhizoma Cynanchi Stauntonii), 3 *liang* of Gancao (甘草，licorice，Radix Glycyrrhizae Praeparata), 3 *liang* of Huangqin (黄芩，scutellaria，Radix Scutellariae), 3 *liang* of Renshen (人参，ginseng，Radix Ginseng) and 3 *liang* of Guizhi (桂枝，cinnamon twig，Ramulus Cinnamomi).

These nine ingredients are chewed and boiled in Zeqi (泽漆，sun spurge，Herba Euphorbiae Helioscopiae) juice to get 5 *sheng*. [The decoction is] taken warm 5 *ge* [each time] and finished at night.

【原文】

（十）

大逆上气，咽喉不利，止逆下气者，麦门冬汤主之。

麦门冬汤方

麦门冬（七升） 半夏（一升） 人参（二两） 甘草（二两） 粳米（三合） 大枣（十二枚）

六味，以水一斗二升，煮取六升。温服一升，日三、夜一服。

【今译】

大逆上气，咽喉干燥不利，可通过止逆下气治疗，用麦门冬汤主治。

【原文】

（十一）

肺痈，喘不得卧，葶苈大枣泻肺汤主之。

葶苈大枣泻肺汤方

葶苈（熬令黄色，捣丸如弹丸大） 大枣（十二枚）

右先以水三升，煮枣取二升，去枣，内葶苈，煮取一升，顿服。

【今译】

肺痈，咳喘不得卧，用葶苈大枣泻肺汤主治。

Volume 1

Line 7. 10

[The disease characterized by] great upward counterflow of qi and inhibited throat [can be treated by] stopping counterflow and descending qi. The appropriate [formula is] Maimendong Decoction (麦门冬汤, ophiopogon decoction).

Maimendong Decoction (麦门冬汤, ophiopogon decoction) [is composed of] 7 *sheng* of Maimendong (麦门冬, ophiopogon, Radix Ophiopogonis), 1 *sheng* of Banxia (半夏, pinellia, Rhizoma Pinelliae), 2 *liang* of Renshen (人参, ginseng, Radix Ginseng), 2 *liang* of Gancao (甘草, licorice, Radix Glycyrrhizae Praeparata), 3 *ge* of Jingmi (粳米, polished round-grained rice, Semen Oryzae Nonglutinosae) and 12 pieces of Dazao (大枣, jujube, Fructus Ziziphus Jujubae).

These six ingredients are decocted in 1 *dou* and 2 *sheng* of water to get 6 *sheng* [after] boiling. [The decoction is] taken warm 1 *sheng* [each time], thrice a day and once at night.

Line 7. 11

Lung abscess with panting and inability to sleep [can be] treated by Tingli Dazao Xiefei Decoction (葶苈大枣泻肺汤, tingli and jujube decoction for draining the lung).

Tingli Dazao Xiefei Decoction (葶苈大枣泻肺汤, tingli and jujube decoction for draining the lung) [is composed of] Tingli (葶苈, lepidium/descurainiae, Semen Lepidii seu Descurainiae) (boil till yellow and pound and make into pills the size of pellets)and 12 pieces of Dazao (大枣, jujube, Fructus Ziziphus Jujubae).

3 *sheng* of water is used. Dazao (大枣, jujube, Fructus Ziziphus Jujubae) is boiled first to get 2 *sheng*. [After] removal of the jujube, Tingli (葶苈, lepidium/descurainiae, Semen Lepidii seu Descurainiae) is boiled in [it] to get 1 *sheng*. [The decoction is] taken in one dose.

【原文】

(十二)

咳而胸满,振寒脉数,咽干不渴,时出浊唾腥臭,久久吐脓如米粥者,为肺痈,桔梗汤主之。

桔梗汤方亦治血痹。

桔梗(一两) 甘草(二两)

右二味,以水三升,煮取一升。分温再服,则吐脓血也。

【今译】

咳嗽而胸满,振寒而脉数,咽干而不渴,不时吐出浊唾腥臭,时常吐脓血痰,状如米粥,为肺痈,宜用桔梗汤主治。

【原文】

(十三)

咳而上气,此为肺胀,其人喘,目如脱状,脉浮大者,越婢加半夏汤主之。

越婢加半夏汤方

麻黄(六两) 石膏(半斤) 生姜(三两) 大枣(十五枚) 甘草(二两) 半夏(半升)

右六味,以水六升,先煮麻黄,去上沫,内诸药,煮取三升,分温三服。

【今译】

咳嗽而气逆,此为肺胀,患者气喘,两目突出如脱状,脉浮大,宜用越婢加半夏汤主治。

【英译】
Line 7. 12
［The disease, characterized by］ cough with chest fullness, quivering with rapid pulse, dry throat without thirst, occasional spitting of turbid sputum, frequent vomiting of pus and blood like porridge, is lung abscess. ［It can be］ treated by Jiegeng Decoction （桔梗汤, platycodon grandiflorum Decoction）.

Jiegeng Decoction （桔梗汤, platycodon grandiflorum Decoction） can also treat blood impediment.

Jiegeng Decoction （桔梗汤, platycodon grandiflorum Decoction） ［is composed of］ 1 *liang* of Jiegeng（桔梗, platycodon grandiflorum, Radix Platycodi） and 2 *liang* of Gancao （甘草, licorice, Radix Glycyrrhizae Praeparata）.

These two ingredients are decocted in 3 *sheng* of water to get 1 *sheng* ［after］ boiling. ［The decoction is］ divided into two ［doses］ and taken warm ［each time］. ［After taking the decoction, the patient will］ vomit pus and blood.

【英译】
Line 7. 13
［The disease with the symptoms and signs of］ cough and upward counterflow of qi is lung distension ［marked by］ panting, protrusion of eyes and floating and large pulse. ［It can be treated by］ Yuebi Decoction （越婢汤, decoction for effusing the spleen） added with Banxia （半夏, pinellia, Rhizoma Pinelliae）.

Yuebi Decoction （越婢汤, decoction for effusing the spleen） added with Banxia （半夏, pinellia, Rhizoma Pinelliae） ［is composed of］ 6 *liang* of Mahuang （麻黄, ephedra, Herba Ephedrae）, 0.5 *jin* of Shigao （石膏, gypsum, Gypsum Fibrosum）, 3 *liang* of Shengjiang （生姜, fresh ginger, Rhizoma Zingiberis Recens）, 15 pieces of Dazao （大枣, jujube, Fructus Ziziphus Jujubae）, 2 *liang* of Gancao （甘草, licorice, Radix Glycyrrhizae Praeparata） and 0.5 *jin* of Banxia （半夏, pinellia, Rhizoma Pinelliae）.

These six ingredients are decocted in 6 *sheng* of water. Mahuang （麻黄, ephedra, Herba Ephedrae） is boiled first. ［After］ removal of the foam, all the other ingredients are put into ［it］ to boil and get 3 *sheng*. ［The decoction is］ divided into three ［doses］ and taken warm.

【原文】

(十四)

肺胀,咳而上气,烦躁而喘,脉浮者,心下有水,小青龙加石膏汤主之。

小青龙加石膏汤方

麻黄 芍药 桂枝 细辛 甘草 干姜(各三两) 五味子 半夏(各半升) 石膏(二两)

右九味,以水一斗,先煮麻黄,去上沫,内诸药,煮取三升。强人服一升,羸者减之,日三服,小儿服四合。

【今译】

肺胀,咳嗽而上气,烦躁而咳喘,脉象浮,心下有水,用小青龙加石膏汤主治。

附方

【原文】

《外台》炙甘草汤治肺痿涎唾多,心中温温液液者。

《千金》甘草汤

甘草

右一味,以水三升,煮减半,分温三服。

【今译】

《外台秘要》中的炙甘草汤,治疗肺痿吐涎唾多,心中泛泛欲吐。

【英译】

Line 7. 14

Lung distension [disease, marked by] cough, upward counterflow of qi, vexation, panting, floating pulse and edema under the heart, [can be treated by] Xiao Qinglong [Decoction] (小青龙汤, minor blue loong decoction) added with Shigao Decoction (石膏汤, gypsum decoction).

Xiao Qinglong [Decoction] (小青龙汤, minor blue loong decoction) added with Shigao Decoction (石膏汤, gypsum decoction) [is composed of] 3 *liang* of Mahuang (麻黄, ephedra, Herba Ephedrae), 3 *liang* of Shaoyao (芍药, peony, Radix Paeoniae), 3 *liang* of Guizhi (桂枝, cinnamon twig, Ramulus Cinnamomi), 3 *liang* of Xixin (细辛, asarum, Herba Asari), 3 *liang* of Gancao (甘草, licorice, Radix Glycyrrhizae Praeparata), 3 *liang* of Ganjiang (干姜, dried ginger, Rhizoma Zingiberis), 0. 5 *sheng* of Wuweizi (五味子, schisandra, Fructus Schisandrae), 0. 5 *sheng* of Banxia (半夏, pinellia, Rhizoma Pinelliae) and 2 *liang* of Shigao (石膏, gypsum, Gypsum Fibrosum).

These nine ingredients are decocted in 1 *dou* of water. Mahuang (麻黄, ephedra, Herba Ephedrae) is boiled first. [After] removal of the foam, all the other ingredients are put into [it] to boil and get 3 *sheng*. Strong patients can take 1 *sheng* [each time], weak patients can take less, and three times a day. For children, 4 *ge* is taken [each time].

Applended formulas

【英译】

Zhi Gancao Decoction (炙甘草汤, fried licorice decoction) [from the book entitled] *Waitai Miyao* (《外台秘要》, *The Medical Secrets of an Official Named Wang Tao*), [used] to treat lung wilting [marked by] frequent copious drool and spittle as well as pervasive nausea.

Zhi Gancao Decoction (炙甘草汤, fried licorice decoction) [is just composed of] Gancao (甘草, licorice, Radix Glycyrrhizae Praeparata).

This ingredient is decocted in 3 *sheng* of water and reduced half [after] boiling. [The decoction is] divided into three [doses] and taken warm.

【原文】

《千金》生姜甘草汤治肺痿咳唾涎沫不止，咽燥而渴。

生姜（五两）　人参（二两）　甘草（四两）　大枣（十五枚）

右四味，以水七升，煮取三升，分温三服。

【今译】

《千金方》中的生姜甘草汤，治疗肺痿，咳嗽唾吐涎沫不止，咽喉干燥而口渴。

【原文】

《千金》桂枝去芍药加皂荚汤治肺痿吐涎沫。

桂枝　生姜（各三两）　甘草（二两）　大枣（十枚）　皂荚（一枚，去皮子，炙焦）

右五味，以水七升，微微火煮取三升，分温三服。

【今译】

《千金方》中的桂枝去芍药加皂荚汤，治疗肺痿吐唾涎沫。

【英译】

Shengjiang Gancao Decoction (生姜甘草汤, fresh ginger and licorice decoction) [from the book entitled] *Qianjin Formulas* (《千金方》, *Thousand Golden Formulas*), [is used] to treat lung wilting [marked by] cough, nausea, incessant spitting, dry throat and thirst.

Shengjiang Gancao Decoction (生姜甘草汤, fresh ginger and licorice decoction) [is composed of] 5 *liang* of Shengjiang (生姜, fresh ginger, Rhizoma Zingiberis Recens), 2 *liang* of Renshen (人参, ginseng, Radix Ginseng), 4 *liang* of Gancao (甘草, licorice, Radix Glycyrrhizae Praeparata) and 15 pieces of Dazao (大枣, jujube, Fructus Ziziphus Jujubae).

These four ingredients are decocted in 7 *sheng* of water to get 3 *sheng* [after] boiling. [The decoction is] divided into three [doses] and taken warm.

【英译】

Guizhi Decoction (桂枝汤, cinnamon twig decoction) with removal of Shaoyao (芍药, peony, Radix Paeoniae) and addition of Zaojia (皂荚, gelditsia, Fructus Gleditsiae) [from the book entitled] *Qianjin Formulas* (《千金方》, *Thousand Golden Formulas*), [is used] to treat lung wilting with vomiting and spittle.

Guizhi Decoction (桂枝汤, cinnamon twig decoction) [is composed of] 3 *liang* of Guizhi (桂枝, cinnamon twig, Ramulus Cinnamomi), 3 *liang* of Shengjiang (生姜, fresh ginger, Rhizoma Zingiberis Recens), 2 *liang* of Gancao (甘草, licorice, Radix Glycyrrhizae Praeparata), 10 pieces of Dazao (大枣, jujube, Fructus Ziziphus Jujubae) and 1 piece of Zaojia (皂荚, gelditsia, Fructus Gleditsiae)(remove the bark and seeds and scorch).

These five ingredients are decocted in 7 *sheng* of water to get 3 *sheng* [after] boiling over mild flame. [The decoction is] divided into three [doses] and taken warm.

【原文】

《外台》桔梗白散治咳而胸满,振寒,脉数,咽干不渴,时出浊唾腥臭,久久吐脓如米粥者,为肺痈。

桔梗　贝母(各三分)　巴豆(一分,去皮,熬,研如脂)

右三味,为散,强人饮服半钱匕,羸者减之。病在膈上者吐脓血,膈下者泻出。若下多不止,饮冷水一杯则定。

【今译】

《外台秘要》中的桔梗白散,治疗咳嗽而胸满,周身振寒,脉象数,咽干而口不渴,时时出现浊唾腥臭,常常吐脓痰,状若米粥,此为肺痈。

【原文】

《千金》苇茎汤治咳有微热烦满,胸中甲错,是为肺痈。

苇茎(二升)　薏苡仁(半升)　桃仁(五十枚)　瓜瓣(半升)

右四味,以水一斗,先煮苇茎得五升,去滓,内诸药,煮取二升。服一升,再服,当吐如脓。

【今译】

《千金方》中的苇茎汤,治疗咳嗽,有微热,烦闷,腹满,胸中甲错,此属肺痈。

【英译】

Jiegeng Bai Powder（桔梗白散，white platycodon grandiflorum powder）[from the book entitled] *Waitai Miyao* (《外台秘要》，*The Medical Secrets of an Official Named Wang Tao*) [can be used] to treat [the disease characterized by] cough with chest fullness, quivering with rapid pulse, dry throat with thirst, occasional spitting of turbid sputum, frequent vomiting of pus like porridge, [which] is lung abscess.

Jiegeng Bai Powder（桔梗白散，white platycodon grandiflorum powder）[is composed of] 3 *fen* of Jiegeng（桔梗，platycodon grandiflorum, Radix Platycodi）, 3 *fen* of Beimu（贝母，fritillaria, Bulbus Fritillariae Thunbergii) and 1 *fen* of Badou（巴豆，croton, Fructus Crotonis）(remove the peel, simmer and grind as paste).

These three ingredients are made into powder. Strong patients take half a *qianbi* [each time] and weak patients take less. [If the disease is located] above the diaphragm, there will be vomiting of pus and blood. [If the disease is located] below the diaphragm, there will be diarrhea. If diarrhea is incessant, drinking a cup of cold water will cease it.

【英译】

Line 7

Weijing Decoction（苇茎汤，phragmites stem decoction）[from the book entitled] *Qianjin Formulas* (《千金方》，*Thousand Golden Formulas*), [can be used] to treat [the disease marked by] cough, mild fever, vexation, abdominal fullness, scaly skin over the chest, [which] is lung abscess.

[Weijing Decoction（苇茎汤，phragmites stem decoction）is composed of] 2 *sheng* of Weijing（苇茎，phragmites stem, Rhizoma Phragmitis）, 0.5 *jin* of Yiyiren（薏苡仁，coix, Semen Coicis）, 50 pieces of Taoren（桃仁，peach kernel, Semen Persicae) and 0.5 *jin* of Guaban（瓜瓣，wax gourd seed）.

These four ingredients are decocted in 1 *dou* of water. Weijing（苇茎，phragmites stem, Rhizoma Phragmitis) is boiled first to get 5 *sheng*. The dregs are removed and all the other ingredients are put into [it] to boil and get 2 *sheng*. [The patient] takes 1 *sheng* first. [When] the second 1 *sheng* is taken, [there will be] vomiting [of sputum] like pus.

【原文】

（十五）

肺痈胸满胀，一身面目浮肿，鼻塞清涕出，不闻香臭酸辛，咳逆上气，喘鸣迫塞，葶苈大枣泻肺汤主之。

【今译】

肺痈胸满胀，患者全身及面目浮肿，鼻塞流清涕，闻不出香臭酸辛等味道，咳嗽逆喘上气，喉中喘鸣堵塞，用葶苈大枣泻肺汤主治。

Volume 1

【英译】

Line 7. 15

Lung abscess [disease is characterized by] chest fullness and distension, puffy dropsy of the whole body including face and eyes, stuffy nose with clear snivel, inability to smell fragrant, fetor, sour and acrid tastes, cough with upward counterflow of qi, panting with rale and congestion. [It can be] treated by Tingli Dazao Xiefei Decoction (葶苈大枣泻肺汤, tingli and jujube decoction for draining the lung).

奔豚气病脉证治第八

【原文】

（一）

师曰：病有奔豚，有吐脓，有惊怖，有火邪，此四部病，皆从惊发得之。

师曰：奔豚病，从少腹起，上冲咽喉，发作欲死，复还止，皆从惊恐得之。

【今译】

老师说：奔豚、吐脓、惊怖、火邪等四种疾病，都是因惊恐诱发而成。

老师说：奔豚病发作时，首先从少腹开始，上冲到咽喉，令患者有欲死之感。发作之后，气又复还。这都是因惊恐而诱发。

Volume 1

Chapter 8
Running Piglet Disease:
Pulses, Syndromes/Patterns and Treatment

【英译】

Line 8. 1

The master said: Running piglet, spitting of pus, fright and pathogenic fire are four types of diseases all caused by fright.

The master said: Running piglet starts from the lower abdomen, surging upwards to the throat, making [the patient feel] about to die. [But when qi] returns, [the disease] ceases. All this results from fright.

【原文】

（二）

奔豚，气上冲胸，腹痛，往来寒热，奔豚汤主之。

奔豚汤方

甘草、芎藭、当归（各二两）　半夏（四两）　黄芩（二两）　生葛（五两）　芍药（二两）　生姜（四两）　甘李根白皮（一升）

右九味，以水二斗，煮取五升。温服一升，日三、夜一服。

【今译】

奔豚发作时，气上冲于胸，导致腹痛，往来寒热，宜用奔豚汤主治。

【英译】

Line 8.2

[When] running piglet [has occurred], qi is surging upwards [from the lower abdomen] to the chest，[leading to] abdominal pain and alternate cold and heat. [It can be] treated by Bentun Decoction (奔豚汤，running piglet decoction).

Bentun Decoction (奔豚汤，running piglet decoction) [is composed of] 2 *liang* of Gancao (甘草，licorice，Radix Glycyrrhizae Praeparata)，2 *liang* of Xiongqiong (芎䓖，xiongqiong，Rhizoma Chuanxiong)，2 *liang* of Danggui (当归，Chinese angelica，Radix Angelicae Sinensis)，4 *liang* of Banxia (半夏，pinellia，Rhizoma Pinelliae)，2 *liang* of Huangqin (黄芩，scutellaria，Radix Scutellariae) of Shengge (生葛，raw pueraria，Radix Puerariae Cruda)，2 *liang* of Shaoyao (芍药，peony，Radix Paeoniae)，4 *liang* of Shengjiang (生姜，fresh ginger，Rhizoma Zingiberis Recens) and 1 *sheng* of Ganligen Baipi (甘李根白皮，plum root bark，Cortex Pruni Salicinae Radicis).

These nine ingredients are decocted in 2 *dou* of water to get 5 *sheng* [after] boiling. [The decoction is] taken warm 1 *sheng* [each time]，thrice a day and once at night.

【原文】

(三)

发汗后,烧针令其汗,针处被寒,核起而赤者,必发奔豚,气从少腹上至心,灸其核上各一壮,与桂枝加桂汤主之。

桂枝加桂汤方

桂枝(五两)　芍药(三两)　甘草(二两,炙)　生姜(三两)　大枣(十二枚)

右五味,以水七升,微火煮取三升,去滓,温服一升。

【今译】

使用发汗法后病仍然不解,又用烧针再发其汗,导致寒气从烧针处侵入人体,致使针刺处红肿如核,必然会引发奔豚,气从少腹部上冲至心胸,在其红肿之处各灸一壮,再用桂枝加桂汤主治。

【英译】

Line 8.3

[When the disease is not resolved] after [application of] diaphoresis and [if acupuncture with] heated needle [is used] again to promote sweating, [it will lead to invasion of pathogenic] cold into the region needled, causing red lumps like fruit kernels. [As a result,] running piglet will inevitably occur and qi will surge upwards from the lower abdomen to the heart. [To resolve it,] one cone is [used] to heat the top of one lump. Guizhi Decoction（桂枝汤，cinnamon twig decoction）added with extra Guizhi（桂枝，cinnamon twig, Ramulus Cinnamomi）[is used together with moxibustion] to treat it.

Guizhi Decoction（桂枝汤，cinnamon twig decoction）added with extra Guizhi（桂枝，cinnamon twig, Ramulus Cinnamomi）[is composed of] 5 *liang* of Guizhi（桂枝，cinnamon twig, Ramulus Cinnamomi），3 *liang* of Shaoyao（芍药，peony, Radix Paeoniae），2 *liang* of Gancao（甘草，licorice, Radix Glycyrrhizae Praeparata）（broil），3 *liang* of Shengjiang（生姜，fresh ginger, Rhizoma Zingiberis Recens）and 12 pieces of Dazao（大枣，jujube, Fructus Ziziphus Jujubae）.

These five ingredients are decocted in 7 *sheng* of water to get 3 *sheng* [after] boiling in mild fire. The dregs are removed and [the decoction is] taken warm 1 *sheng* [each time].

【原文】

（四）

发汗后，脐下悸者，欲作奔豚，茯苓桂枝甘草大枣汤主之。

茯苓桂枝甘草大枣汤方

茯苓（半斤）　甘草（二两，炙）　大枣（十五枚）　桂枝（四两）

右四味，以甘澜水一斗，先煮茯苓，减二升，内诸药，煮取三升，去滓。温服一升，日三服。

【今译】

使用发汗法后，脐下出现悸动的，奔豚将要发作，宜用茯苓桂枝甘草大枣汤主治。

【英译】

Line 8.4

After [application of] diaphoresis, there is palpitation below the umbilicus, indicating that running piglet is going to occur. Fuling Guizhi Gancao Dazao Decoction (茯苓桂枝甘草大枣汤, poria, cinnamon twig, licorice and jujube decoction) [can be used] to treat it.

Fuling Guizhi Gancao Dazao Decoction (茯苓桂枝甘草大枣汤, poria, cinnamon twig, licorice and jujube decoction) [is composed of] 0.5 *jin* of Fuling (茯苓, poria, Poria), 2 *liang* of Gancao (甘草, licorice, Radix Glycyrrhizae Praeparata)(broil), 15 pieces of Dazao (大枣, jujube, Fructus Ziziphus Jujubae) and 4 *liang* of Guizhi (桂枝, cinnamon twig, Ramulus Cinnamomi).

These four ingredients are decocted in 1 *dou* of ganlan water (甘澜水, the water that is poured and splashed repeatedly in a pot). Fuling (茯苓, poria, Poria) is boiled first to get 2 *sheng*. [Then] all the other ingredients are put into [it] to boil and get 3 *sheng*. The dregs are removed and [the decoction is] taken warm 1 *sheng* [each time] and three times a day.

胸痹心痛短气病脉证治第九

【原文】

（一）

师曰：夫脉当取太过不及，阳微阴弦，即胸痹而痛。所以然者，责其极虚也。今阳虚知在上焦，所以胸痹、心痛者，以其阴弦故也。

【今译】

老师说：诊脉时应依据太过与不及，寸口脉微，尺脉弦，就是胸痹心痛病的表现。之所以如此，是因为其气极虚所致。现在通过诊断可知阳虚是在上焦，所以产生了胸痹、心痛等症状，是因为患者尺部脉弦所致。

【原文】

（二）

平人无寒热，短气不足以息者，实也。

【今译】

表面上健康的人，无恶寒发热症状，但呼吸窘迫，难以相续，属于实证。

Chapter 9
Chest Impediment, Heart Pain and Shortness of Breath Disease: Pulses, Syndromes/Patterns and Treatment

【英译】

Line 9.1

The master said: [Diagnosis by means of taking] pulse should depend on exuberance and insufficiency. [When] yang [pulse] (pulse in the cunkou region) is faint and yin [pulse] (pulse in the chi region) is taut, [it] indicates chest impediment and pain. The reason is that qi is extremely weak. Now [through examination, it is] known that yang deficiency is in the upper energizer. That is why chest impediment and pain are caused because yin [pulse] (pulse in the chi region) is taut.

【英译】

Line 9.2

People, who are physically healthy without aversion to cold and fever, but with shortness of breath and hypopnea, [actually suffer from] excess [syndrome/pattern].

【原文】

（三）

胸痹之病,喘息咳唾,胸背痛,短气,寸口脉沉而迟,关上小紧数,栝蒌薤白白酒汤主之。

栝蒌薤白白酒汤方

栝蒌实（一枚,捣） 薤白（半斤） 白酒（七升）

右三味,同煮,取二升,分温再服。

【今译】

患胸痹之病的人,呼吸急促,咳嗽吐痰,胸背疼痛,短气,寸口脉沉而迟,关上脉细小紧数,用栝蒌薤白白酒汤主治。

【原文】

（四）

胸痹不得卧,心痛彻背者,栝蒌薤白半夏汤主之。

栝蒌薤白半夏汤方

栝蒌实（一枚） 薤白（三两） 半夏（半斤） 白酒（一斗）

右四味,同煮,取四升。温服一升,日三服。

【今译】

胸痹不得平卧,心痛透彻到背的患者,用栝蒌薤白半夏汤主之。

Volume 1

【英译】

Line 9.3

Chest impediment [is characterized by] panting, spitting, nausea, pain in the chest and back, shortness of breath, sunken and slow pulse in the cunkou [region], small, tight and rapid pulse in the guan [region]. Gualou Xiebai Baijiu Decoction (栝蒌薤白白酒汤, trichosanthes fruit, long-stamen onion and white wine decoction) [can be used] to treat it.

Gualou Xiebai Baijiu Decoction (栝 蒌 薤 白 白 酒 汤, trichosanthes fruit, long-stamen onion and white wine decoction) [is composed of] 1 piece of Gualoushi (栝蒌实, trichosanthes fruit, Fructus Trichosanthis) (pound), 0.5 *jin* of Xiebai (薤白, long-stamen onion, Bulbus Alli Macrostemonis) and 7 *sheng* of Baijiu (白酒, white liquor, Vino Alba).

These three ingredients are boiled to get 2 *sheng* [of water]. [The decoction is] divided into two [doses] and taken warm.

【英译】

Line 9.4

Chest impediment [marked by] difficulty to lie down and heart pain extending to the back [can be] treated by Gualou Xiebai Banxia Decoction (栝 蒌 薤 白 半 夏 汤, trichosanthes fruit, long-stamen onion and pinellia decoction).

Gualou Xiebai Banxia Decoction (栝蒌薤白半夏汤, trichosanthes fruit, long-stamen onion and pinellia decoction)[is composed of] 1 piece of Gualoushi (栝蒌实, trichosanthes fruit, Fructus Trichosanthis), 3 *liang* of Xiebai (薤白, long-stamen onion, Bulbus Alli Macrostemonis), 0.5 *jin* of Banxia (半夏, pinellia, Rhizoma Pinelliae) and 1 *dou* of Baijiu (白酒, white liquor, Vino Alba).

These four ingredients are boiled together to get 4 *sheng* [after] boiling. [The decoction is] taken warm 1 *sheng* [each time] and three times a day.

【原文】

(五)

胸痹心中痞,留气结在胸,胸满,胁下逆抢心,枳实薤白桂枝汤主之,人参汤亦主之。

枳实薤白桂枝汤方

枳实(四枚) 厚朴(四两) 薤白(半斤) 桂枝(一两) 栝蒌(一枚,捣)

右五味,以水五升,先煮枳实、厚朴,取二升,去滓,内诸药,煮数沸,分温三服。

人参汤方

人参、甘草、干姜、白术(各三两)

右四味,以水八升,煮取三升。温服一升,日三服。

【今译】

胸痹病,心中痞塞,气留结在胸,导致胸满,胁下气逆上冲于心,用枳实薤白桂枝汤主治,人参汤也可主治。

Volume 1

【英译】

Line 9.5

[In] chest impediment [disease], [there are symptoms and signs of] lump in the heart, accumulation of qi in the chest, chest fullness, counterflow of qi below the rib-side surging upwards to the heart. Zhishi Xiebai Guizhi Decoction (枳实薤白桂枝汤, processed unripe bitter orange, long-stamen onion and cinnamon twig decoction) [can be used] to treat it. Renshen Decoction (人参汤, ginseng decoction) [can also be used] to treat it.

Zhishi Xiebai Guizhi Decoction (枳实薤白桂枝汤, processed unripe bitter orange, long-stamen onion and cinnamon twig decoction) [is composed of] 4 pieces of Zhishi (枳实, processed unripe bitter orange, Fructus Aurantii Immaturus), 4 *liang* of Houpo (厚朴, magnolia bark, Cortex Magnoliae Officinalis), 0.5 *jin* of Xiebai (薤白, long-stamen onion, Bulbus Alli Macrostemonis), 1 *liang* of Guizhi (桂枝, cinnamon twig, Ramulus Cinnamomi) and 1 piece of Gualou (栝蒌, trichosanthes fruit, Fructus Trichosanthis)(pound).

These five ingredients are decocted in 5 *sheng* of water. Zhishi (枳实, processed unripe bitter orange, Fructus Aurantii Immaturus) and Houpo (厚朴, magnolia bark, Cortex Magnoliae Officinalis) are boiled first to get 2 *sheng*. The dregs are removed and all the other ingredients are put into [it] to boil for several times. [The decoction is] divided into three [doses] and taken warm.

Renshen Decoction (人参汤, ginseng decoction) [is composed of] 3 *liang* of Renshen (人参, ginseng, Radix Ginseng), 3 *liang* of Gancao (甘草, licorice, Radix Glycyrrhizae Praeparata), 3 *liang* of Ganjiang (干姜, dried ginger, Rhizoma Zingiberis) and 3 *liang* of Baizhu (白术, rhizome of largehead atractylodes, Rhizoma Atractylodis Macrocephalae).

These four ingredients are decocted in 8 *sheng* of water to get 3 *sheng* [after] boiling. [The decoction is] taken warm 1 *sheng* [each time] and three times a day.

【原文】

(六)

胸痹,胸中气塞,短气,茯苓杏仁甘草汤主之,橘枳姜汤亦主之。

茯苓杏仁甘草汤方

茯苓(三两)　杏仁(五十个)　甘草(一两)

右三味,以水一斗,煮取五升。温服一升,日三服,不差,更服。

橘枳姜汤方

橘皮(一斤)　枳实(三两)　生姜(半斤)

右三味,以水五升,煮取二升,分温再服。

【今译】

　　胸痹病患者,胸中之气痞塞,短气,宜用茯苓杏仁甘草汤主治,也可用橘枳姜汤主治。

【原文】

(七)

胸痹缓急者,薏苡附子散主之。

薏苡附子散方

薏苡仁(十五两)　大附子(十枚,炮)

右二味,杵为散,服方寸匕,日三服。

【今译】

　　胸痹病发作,病情危急的,宜用薏苡附子散主治。

【英译】

Line 9.6

Chest impediment [characterized by] stagnation of qi in the chest and shortness of breath [can be] treated by Fuling Xingren Gancao Decoction (茯苓杏仁甘草汤, poria, apricot kernel and licorice decoction). Juzhi Jiang Decoction (橘枳姜汤, tangerine peel, processed unripe bitter orange and fresh ginger decoction) [can also be used] to treat it.

Fuling Xingren Gancao Decoction (茯苓杏仁甘草汤, poria, apricot kernel and licorice decoction) [is composed of] 3 *liang* of Fuling (茯苓, poria, Poria), 50 pieces of Xingren (杏仁, apricot kernel, Semen Armeniacae Amarum) and 1 *liang* of Gancao (甘草, licorice, Radix Glycyrrhizae Praeparata).

These three ingredients are decocted in 1 *dou* of water to get 5 *sheng* [after] boiling. [The decoction is] taken warm 1 *sheng* [each time] and three times a day. [If the disease is] not cured, [the decoction should be] taken again.

Juzhi Jiang Decoction (橘枳姜汤, tangerine peel, processed unripe bitter orange and fresh ginger decoction) [is composed of] 1 *jin* of Jupi (橘皮, tangerine peel, Pericarpium Citri Reticulatae), 3 *liang* of Zhishi (枳实, processed unripe bitter orange, Fructus Aurantii Immaturus) and 0.5 *jin* of Shengjiang (生姜, fresh ginger, Rhizoma Zingiberis Recens).

These three ingredients are decocted in 5 *sheng* of water to get 2 *sheng* [after] boiling. [The decoction is] divided into two [doses] and taken warm.

【英译】

Line 9.7

Chest impediment [disease], acute [right after occurrence], [should be] treated by Yiyi Fuzi Powder (薏苡附子散, aconite and coix powder).

Yiyi Fuzi Powder (薏苡附子散, aconite and coix powder) [is composed of] 15 *liang* of Yiyiren (薏苡仁, coix, Semen Coicis) and 10 pieces of big Fuzi (附子, aconite, Radix Aconiti Lateralis Preparata)(fry heavily).

These two ingredients are grated into powder. [The powder is taken] 1 *fangcunbi* [each time] and three times a day.

【原文】

(八)

心中痞,诸逆心悬痛,桂枝生姜枳实汤主之。

桂姜枳实汤方

桂枝、生姜(各三两) 枳实(五枚)

右三味,以水六升,煮取三升,分温三服。

【今译】

心中痞满,停滞心下的诸多病邪向上冲逆,导致心胸郁闷疼痛,用桂枝生姜枳实汤主治。

【原文】

(九)

心痛彻背,背痛彻心,乌头赤石脂丸主之。

乌头赤石脂丸方

蜀椒(一两。一法二分) 乌头(一分,炮) 附子(半两,炮。一法一分) 干姜(一两。一法一分) 赤石脂(一两。一法二分)

右五味,末之,蜜丸如梧子大。先食服一丸,日三服。

【今译】

心中疼痛,透彻于背,背部疼痛,透彻于心,可用乌头赤石脂丸主治。

【英译】

Line 9.8

[The disease marked by] stagnation in the heart, various [pathogenic factors] in reversal surge upwards to the heart and suspending pain. [can be] treated by Guijiang Zhishi Decoction (桂姜枳实汤, cinnamon twig, ginger and processed unripe bitter orange decoction).

Guijiang Zhishi Decoction (桂姜枳实汤, cinnamon twig, ginger and processed unripe bitter orange decoction) [is composed of] 3 *liang* of Guizhi (桂枝, cinnamon twig, Ramulus Cinnamomi), 3 *liang* of Shengjiang (生姜, fresh ginger, Rhizoma Zingiberis Recens) and 5 pieces of Zhishi (枳实, processed unripe bitter orange, Fructus Aurantii Immaturus).

These three ingredients are decocted in 6 *sheng* of water to get 3 *sheng* [after] boiling. [The decoction is] divided into three [doses] and taken warm.

【英译】

Line 9.9

[The disease characterized by] heart pain involving the back and back pain involving the heart [can be] treated by Wutou Chishizhi Pill (乌头赤石脂丸, aconite and halloysite Pill).

Wutou Chishizhi Pill (乌头赤石脂丸, aconite and halloysite Pill) [is composed of] 1 *liang* of Shujiao (蜀椒, zanthoxylum, Pericarpium Zanthoxyli)(or 2 *fen*), 1 *fen* of Wutou (乌头, aconite, Radix aconite)(fry heavily), 0.5 *liang* of Fuzi (附子, aconite, Radix Aconiti Lateralis Preparata)(fry heavily, or 1 *fen*), 1 *liang* of Ganjiang (干姜, dried ginger, Rhizoma Zingiberis)(or 1 *fen*) and 1 *liang* of Chishizhi (赤石脂, halloysite, Halloysitum Rubrum)(or 2 *fen*).

These five ingredients are grated into powder and [mixed with] honey to make pills the size of firmiana seeds. Before eating [food, the patient should] take 1 pill [first] and three times a day.

Appended formula

附方

【原文】

九痛丸治九种心痛。

附子(三两,炮)　生狼牙(一两,炙香)　巴豆(一两,去皮心,熬,研如脂)　人参　干姜　吴茱萸(各一两)

右六味,末之,炼蜜丸如梧子大。酒下,强人初服三丸,日三服,弱者二丸。兼治卒中恶,腹胀痛,口不能言;又治连年积冷,流注心胸痛,并冷冲上气,落马坠车血疾等,皆主之。忌口如常法。

【今译】

九痛丸用以治疗九种心痛。

Volume 1

【英译】

Jiutong Pill（九痛丸, nine pains pill）is used to treat nine [kinds of diseases with] heart pain.

Jiutong Pill（九痛丸, nine pains pill）[is composed of] 3 *liang* of Fuzi（附子, aconite, Radix Aconiti Lateralis Preparata）（fry heavily）, 1 *liang* of Shenglangya（生狼牙, potentilla cryptotaenia root, Radix Potentillae Cryptotaeniae）（broil fragrantly）, 1 *liang* of Badou（巴豆, croton, Fructus Crotonis）（remove the peel and heart, simmer and grind as paste）, 1 *liang* of Renshen（人参, ginseng, Radix Ginseng）, 1 *liang* of Ganjiang（干姜, dried ginger, Rhizoma Zingiberis）and 1 *liang* of Wuzhuyu（吴茱萸, evodia, Fructus Evodiae）.

These six ingredients are pounded into powder and blended with Lianmi（炼蜜, processed honey, Mel Praeparatum）to make pills the size of firmiana seeds. [The pills are] swallowed with wine. Strong patients initially take 3 pills [each time] and three times a day, while weak patients take 2 pills [each time]. [This formula] [can also be used] to treat sudden attack by severe [pathogenic factors] with abdominal distension and pain as well as inability to speak. Furthermore, [it can be used] to treat accumulation of cold for years that flows into the heart and chest, causing pain in the heart and chest, cold swelling, qi surging upward and bleeding like falling from horses or carts. [This formula can be used] to treat all [these pathological conditions]. Dietary contraindications are the same as usual.

腹满寒疝宿食病脉证治第十

【原文】

（一）

趺阳脉微弦,法当腹满,不满者必便难,两胠疼痛,此虚寒从下上也,当以温药服之。

【今译】

趺阳脉(脾胃之脉)若微弦,应当有腹部胀满的症状,如果没有腹部胀满者,则必然出现大便困难,两胁疼痛,这是虚寒从下犯上所致,应当通过服用温药治疗。

【原文】

（二）

病者腹满,按之不痛为虚,痛者为实,可下之。舌黄未下者,下之黄自去。

【今译】

病人腹部胀满,按压而无疼痛感的为虚,有疼痛感的为实,可用下法治疗。如果病人舌黄而没有使用下法治疗的,用了下法治疗黄舌苔就会自然消解。

Chapter 10
Abdominal Fullness, Cold Hernia and Food Retention Disease: Pulses, Syndromes/Patterns and Treatment

【英译】

Line 10. 1

[If] fuyang (pulse of the spleen and stomach) is faint and taut, there should be abdominal fullness. [If] there is no abdominal fullness, there must be difficulty in defecation and pain at the hypochondrium due to deficiency-cold surging up from the lower to the upper. [It] can [be treated by] taking medicinals warm [in nature].

【英译】

Line 10. 2

[In] the patient with abdominal fullness, no pain when pressed indicates deficiency [syndrome/pattern] and pain when pressed indicates excess [syndrome/pattern], [which] can be [treated by] purgation. [If] the tongue [fur] is yellow before [application of] purgation, yellow [fur] will disappear when purged.

【原文】

（三）

腹满时减，复如故，此为寒，当与温药。

【今译】

患者腹部胀满，时有减轻，但又胀满如故，这是寒邪所致，应当用温药治疗。

【原文】

（四）

病者痿黄，躁而不渴，胸中寒实而利不止者，死。

【今译】

病人肌肤痿黄，烦躁而口中不渴，寒实之邪结于胸中，若下利不止，就会导致死亡。

【原文】

（五）

寸口脉弦者，即胁下拘急而痛，其人啬啬恶寒也。

【今译】

寸口之脉若弦，患者胁下则拘急疼痛，瑟瑟发抖而恶寒。

Volume 1

【英译】

Line 10.3

[There are cases where] abdominal [distension and] fullness is periodically alleviated but soon returns as before. This is [caused by pathogenic] cold and should [be treated by] medicinals warm [in nature].

【英译】

Line 10.4

[When] a patient [has the symptoms and signs of] withered and yellow skin and vexation without thirst, [it is due to] cold-excess [binding] in the chest. [If there is] incessant diarrhea, [it will cause] death.

【英译】

Line 10.5

[If] the pulse in the cunkou [region] is taut, [there will be] spasm and pain below the hypochondrium, quivering and aversion to cold.

【原文】

（六）

夫中寒家，喜欠，其人清涕出，发热色和者，善嚏。

【今译】

素体虚寒之人，时常呵欠。如果鼻流清涕，发热但面色如常，易打喷嚏。

【原文】

（七）

中寒，其人下利，以里虚也，欲嚏不能，此人肚中寒。

【今译】

素体虚寒之人，时有下利，是因为里虚所致，想打喷嚏但却不能，这是因为患者腹中有寒。

【原文】

（八）

夫瘦人绕脐痛，必有风冷，谷气不行，而反下之，其气必冲。不冲者，心下则痞。

【今译】

瘦弱的患者，如果脐部周围疼痛，必然是风冷之邪所致，因而谷气停滞，大便不通。如果反而使用下法治疗，必然引起气逆上冲。如果气不上冲，就会结于心下，导致痞满。

Volume 1

【英译】

Line 10.6

Patients with cold in the center tend to yawn. [If there is] clear snivel with fever and normal complexion, [they] tend to sneeze.

【英译】

Line 10.7

[If] the patient with cold in the center has diarrhea, [it is] due to internal deficiency. [If the patient] wants to sneeze but is unable to do so, [it is due to] cold in the patient's abdomen.

【英译】

Line 10.8

[In] emaciated patients, [if there is] pain around the umbilicus, there must be wind-cold, [consequently causing] indigestion [and constipation]. [If treated by] purgation, qi will surge upwards. [If qi] does not surge, [it will bind] below the heart and [accumulate into] lump.

【原文】

（九）

病腹满，发热十日，脉浮而数，饮食如故，厚朴七物汤主之。

厚朴七物汤方

厚朴（半斤）　甘草　大黄（各三两）　大枣（十枚）　枳实（五枚）

桂枝（二两）　生姜（五两）

右七味，以水一斗，煮取四升，温服八合，日三服。呕者，加半夏五合，下利去大黄；寒多者，加生姜至半斤。

【今译】

病人腹部胀满，发热十多日，脉象浮数，饮食如常，用厚朴七物汤主治。

【原文】

（十）

腹中寒气，雷鸣切痛，胸胁逆满，呕吐，附子粳米汤主之。

附子粳米汤方

附子（一枚，炮）　半夏（半升）　甘草（一两）　大枣（十枚）　粳米（半升）

右五味，以水八升，煮米熟汤成，去滓。温服一升，日三服。

【今译】

患者腹中有寒气，就会引起腹中雷鸣剧痛，胸胁逆满，呕吐，宜用附子粳米汤主治。

Volume 1

【英译】

Line 10.9

[There are cases where] the patient with abdominal [distension and] fullness has fever for over ten days, the pulse is floating and rapid but drinking [water] and eating [food] are normal. Houpo Qiwu Decoction (厚朴七物汤, magnolia bark and seven medicinals decoction) [can be used] to treat it.

Houpo Qiwu Decoction (厚朴七物汤, magnolia bark and seven medicinals decoction) [is composed of] 0. 5 *jin* of Houpo (厚朴, magnolia bark, Cortex Magnoliae Officinalis), 3 *liang* of Gancao (甘草, licorice, Radix Glycyrrhizae Praeparata), 3 *liang* of Dahuang (大黄, rhubarb, Radix et Rhizoma Rhei), 10 pieces of Dazao (大枣, jujube, Fructus Ziziphus Jujubae), 5 pieces of Zhishi (枳实, processed unripe bitter orange, Fructus Aurantii Immaturus), 2 *liang* of Guizhi (桂枝, cinnamon twig, Ramulus Cinnamomi) and 5 *liang* of Shengjiang (生姜, fresh ginger, Rhizoma Zingiberis Recens).

These seven ingredients are decocted in 1 *dou* of water to get 4 *sheng* [after] boiling. [The decoction is] taken warm 8 *ge* [each time] and three times a day. For vomiting, 5 *ge* of Banxia (半夏, pinellia, Rhizoma Pinelliae) is added; for diarrhea, Dahuang (大黄, rhubarb, Radix et Rhizoma Rhei) is removed; for excessive cold, Shengjiang (生姜, fresh ginger, Rhizoma Zingiberis Recens) is increased to 0. 5 *jin*.

【英译】

Line 10. 10

[If there is] cold qi in the abdomen, [it will cause] thunderous borborygmus, acute abdominal pain, counterflow and fullness in the chest and rib-side, and retching and vomiting. [It can be] treated by Fuzi Jingmi Decoction (附子粳米汤, aconite and polished round-grained rice decoction).

Fuzi Jingmi Decoction (附子粳米汤, aconite and polished round-grained rice decoction) [is composed of] 1 piece of Fuzi (附子, aconite, Radix Aconiti Lateralis Preparata)(fry heavily), 0. 5 *sheng* of Banxia (半夏, pinellia, Rhizoma Pinelliae), 1 *liang* of Gancao (甘草, licorice, Radix Glycyrrhizae Praeparata), 10 pieces of Dazao (大枣, jujube, Fructus Ziziphus Jujubae) and 0. 5 *sheng* of Jingmi (粳米, polished round-grained rice, Semen Oryzae Nonglutinosae).

These five ingredients are decocted in 8 *sheng* of water and the rice is well cooked to finish the decoction. The dregs are removed and [the decoction is] taken warm 1 *sheng* [each time] and three times a day.

【原文】

(十一)

痛而闭者,厚朴三物汤主之。

厚朴三物汤方

厚朴(八两)　大黄(四两)　枳实(五枚)

右三味,以水一斗二升,先煮二味,取五升,内大黄,煮取三升。温服一升,以利为度。

【今译】

患者腹中胀痛,大便不通,用厚朴三物汤主治。

【原文】

(十二)

按之心下满痛者,此为实也,当下之,宜大柴胡汤。

大柴胡汤方

柴胡(半斤)　黄芩(三两)　芍药(三两)　半夏(半升,洗)　枳实(四枚,炙)　大黄(二两)　大枣(十二枚)　生姜(五两)

右八味,以水一斗二升,煮取六升,去滓,再煎。温服一升,日三服。

【今译】

按压患者心下,患者有腹部胀满疼痛之感,此为实证,应当用下法治疗,用大柴胡汤主治。

Volume 1

【英译】

Line 10. 11

［Abdominal distension and］ pain with constipation ［can be］ treated by Houpo Sanwu Decoction（厚朴三物汤，magnolia bark and three medicinals decoction）.

Houpo Sanwu Decoction（厚朴三物汤，magnolia bark and three medicinals decoction）［is composed of］8 *liang* of Houpo（厚朴，magnolia bark，Cortex Magnoliae Officinalis），4 *liang* of Dahuang（大黄，rhubarb，Radix et Rhizoma Rhei）and 5 pieces of Zhishi（枳实，processed unripe bitter orange，Fructus Aurantii Immaturus）.

These three ingredients are decocted in 1 *dou* and 2 *sheng* of water. Two ingredients are decocted first to get 5 *sheng* ［after］ boiling. ［Then］Dahuang（大黄，rhubarb，Radix et Rhizoma Rhei）is put into ［it］ to boil and get 3 *sheng*. ［The decoction is］ taken warm 1 *sheng* ［each time］ till defecation is normalized.

【英译】

Line 10. 12

［Abdominal］ fullness and pain under pressure indicates excess ［syndrome/pattern］ and should ［be treated by］ purgation. Da Chaihu Decoction（大柴胡汤，major bupleurum decoction）is the appropriate ［formula for treating it］.

Da Chaihu Decoction（大柴胡汤，major bupleurum decoction）［is composed of］0.5 *jin* of Chaihu（柴胡，bupleurum，Radix Bupleuri），3 *liang* of Huangqin（黄芩，scutellaria，Radix Scutellariae），3 *liang* of Shaoyao（芍药，peony，Radix Paeoniae），0.5 *sheng* of Banxia（半夏，pinellia，Rhizoma Pinelliae)(wash），4 pieces of Zhishi（枳实，processed unripe bitter orange，Fructus Aurantii Immaturus)(broil），2 *liang* of Dahuang（大黄，rhubarb，Radix et Rhizoma Rhei），12 pieces of Dazao（大枣，jujube，Fructus Ziziphus Jujubae）and 5 *liang* of Shengjiang（生姜，fresh ginger，Rhizoma Zingiberis Recens）.

These eight ingredients are decocted in 1 *dou* and 2 *sheng* of water to get 6 *sheng* ［after］ boiling. ［After］ removal of dregs，［it is］ boiled again. ［The decoction is］ taken warm 1 *sheng* ［each time］ and three times a day.

【原文】

(十三)

腹满不减,减不足言,当须下之,宜大承气汤。

大承气汤方

大黄(四两,酒洗)　厚朴(半斤,去皮,炙)　枳实(五枚,炙)　芒硝(三合)

右四味,以水一斗,先煮二物,取五升,去滓,内大黄,煮取二升,内芒硝,更上火微一二沸。分温再服,得下,余勿服。

【今译】

患者腹部胀满,持续不减,即便有所减轻,但也微不足道,应当用攻下法治疗,宜用大承气汤主治。

【原文】

(十四)

心胸中大寒痛,呕不能饮食,腹中寒,上冲皮起,出见有头足,上下痛而不可触近,大建中汤主之。

大建中汤方

蜀椒(二合,去汗)　干姜(四两)　人参(二两)

右三味,以水四升,煮取二升,去滓,内胶饴一升,微火煎取一升半。分温再服,如一炊顷,可饮粥二升,后更服,当一日食糜,温覆之。

【今译】

患者心胸中寒邪盛,引起剧烈疼痛,呕吐不能饮食,腹中寒气上冲服壁,出见有头足样块状物,上下疼痛,不可用手触近,用大建中汤主治。

Volume 1

【英译】

Line 10. 13

[There are cases where] abdominal fullness is difficult to alleviate, and [even if] alleviated a little, [it is] still very serious. [To treat it,] purgation should be used. The appropriate [formula is] Da Chengqi Decoction (大承气汤, major decoction for harmonizing qi).

Da Chengqi Decoction (大承气汤, major decoction for harmonizing qi) [is composed of] 4 *liang* of Dahuang (大黄, rhubarb, Radix et Rhizoma Rhei) (wash in wine), 0. 5 *jin* of Houpo (厚朴, magnolia bark, Cortex Magnoliae Officinalis) (remove the bark and broil), 5 pieces of Zhishi (枳实, processed unripe bitter orange, Fructus Aurantii Immaturus) (broil) and 3 *ge* of Mangxiao (芒硝, mirabilite, Mirabilitum).

These four ingredients are decocted in 1 *dou* of water. Two ingredients are boiled first to get 5 *sheng*. The dregs are removed and Dahuang (大黄, rhubarb, Radix et Rhizoma Rhei) is put into [it] to boil and get 2 *sheng*. [Finally] Mangxiao (芒硝, mirabilite, Mirabilitum) is put into [it] to boil once or twice under mild fire. [The decoction is] divided into two [doses] and taken warm. [If] defecation is promoted, [the patient should] stop taking the rest [of the decoction].

【英译】

Line 10. 14

[When there is] severe cold and pain in the heart and chest, [it will cause] retching, inability to drink and eat, cold in the abdomen that surges upward to the [abdominal fleshes and] skin with protrusion like head and foot, and pain in the upper and lower that cannot be pressed. Da Jianzhong Decoction (大建中汤, major decoction for strengthening the middle) [can be used] to treat it.

Da Jianzhong Decoction (大建中汤, major decoction for strengthening the middle) [is composed of] 2 *ge* of Shujiao (蜀椒, zanthoxylum, Pericarpium Zanthoxyli) (remove sweating), 4 *liang* of Ganjiang (干姜, dried ginger, Rhizoma Zingiberis) and 2 *liang* of Renshen (人参, ginseng, Radix Ginseng).

These three ingredients are decocted in 4 *sheng* of water to get 2 *sheng* [after] boiling. The dregs are removed and 1 *sheng* of Jiaoyi (胶饴, gelly glue) is put into [it] to boil over mild fire to get 1. 5 *sheng*. [The decoction is] divided into two [doses] and taken warm. [After a period of] the time for cooking a meal, [the patient] can take 2 *sheng* of porridge, and then take a dose [of decoction]. [The patient] should take gruel the whole day and [cover himself with clothes or quilt in order to] warm [himself].

【原文】

(十五)

胁下偏痛,发热,其脉紧弦,此寒也,以温药下之,宜大黄附子汤。

大黄附子汤方

大黄(三两)　附子(三枚,炮)　细辛(二两)

右三味,以水五升,煮取二升,分温三服。若强人煮二升半,分温三服。服后如人行四五里,进一服。

【今译】

患者胁下一侧疼痛,发热,脉象紧弦,是寒邪所致,应以温药下法治疗,宜用大黄附子汤主治。

【原文】

(十六)

寒气厥逆,赤丸主之。

赤丸方

茯苓(四两)　乌头(二两,炮)　半夏(四两,洗。一方用桂)　细辛(一两)

右四味,末之,内真朱为色,炼蜜丸如麻子大。先食酒饮下三丸,日再、夜一服;不知,稍增之,以知为度。

【今译】

寒气过盛,造成四肢厥逆,宜用赤丸主治。

Volume 1

【英译】

Line 10. 15

［The symptoms and signs of］ lateral pain below the hypochondrium, fever, and tight and taut pulse indicate cold. ［It］ should ［be treated by］ purgation with medicinals warm ［in property］. The appropriate ［formula is］ Dahuang Fuzi Decoction (大黄附子汤, rhubarb and aconite decoction).

Dahuang Fuzi Decoction (大黄附子汤, rhubarb and aconite decoction) ［is composed of］ 3 *liang* of Dahuang (大黄, rhubarb, Radix et Rhizoma Rhei), 3 pieces of Fuzi (附子, aconite, Radix Aconiti Lateralis Preparata)(fry heavily)and 2 *liang* of Xixin (细辛, asarum, Herba Asari).

These three ingredients are decocted in 5 *sheng* of water to get 2 *sheng* ［after］ boiling. ［The decoction is］ divided into three ［doses］ and taken warm. For the strong patient, 2.5 *sheng* ［of decoction］ is boiled, divided into three ［doses］ and taken warm. After taking ［the first dose］, ［the patient should wait for the time it takes for him］ to walk four or five li (about 2 or 2.5 kilometers) and then take the second ［dose］.

【英译】

Line 10. 16

Exuberant cold qi ［will cause］ reversal cold ［of limbs］, which ［can be］ treated by Chi Pill (赤丸, red pill).

Chi Pill (赤丸, red pill) ［is composed of］ 4 *liang* of Fuling (茯苓, poria, Poria), 2 *liang* of Wutou (乌头, aconite, Radix aconite)(fry heavily), 4 *liang* of Banxia (半夏, pinellia, Rhizoma Pinelliae) (wash, another edition uses cinnamon twig)and 1 *liang* of Xixin (细辛, asarum, Herba Asari).

These four ingredients are grated into powder. Zhenzhu (真朱, cinnabar, Cinnabaris) is added and blended with Lianmi (炼蜜, processed honey, Mel Praeparatum) to make pills the size of hemp seeds. Before eating food, ［the patient should］ take 3 pills with wine, twice a day and once at night. ［If there is］ no effect, ［the dose should］ gradually increase till there is effect.

【原文】

（十七）

腹痛，脉弦而紧，弦则卫气不行，即恶寒，紧则不欲食，邪正相搏，即为寒疝，绕脐痛。若发则白汗出，手足厥冷，其脉沉弦者，大乌头煎主之。

大乌头煎方

乌头（大者五枚，熬，去皮，不㕮咀）

右以水三升，煮取一升，去滓，内蜜二升，煎令水气尽，取二升。强人服七合，弱人服五合。不差，明日更服，不可一日再服。

【今译】

患者腹痛，脉象弦紧，脉弦说明卫气不能运行，因此导致恶寒；脉紧说明患者不欲食，邪气与正气搏击，就会导致寒疝，引起脐部周围疼痛。如果剧烈发作就会出现冷汗，手足厥冷，脉象沉弦，用大乌头煎主治。

【原文】

（十八）

寒疝腹中痛，及胁痛里急者，当归生姜羊肉汤主之。

当归生姜羊肉汤方

当归（三两）　生姜（五两）　羊肉（一斤）

右三味，以水八升，煮取三升，温服七合，日三服。若寒多者，加生姜成一斤；痛多而呕者，加橘皮二两、白术一两。加生姜者，亦加水五升，煮取三升二合，服之。

【今译】

寒疝患者，若腹中疼痛，且两胁作痛，里急后重的，应当以归生姜羊肉汤主治。

Volume 1

【英译】
Line 10. 17

[In] abdominal pain, sometimes there is taut and tight pulse. Taut [pulse] indicates failure of defense qi to move, [and therefore] causing aversion to cold; tight [pulse] indicates no desire to eat food. [When] pathogenic [qi] and healthy [qi] are contending with each other, it will cause cold hernia and pain around the umbilicus. If the occurrence is acute, [there will be] cold sweating, reversal cold of hands and feet, sunken and taut pulse. Da Wutou Decoction (大乌头煎, major aconite decoction) [can be used to] treat it.

Da Wutou Decoction (大乌头煎, major aconite decoction) [is composed of] 5 pieces of Wutou (乌头, aconite, Radix aconite) (big, simmer, remove peel, do not chew).

This ingredient is decocted in 3 *sheng* of water to get 1 *sheng* [after] boiling. [After] removal of the dregs, 2 *sheng* of honey is added. [The decoction is] boiled [again] to get 2 *sheng* till all water has evaporated. For strong patients, 7 *ge* is taken [each time]; for weak patients, 5 *ge* is taken [each time]. [If the disease is] not alleviated, take [another dose] next day. Two [doses] cannot be taken in one day.

【英译】
Line 10. 18

Cold hernia with abdominal pain, costal pain and tenesmus should be treated by Danggui Shengjiang Decoction (当归生姜汤, Chinese angelica and fresh ginger decoction).

Danggui Shengjiang Decoction (当归生姜汤, Chinese angelica and fresh ginger decoction) [is composed of] 3 *liang* of Danggui (当归, Chinese angelica, Radix Angelicae Sinensis), 5 *liang* of Shengjiang (生姜, fresh ginger, Rhizoma Zingiberis Recens) and 1 *jin* of Yangrou (羊肉, goat meat, Caprae seu Ovis Caro).

These three ingredients are decocted in 8 *sheng* of water to get 3 *sheng*. [The decoction is] taken warm 7 *sheng* [each time] and three times a day. For excessive cold, Shengjiang (生姜, fresh ginger, Rhizoma Zingiberis Recens) increases to 1 *jin*; for incessant pain with nausea, 2 *liang* of Jupi (橘皮, tangerine peel, Pericarpium Citri Reticulatae) and 1 *liang* of Baizhu (白术, rhizome of largehead atractylodes, Rhizoma Atractylodis Macrocephalae) are added. To add Shengjiang (生姜, fresh ginger, Rhizoma Zingiberis Recens), 5 more *sheng* of water should be added to boil and get 3 *sheng* and 2 *ge* [for patients] to take.

【原文】

(十九)

寒疝腹中疼痛,逆冷,手足不仁,若身疼痛,灸、刺、诸药不能治,抵当乌头桂枝汤主之。

乌头桂枝汤方

乌头

右一味,以蜜二斤,煎减半,去滓,以桂枝汤五合解之,得一升后,初服二合;不知,即取三合;又不知,复加至五合。其知者,如醉状,得吐者,为中病。

桂枝汤方

桂枝(三两,去皮)　芍药(三两)　甘草(二两,灸)　生姜(三两)
大枣(十二枚)

右五味,剉,以水七升,微火煮取三升,去滓。

【今译】

寒疝患者腹中疼痛,且周身逆冷,手足麻木不仁。如果身体疼痛,就不能用灸法、刺法及其他药物治疗,用抵当乌头桂枝汤主治。

【英译】

Line 10. 19

Cold hernia ［is marked by］ abdominal pain，reversal cold，numbness of hands and feet. If there is generalized pain，moxibustion，acupuncture and other medicinals cannot be used to treat. ［The appropriate formulas used］ to treat are Wutou Decoction（乌头汤，aconite decoction）and Guizhi Decoction（桂枝汤，cinnamon twig decoction）.

Wutou Decoction（乌头汤，aconite decoction）is only composed of Wutou（乌头，aconite，Radix aconite）.

This ingredient is boiled with 2 *jin* of honey to reduce half of it. ［After］ removal of dregs，it is blended with Guizhi Decoction（桂枝汤，cinnamon twig decoction）to get 1 *sheng*. ［The patient should］ take 1 *ge* at first and then 2 *ge*. ［If there is］ no effect，［the patient should］ take 3 *ge*. ［If］ there is still no effect，［the patient should］ take 5 *ge* more. ［When］ there is effect，［the patient appears］ like being drunken. ［If the patient］ vomits，［it indicates that］ the disease is resolved.

Guizhi Decoction（桂枝汤，cinnamon twig decoction）［is composed of］ 3 liang of Guizhi（桂枝，cinnamon twig，Ramulus Cinnamomi）（remove the bark），3 liang of Shaoyao（芍药，Peony，Radix Paeoniae），2 liang of Gancao（甘草，licorice，Radix Glycyrrhizae Praeparata）（broil），3 liang of Shengjiang（生姜，fresh ginger，Rhizoma Zingiberis Recens）and 12 pieces of Dazao（大枣，jujube，Fructus Ziziphus Jujubae）. These five ingredients are cut and decocted in 7 sheng of water to get 3 sheng ［after］ boiling with mild fire. The dregs are removed.

【原文】

(二十)

其脉数而紧乃弦,状如弓弦,按之不移。脉数弦者,当下其寒;脉紧大而迟者,必心下坚;脉大而紧者,阳中有阴,可下之。

【今译】

患者脉象数而紧的,就是脉弦,其形状如弓弦般硬直,按压也不移动。如果脉象数而弦的,应当用下法祛除其寒;如果脉象紧大且迟的,其心下一定坚硬;如果脉象大而紧的,阳中就有阴,可以使用温下法治疗。

【原文】

《外台》乌头汤治寒疝腹中绞痛,贼风入攻五脏,拘急不得转侧,发作有时,使人阴缩,手足厥逆。方见上。

【今译】

《外台秘要》中的乌头汤可用以治疗寒疝腹中绞痛,贼风攻入五脏,导致腹中拘急而不能转侧,发作有时,使生殖器受寒而上缩,手足厥逆。治疗所用之方上面已经谈到。

Volume 1

【英译】

Line 10.20

[If] the pulse is rapid, tight and taut, it means taut pulse that will not move when pressed. [When] the pulse is rapid and taut, cold should be eliminated by purgation; [if] the pulse is tight, large and slow, there must be hard lump below the heart; [if] the pulse is large and tight, [it indicates that] there is yin in yang and can [be treated by] purgation.

【英译】

Wutou Decoction (乌头汤, aconite decoction) [from the book entitled] *Waitai Miyao* (《外台秘要》, *The Medical Secrets of an Official Named Wang Tao*) [is used] to treat cold hernia [marked by] abdominal pain, invasion of pathogenic wind into the five zang-organs, spasm of limbs and difficulty to turn. [Such a disease] occurs occasionally, causing contracted genitals and reversal cold of hands and feet. *Waitai Miyao* (《外台秘要》, *The Medical Secrets of an Official Named Wang Tao*) is already mentioned above.

【原文】

《外台》柴胡桂枝汤方治心腹卒中痛者。

柴胡（四两） 黄芩 人参 芍药 桂枝 生姜（各一两半） 甘草（一两） 半夏（二合半） 大枣（六枚）

右九味，以水六升，煮取三升。温服一升，日三服。

【今译】

《外台秘要》中的柴胡桂枝汤方，可用以治疗因外邪突袭所致的心腹疼痛。

【原文】

《外台》走马汤治中恶心痛腹胀，大便不通。

巴豆（二枚，去皮心，熬） 杏仁（二枚）

右二味，以绵缠，捶令碎，热汤二合，捻取白汁饮之，当下。老小量之。通治飞尸、鬼击病。

【今译】

《外台秘要》中的走马汤，用以治疗中恶病，心痛腹胀，大便不通。

【英译】

Chaihu Guizhi Decoction （柴胡桂枝汤，bupleurum and cinnamon twig decoction）［from the book entitled］ *Waitai Miyao* (《外台秘要》, *The Medical Secrets of an Official Named Wang Tao*) ［is used］ to treat sharp abdominal pain.

Chaihu Guizhi Decoction (柴胡桂枝汤，bupleurum and cinnamon twig decoction) ［is composed of］ 4 *liang* of Chaihu（柴胡，bupleurum, Radix Bupleuri），1.5 *liang* of Huangqin （黄芩，scutellaria，Radix Scutellariae），1.5 *liang* of Renshen （人参，ginseng，Radix Ginseng），1.5 *liang* of Shaoyao（芍药，peony，Radix Paeoniae），1.5 *liang* of Guizhi（桂枝，cinnamon twig，Ramulus Cinnamomi），1.5 *liang* of Shengjiang（生姜，fresh ginger，Rhizoma Zingiberis Recens），1 *liang* of Gancao（甘草，licorice，Radix Glycyrrhizae Praeparata），2.5 *ge* of Banxia（半夏，pinellia，Rhizoma Pinelliae）and 6 pieces of Dazao（大枣，jujube，Fructus Ziziphi Jujubae）.

These nine ingredients are decocted in 6 *sheng* of water to get 3 *sheng* ［after］ boiling. ［The decoction is］ taken warm 1 *sheng* ［each time］ and three times a day.

【英译】

Zouma Decoction（走马汤，running horse decoction）［from the book entitled］ *Waitai Miyao* (《外台秘要》, *The Medical Secrets of an Official Named Wang Tao*) ［is used］ to treat ［the disease characterized by］ nausea，heart pain，abdominal distension and constipation.

Zouma Decoction （走马汤，running horse decoction） ［is composed of］ 2 pieces of Badou（巴豆，croton，Fructus Crotonis）（remove the bark and simmer）and 2 pieces of Xingren（杏仁，apricot kernel，Semen Armeniacae Amarum）.

These two ingredients are wrapped in sack，pounded and mixed with 2 *ge* of hot water to remove white liquid. ［The decoction］ is taken for promoting defection. The dose is decided according to the age of patients. It is usually used to treat ［disease like］ a flying corpse or attack by a ghost.

【原文】

(二十一)

问曰：人病有宿食，何以别之？师曰：寸口脉浮而大，按之反涩，尺中亦微而涩，故知有宿食，大承气汤主之。

【今译】

问：病人有食物积滞不化，如何辨别呢？

老师说：其临床表现为，寸口脉浮大，按压时反而出现涩象，尺脉也是微而涩，所以就可以知道有食物积滞不化，用大承气汤主治。

【原文】

(二十二)

脉数而滑者，实也，此有宿食，下之愈，宜大承气汤。

【今译】

脉象数而滑的，是实证，是由食物积滞不化所致，用下法可以治愈，宜用大承气汤主治。

【英译】

Line 10.21

Question: How to differentiate undigested food 〔in the stomach〕 of the patient?

The master said: 〔The clinical manifestations are〕 floating and large pulse in the cunkou 〔region that appears〕 rough 〔when〕 pressed, faint and rough 〔pulse in〕 the chi 〔region〕. That is why 〔it can be〕 known 〔that〕 there is undigested food 〔in the stomach〕. Da Chengqi Decoction (大承气汤, major decoction for harmonizing qi) 〔can be used〕 to treat it.

【英译】

Line 10.22

Rapid and slippery pulse 〔indicates〕 excess 〔syndrome/pattern〕 due to undigested food 〔in the stomach〕. 〔It can be〕 cured by purgation. The appropriate 〔formula for treating it is〕 Da Chengqi Decoction (大承气汤, major decoction for harmonizing qi).

【原文】

(二十三)

下利不饮食者,有宿食也,当下之,宜大承气汤。

大承气汤方:见前痉病中。

【今译】

患者有腹泻而不思饮食的,是食物积滞不化,应当以下法治疗,宜用大承气汤主治。

【原文】

(二十四)

宿食在上脘,当吐之,宜瓜蒂散。

瓜蒂散方

瓜蒂(一枚,熬黄) 赤小豆(一分,煮)

右二味,杵为散,以香豉七合煮取汁,和散一钱匕,温服之。不吐者,少加之,以快吐为度而止。亡血及虚者,不可与之。

【今译】

患者有积滞不化的食物停留在胃之上,应当用吐法治疗,宜用瓜蒂散主治。

Volume 1

【英译】

Line 10.23

Diarrhea without desire to drink ［water］ and eat ［food］ indicates excess ［syndrome/pattern］ due to undigested food ［in the stomach］. ［It can be］ cured by purgation. The appropriate ［formula for treating it is］ Da Chengqi Decoction (大承气汤，major decoction for harmonizing qi).

【英译】

Line 10.24

［When］ undigested food ［is stagnated］ in the upper duct of the stomach，Guadi Powder (瓜蒂散，melon stalk powder) ［can be used］ to treat it.

Guadi Powder (瓜蒂散，melon stalk powder) ［is composed of］ 1 piece of Guadi (瓜蒂，melon stalk，Pedicellus Melo) (simmer yellow) and 1 *fen* of Chixiaodou (赤小豆，rice bean，Semen Phaseoli) (boil).

These two ingredients are grated into powder. 7 *ge* of fermented soybean is boiled to get juice. ［The juice］ and powder are ［mixed into］ one *qianbi* and taken warm. ［If there is］ no vomiting，take a little ［powder］. ［When there is］ vomiting，stop taking ［the powder］. Those ［suffering from］ bleeding and deficiency cannot take it.

【原文】

(二十五)

脉紧如转索无常者,有宿食也。

【今译】

脉象紧的就像转动中的绳索一样,变化无常,说明有食物积滞不化。

【原文】

(二十六)

脉紧,头痛风寒,腹中有宿食不化也。

【今译】

脉象紧,头痛,有风寒,说明腹中有食物积滞不化的症状。

Volume 1

【英译】

Line 10.25

The pulse that is as tight as a turning thread without any changes [indicates that] there is undigested food [in the stomach].

【英译】

Line 10.26

Tight pulse，headache and retention of wind-cold [indicate that] there is undigested food [in the stomach].

卷中

五脏风寒积聚病脉证并治第十一

【原文】

（一）

肺中风者，口燥而喘，身运而重，冒而肿胀。

【今译】

肺受风邪侵袭后，导致口燥，气喘，身体颤动而沉重，头昏冒，身体肿胀。

【原文】

（二）

肺中寒，吐浊涕。

【今译】

肺脏遭受了寒邪的侵袭后，导致患者呕吐稠浊黏液。

Volume 2

Chapter 11
Accumulation of Wind and Cold in the Five Zang-Organs Disease: Pulses, Syndromes/Patterns and Treatment

【英译】

Line 11. 1

[After] invasion of wind into the lung, [there are symptoms and signs of] dryness of the mouth, panting, quivering and heaviness of the body, dizziness, swelling and distension of the body.

【英译】

Line 11.2

Invasion of cold into the lung [will cause] vomiting of turbid saliva.

【原文】

（三）

肺死脏，浮之虚，按之弱如葱叶，下无根者，死。

【今译】

因肺气将绝而出现的真脏脉，浮虚无力，按压时感到虚弱的像葱叶一样，空而无根，为死证。

【原文】

（四）

肝中风者，头目瞤，两胁痛，行带伛，令人嗜甘。

【今译】

肝脏遭受风邪的侵袭，导致头部颤动，眼皮跳动，两胁疼痛，行走时弯腰驼背带伛，使患者喜欢吃甘甜饮食。

Volume 2

【英译】

Line 11.3

True visceral pulse of the lung is floating and weak. [When] pressed, [it is felt] as weak as scallion leaf without root. [It is a sign of] death.

【英译】

Line 11.4

Invasion of wind into the liver [causes] quivering of the head and eyes, pain in the hypochondrium, hunched back when walking and predilection of sweet [food].

【原文】

（五）

肝中寒者,两臂不举,舌本燥,喜太息,胸中痛,不得转侧,食则吐而汗出也。

【今译】

肝脏遭受寒邪的侵袭,导致两臂不能不举,舌本干燥,常常太息,胸中疼痛,不能转侧,用餐后即呕吐而汗出。

【原文】

（六）

肝死脏,浮之弱,按之如索不来,或曲如蛇行者,死。

【今译】

肝的真脏脉浮而弱,按压时感到像绳索空悬一样,摸之即去,不能复来,或者脉象曲,就像蛇在蠕动一样,是死证。

【英译】

Line 11.5

Invasion of cold into the liver [causes] inability of the arms to raise, dryness of the tongue root, frequent sighing, pain in the chest, inability to turn [the body] and vomiting and sweating [after] eating.

【英译】

Line 11.6

True visceral pulse of the liver is floating and weak. [When] pressed, [it is felt] like [a piece of flying] rope [that cannot] come down, or like a moving snake. [It is a sign of] death.

【原文】

（七）

肝着，其人常欲蹈其胸上，先未苦时，但欲饮热，旋覆花汤主之。

旋覆花汤方

旋覆花三两　葱十四茎　新绛少许

上三味，以水三升，煮取一升，顿服之。

【今译】

肝着病人，经常要按压其胸部，一开始病情不重，主要饮用热汤即可，可用旋覆花汤主治。

【原文】

（八）

心中风者，翕翕发热，不能起，心中饥，食即呕吐。

【今译】

心中遭受风邪侵袭，引起轻微发热，不能起立行动，心中饥饿，但用食即呕吐。

Volume 2

【英译】

Line 11.7

[In] liver stagnancy, the patient frequently presses his chest [with his hands]. At the beginning, [the disease is] not very serious and [can be resolved after] drinking hot water. [It can be] treated by Xuanfuhua Decoction（旋覆花汤，inula flower decoction）.

Xuanfuhua Decoction（旋覆花汤，inula flower decoction）[is composed of] 3 *liang* of Xuanfuhua（旋覆花，inula flower，Flos Insulae），14 pieces of Cong（葱，scallion，Herba Alli Fistulosi）and a little Xinjiang（新绛，fresh madder，Radix Rubiae Recens）.

These three ingredients are decocted in 3 *sheng* of water to get 1 *sheng* [after] boiling. [The decoction is] taken once the whole.

【英译】

Line 11.8

[When] there is pathogenic wind in the heart，[it will cause] light fever，difficult to stand up，hunger and vomiting after eating.

【原文】

（九）

心中寒者，其人苦病心如噉蒜状，剧者心痛彻背，背痛彻心，譬如蛊注。其脉浮者，自吐乃愈。

【今译】

心脏遭受寒邪侵袭，患者感到痛苦，就像吃了大蒜似的感受，疼痛剧烈的心痛牵引到背，背痛则牵引到心，就像蛊注病中的蛊虫啃咬一样。其脉象浮的，服药而自吐的就能痊愈。

【原文】

（十）

心伤者，其人劳倦，即头面赤而下重，心中痛而自烦，发热，当脐跳，其脉弦，此为心脏伤所致也。

【今译】

心脏遭受损伤的患者，劳动时感到疲倦，出现头面发红，身体下部沉重，心中疼痛，自感心烦不安，发热，脐部有动感跳，脉象弦，这是心脏损伤所致。

Volume 2

【英译】

Line 11.9

Invasion of cold into the heart [causes] suffering in the heart like eating garlic. [When there is] sharp pain in the heart, [it will] involve the back, [When there is sharp] pain in the back, [it will] involve the heart like poisonous insects. [If] the pulse is floating, [the disease will] heal [when there is] spontaneous vomiting.

【英译】

Line 11.10

[When suffering from] heart damage, the patient feels tired when working [with the symptoms and signs of] red head and face, heaviness of the lower part of the body, pain in the heart, vexation, fever, beating around the umbilicus and taut pulse. This is due to injury of the heart.

【原文】

(十一)

心死脏,浮之实如麻豆,按之益躁疾者,死。

【今译】

心死脏的脉象,轻按即坚实如麻豆一样,重按时脉象更加躁动疾速的,是死证。

【原文】

(十二)

邪哭使魂魄不安者,血气少也;血气少者属于心,心气虚者,其人则畏,合目欲眠,梦远行而精神离散,魂魄妄行。阴气衰者为癫,阳气衰者为狂。

【今译】

因邪之侵袭而致患者啼哭而魂魄不安的,是血气少的缘故;血气少属于心疾,心气虚的,患者则有畏惧之感,时常闭合双目欲睡,梦中自己远行而精神离散,魂魄散乱妄行。阴气衰的为癫病,阳气衰的为狂病。

【英译】

Line 11. 11

True visceral pulse of the heart is floating and hard like pellet or bean [when pressed lightly]. [If it is] agitated and beating fast [when] pressed [heavily], [it is a sign of] death.

【英译】

Line 11. 12

[The patient who is] crying [when attacked by] pathogenic [factors] with disquiet of the ethereal soul and corporeal soul [is due to] scantiness of blood and qi. Scantiness of blood and qi belongs to heart [disease]. [When] heart qi is deficient, the patient will feel fearful, closing the eyes with the desire to sleep, going far away in dream with dispersion of spirit and frenetic movement of the ethereal soul and corporeal soul. Decline of yin qi indicates epilepsy and decline of yang qi indicates mania.

【原文】

(十三)

脾中风者,翕翕发热,形如醉人,腹中烦重,皮目瞤瞤而短气。

【今译】

脾脏遭受风邪的侵袭,引发微微发热,形状如醉人一样,腹中烦闷沉重,眼皮跳动而短气。

【原文】

(十四)

脾死脏,浮之大坚,按之如覆杯洁洁状如摇者,死。

【今译】

脾死脏的脉象,浮大而坚,按压时感觉像倒翻的水杯一样,摇动不定,是死证。

【英译】

Line 11. 13

Invasion of wind into the spleen [causes] slight fever like a drunken person, vexation and heaviness in the abdomen, quivering of the eyelids and shortness of breath.

【英译】

Line 11. 14

True visceral pulse of the spleen is floating, large and hard. [When] pressed, [it is felt] like upturned cup, shaking [and disquiet]. [It is a sign of] death.

【原文】

（十五）

趺阳脉浮而涩,浮则胃气强,涩则小便数,浮涩相搏,大便则坚,其脾为约,麻子仁丸主之。

麻子仁丸方

麻子仁（二升）　芍药（半斤）　枳实（一斤）　大黄（一斤）　厚朴（一尺）　杏仁（一升）

右六味,末之,炼蜜和丸梧子大。饮服十丸,日三,以知为度。

【今译】

趺阳脉浮而涩,浮脉表明胃气强盛,涩脉表明小便数,浮脉于涩脉相搏,则使大便坚硬,说明脾受制约,宜用麻子仁丸主治。

【原文】

（十六）

肾着之病,其人身体重,腰中冷,如坐水中,形如水状,反不渴,小便自利,饮食如故,病属下焦,身劳汗出,衣里冷湿,久久得之,腰以下冷痛,腹重如带五千钱,甘姜苓术汤主之。

甘草干姜茯苓白术汤方

甘草　白术（各二两）　干姜　茯苓（各四两）

右四味,以水五升,煮取三升。分温三服,腰中即温。

Volume 2

【英译】

Line 11. 15

[There are cases where] Fuyang pulse is floating and rough. Floating [pulse] indicates [that] stomach qi is strong; rough [pulse] indicates [that] urination is frequent; coexistence of floating [pulse] and rough [pulse] indicates hard stool and the straitened spleen. The appropriate [formula] for treating it is Maziren Pill (麻子仁丸,cannabis seed, Semen Cannabis).

Maziren Pill (麻子仁丸,cannabis seed, Semen Cannabis) [is composed of] 2 *sheng* of Maziren (麻子仁,cannabis seed, Semen Cannabis), 0.5 *jin* of Shaoyao (芍药, peony, Radix Paeoniae), 1 *jin* of Zhishi (枳实, processed unripe bitter orange, Fructus Aurantii Immaturus), 1 *jin* of Dahuang (大黄, rhubarb, Radix et Rhizoma Rhei), 1 *chi* of Houpo (厚朴, magnolia bark, Cortex Magnoliae Officinalis) and 1 *sheng* of Xingren (杏仁, apricot kernel, Semen Armeniacae Amarum).

These six ingredients are pounded into powder and blended with Lianmi (炼蜜, processed honey, Mel Praeparatum) to produce pills the size of pellets. 10 pills are taken in water [each time] and three times a day till there is effect.

【英译】

Line 11. 16

[In] kidney stagnancy disease, the patient's body is heavy with cold in the waist like sitting in cold water with the manifestations of edema, but no thirst. [Besides,] urination is spontaneous and the way to eat is normal, [indicating that] the disease is in the lower energizer. [There will be] sweating [when the patient is] physically tired with cold and

【今译】

肾着之病,患者身体沉重,腰中寒冷,就像坐在水中一样,形状如水气病,但反而不渴,小便自利,饮食正常,属下焦之病。患者因体力劳动而出汗,衣服中又冷又湿,时间久了就会得此病,腰以下冷痛,腹部沉重如带有五千个铜钱似的,宜用甘姜苓术汤主治。

dampness in the clothes. [When] enduring for a long time, [there will be] cold pain below the waist and the abdomen [will be] as heavy as five thousands of bronze coins. The appropriate [formula] for treating it is Ganjiang Lingzhu Decoction (甘姜苓术汤, licorice, dried ginger, poria and largehead atractylodes rhizome decoction).

Ganjiang Lingzhu Decoction (甘姜苓术汤, licorice, dried ginger, poria and largehead atractylodes rhizome decoction) [is composed of] 2 *liang* of Gancao (甘草, licorice, Radix Glycyrrhizae Praeparata), 2 *liang* of Baizhu (白术, rhizome of largehead atractylodes, Rhizoma Atractylodis Macrocephalae), 4 *liang* of Ganjiang (干姜, dried ginger, Rhizoma Zingiberis) and 4 *liang* of Fuling (茯苓, poria, Poria).

These four ingredients are decocted in 5 *sheng* of water to get 3 *sheng* [after] boiling. [The decoction is] divided into three [doses] and taken warm. [After taking the decoction,] the waist will be warm.

【原文】

(十七)

肾死脏,浮之坚,按之乱如转丸,益下入尺中者,死。

【今译】

肾死脏之脉,浮而坚,按之则乱得像转丸一样,其脉溢而涌入尺中的,是死证。

【原文】

(十八)

问曰:三焦竭部,上焦竭善噫,何谓也?师曰:上焦受中焦气未和,不能消谷,故能噫耳。下焦竭,即遗溺失便,其气不和,不能自禁制,不须治,久则愈。

【今译】

问:三焦部功能衰退,上焦衰退时患者常嗳气,这是什么原因呢?

老师说:上焦禀受中焦治气,如果胃气未和,就不能消化食物,所以引起嗳气。下焦衰竭,就会引起遗尿,大便失禁,因下焦气不和,所以就不能自制。这种情况不须治疗,时间一长正气就会恢复,病情就会自愈。

Volume 2

【英译】

Line 11. 17

The true visceral pulse of the kidney is floating and hard. [When] pressed, [it is felt] like pills. [When] stretching through to the chi [region], [it is a sign of] death.

【英译】

Line 11. 18

Question: [There are cases where] the triple energizer has declined, [But when] the upper energizer [begins] to decline, [the patient] tends to sigh. What is the reason?

The master said: [When] qi transmits from the upper energizer to the middle energizer and fails to harmonize, [the patient is] unable to digest food, and that is why there is frequent sighing. [When] the lower energizer [begins] to decline, [it will] cause enuresis and incontinence of defecation. [Since] qi is not harmonized, [the patient is] unable to control [the movement] spontaneously. [There is] no need to treat it. [After] a certain period of enduring, [the disease will] heal spontaneously.

【原文】

(十九)

师曰：热在上焦者，因咳为肺痿；热在中焦者，则为坚；热在下焦者，则尿血，亦令淋秘不通。大肠有寒者，多鹜溏；有热者，便肠垢。小肠有寒者，其人下重便血；有热者，必痔。

【今译】

老师说：热邪停滞在上焦，因而引起咳嗽，为肺痿病；热邪停滞在中焦，导致大便坚硬；热邪在下焦，则导致尿血，也可导致小便淋沥涩痛，闭塞不通。大肠有寒邪的，大便溏稀如鸭粪；大肠有热邪的，大便黏液垢腻。小肠有寒邪的，里急后重而便血；小肠有热邪的，必然引起痔疮。

Volume 2

【英译】

Line 11. 19

The master said: [When pathogenic] heat is in the upper energizer, [it will] cause cough and lung wilting; [when pathogenic] heat is in the middle energizer, it is hard; [when pathogenic] heat is in the lower energizer, [there will be] blood in urine and stranguria will be caused. [When] there is cold in the large intestine, [there will be] incessant sloppy stool; [when pathogenic] heat is in the large intestine, [there will be] sticky stool; [when pathogenic] cold is in the small intestine, the patient [will suffer from] tenesmus and bloody stool; [when] there is [pathogenic] heat [in the small intestine], hemorrhoids will be caused.

【原文】

（二十）

问曰：病有积、有聚、有䅟气，何谓也？

师曰：积者，脏病也，终不移；聚者，腑病也，发作有时，展转痛移，为可治；䅟气者，胁下痛，按之则愈，复发，为䅟气。

诸积大法：脉来细而附骨者，乃积也。寸口积在胸中；微出寸口，积在喉中；关上积在脐旁；上关上，积在心下；微下关，积在少腹。尺中，积在气冲；脉出左，积在左；脉出右，积在右；脉两出，积在中央。各以其部处之。

【今译】

问：病有积、有聚、有䅟气的，指的是什么呢？

老师说：积者，指的是五脏之病，始终无法移动；聚者，指的是六腑之病，发作有一定的时间，疼痛展转而移，是可以治疗的；䅟气者，指的是胁下痛，按压则痛消失，但随后又复发为䅟气。

各种积病的诊断大法：脉象细而重按至骨的，是积病。寸口脉细的，积病在胸中；脉象微而出寸口的，积病在喉中；关部脉细的，积病在脐旁；脉细而处于关部之上的，积病在心下；脉微而出于关部下的，积病在少腹。尺脉细的，积病在气冲；脉细而出于左侧的，积病在左侧；脉细而出于右侧的，积病在右侧；脉细出于左右两侧，积病在中央。可根据积病的所致部位进行诊断治疗。

Volume 2

【英译】

Line 11.20

Question: [In] diseases, [there are] accumulations, gatherings and cereal qi. What are they?

The master said: Accumulations [indicate] a disease of zang-organs that never moves; gatherings [indicate] a disease of fu-organs that occurs in a certain time and pain that moves and is curable; cereal qi [indicates] pain below the rib-side that is relieved when pressed, but returns [when it] becomes cereal qi.

The major method [is used to diagnose] various accumulations: The pulse [that is] thin and fixed to the bone [when pressed] indicates accumulations. [When the pulse in] cunkou [region is thin], the accumulation is in the chest; [when] the faint [pulse] moves outside cunkou, [it indicates that] the accumulation is in the throat; [when the pulse is thin and moves to] the upper of guan [region], [it indicates that] the accumulation is in the heart; [when the pulse is] faint [and moves to] the lower of guan [region], [it indicates that] the accumulation is in the lower abdomen. [When] chi [pulse is thin], the accumulation is in Qichong (ST 30). [When] the [thin] pulse moves to the left, the accumulation is in the left; [when] the [thin] pulse is in the right, the accumulation is in the right; [when] the [thin] pulse moves to both sides, the accumulation is in the center. [It] can be treated according to its location in different places.

痰饮咳嗽病脉证并治第十二

【原文】

（一）

问曰：夫饮有四，何谓也？师曰：有痰饮，有悬饮，有溢饮，有支饮。

【今译】

问：饮病有四种，是哪些呢？

老师说：这四种饮病，有水津与阳热之气相搏而引起的痰饮；有水饮聚于胁下，像水囊空悬的悬饮；有水饮满盈，浸渍肌肤，旁溢四肢的溢饮；有水饮支撑于上，发于胸腔心肺之间的支饮。

Volume 2

Chapter 12
Phlegm, Fluid Retention and Cough Disease:
Pulses, Syndromes/Patterns and Treatment

【英译】

Line 12. 1

Question: There are four kinds of fluid retention. What are they?

The master said: They are phlegmatic fluid retention, suspended fluid retention, spilling fluid retention and propping fluid retention.

【原文】

（二）

问曰：四饮何以为异？

师曰：其人素盛今瘦，水走肠间，沥沥有声，谓之痰饮；饮后水流在胁下，咳唾引痛，谓之悬饮；饮水流行，归于四肢，当汗出而不汗出，身体疼重，谓之溢饮；咳逆倚息，短气不得卧，其形如肿，谓之支饮。

【今译】

问：四饮有什么区别呢？

老师说：如果病人平素身体肥胖，如今却消瘦了，就是因为水液走向肠间，发出沥沥之声，称之为痰饮；饮水之后，水流在胁下，出现咳唾痰涎，引起胁下疼痛的，称之为悬饮；饮水后水液流行，渗于四肢，应当出汗但却没有出汗，身体疼重，称之为溢饮；咳嗽气逆，倚床喘息，短气而不得平卧，身体有浮肿之相，称之为支饮。

【英译】

Line 12.2

Question: What is the difference [between] the four kinds of fluid retention?

The master said: [When] a patient is usually fat but now suddenly becomes emaciated and has water running into the intestines with gurgling sound, it is called phlegmatic fluid retention; after drinking, water flows under the rib-side, causing cough, spitting and pain, it is called suspended fluid retention; [after drinking,] water flows into the four limbs, resulting in no sweating when there should be sweating, generalized pain and heaviness, it is called spilling fluid retention; [when there are symptoms and signs of] cough and qi counterflow, propped breathing, shortness of breath, inability to lie down and swollen appearance, it is called propped fluid retention.

【原文】

（三）

水在心，心下坚筑，短气，恶水不欲饮。

【今译】

水饮浸渍于心，心下坚满，短气，恶水，不想饮水。

【原文】

（四）

水在肺，吐涎沫，欲饮水。

【今译】

水浸渍在肺，表现为呕吐涎沫，想饮水。

【原文】

（五）

水在脾，少气身重。

【今译】

水浸渍在脾，气短，身体沉重。

Volume 2

【英译】

Line 12.3

[The manifestations of] water flowing into the heart [include] hardness and fullness below the heart, shortness of breath, aversion to water and no desire to drink water.

【英译】

Line 12.4

[The manifestations of] water flowing into the lung [include] vomiting of drool and foam with desire to drink water.

【英译】

Line 12.5

[The manifestations of] water flowing into the spleen [include] shortness of breath and heaviness of the body.

【原文】

（六）

水在肝，胁下支满，嚏而痛。

【今译】

水浸渍在肝，胁下支撑胀满，打喷嚏时胁肋疼痛。

【原文】

（七）

水在肾，心下悸。

【今译】

水浸渍在肾，心下悸动。

【原文】

（八）

夫心下有留饮，其人背寒冷如手大。

【今译】

心下有水饮停留，病人背部寒冷，范围如手掌大小。

Volume 2

【英译】

Line 12.6

[The manifestations of] water flowing into the liver [include] propped fullness in the hypochondrium and pain when sneezing.

【英译】

Line 12.7

[The manifestations of] water flowing into the kidney [is] palpitation below the heart.

【英译】

Line 12.8

[The manifestations of] water retention in the heart [include] cold in the back [over the region] as large as a hand.

【原文】

（九）

留饮者，胁下痛引缺盆，咳嗽则辄已。

【今译】

体内有留饮的患者，胁下痛牵引缺盆，咳嗽时疼痛更甚。

【原文】

（十）

胸中有留饮，其人短气而渴，四肢历节痛。脉沉者，有留饮。

【今译】

如果胸中有留饮，病人就会有短气而渴，四肢关节疼痛，脉象沉等症状，这是因为留饮所致。

【原文】

（十一）

膈上病痰，满喘咳吐，发则寒热，背痛腰疼，目泣自出，其人振振身瞤剧，必有伏饮。

【今译】

患者膈上有痰，就会产生胸满、气喘、咳嗽、吐痰等症状，发作时则恶寒发热，背痛腰疼，泪水自行流出，身体颤抖，摇动剧烈，这主要是痰饮停滞于内所致。

Volume 2

【英译】

Line 12. 9

[The manifestations of] water retention [in the body include] pain below the hypochondrium stretching into the supraclavicular fossa [which is] exacerbated [by] cough.

【英译】

Line 12. 10

[The manifestations of] water retention in the chest [include] shortness of breath, thirst, pain of joints in the four limbs and sunken pulse due to fluid retention.

【英译】

Line 12. 11

Pathogenic phlegm above the diaphragm [will cause] fullness [in the chest], panting, cough and vomiting. [When it has] occurred, [the manifestations include] aversion to cold, fever, back pain, waist pain, spontaneous tearing, twitching and severe quivering of the body, [indicating that] there must be fluid retention [inside the body].

【原文】

(十二)

夫病人饮水多,必暴喘满。凡食少饮多,水停心下,甚者则悸,微者短气。

脉双弦者,寒也,皆大下后善虚;脉偏弦者,饮也。

【今译】

病人饮水过多,必然突然气喘胀满。凡吃饭少而饮水多的,就会导致水停留于心下,病情严重的则会引起悸动。病情较轻的,则会引起呼吸短促。

两手脉皆弦的,为虚寒证,皆属大度攻下而引起的里虚所致。如果一手之脉偏弦的,就属痰饮之病。

【原文】

(十三)

肺饮不弦,但苦喘短气。

【今译】

肺中有水饮停留,但脉象不弦,只有气喘严重,呼吸短促。

Volume 2

【英译】

Line 12. 12

[When] a patient drinks a lot of water, [it will] inevitably [cause] fulminant panting and fullness. [If a patient] eats less and drinks more, [there will be] retention of water below the heart. [If the case is] severe, [it will cause] palpitation; [if the case is] mild, [it will cause] shortness of breath.

The taut pulses in both sides [indicate] cold [syndrome/pattern] due to deficiency caused by great purgation. The taut pulse in one side [indicates] fluid retention.

【英译】

Line 12. 13

[When there is] fluid retention in the lung, the pulse is not taut, but panting is severe and breath is short.

【原文】

(十四)

支饮亦喘而不能卧,加短气,其脉平也。

【今译】

支饮也有气喘而不能平卧,另外还有呼吸短促的症状,其脉象是平和的。

【原文】

(十五)

病痰饮者,当以温药和之。

【今译】

患痰饮病的,应当用温药调和治疗。

【原文】

(十六)

心下有痰饮,胸胁支满,目眩,苓桂术甘汤主之。

苓桂术甘汤方

茯苓(四两)　桂枝　白术(各三两)　甘草(二两)

右四味,以水六升,煮取三升。分温三服,小便则利。

【今译】

心下有痰饮停留,胸胁支撑胀满,眼睛晕眩的,宜用苓桂术甘汤主治。

【英译】

Line 12. 14

[In] propped fluid retention, [when there is] also panting, inability to lie down and shortness of breath, the pulse is normal.

【英译】

Line 12. 15

[Patients with] phlegmatic fluid retention disease should be harmonized [and treated] by medicinals warm [in property].

【英译】

Line 12. 16

For phlegmatic fluid retention below the heart [with the symptoms and signs of] propping fullness in the chest and rib-side and dizzy vision, Linggui Zhugan Decoction (苓桂术甘汤, poria, cinnamon twig, largehead atractylodes rhizome and licorice decoction) [can be used] to treat it.

Linggui Zhugan Decoction (苓桂术甘汤, poria, cinnamon twig, largehead atractylodes rhizome and licorice decoction) [is composed of] 4 *liang* of Fuling (茯苓, poria, Poria), 3 *liang* of Guizhi (桂枝, cinnamon twig, Ramulus Cinnamomi), 3 *liang* of Baizhu (白术, rhizome of largehead atractylodes, Rhizoma Atractylodis Macrocephalae) and 2 *liang* of Gancao (甘草, licorice, Radix Glycyrrhizae Praeparata).

These four ingredients are decocted in 6 *sheng* of water to get 3 *sheng* [after] boiling. [The decoction is] divided into three [doses] and taken warm. Urination [will be] normalized [after taking the decoction].

【原文】

(十七)

夫短气有微饮,当从小便去之,苓桂术甘汤主之,肾气丸亦主之。

【今译】

呼吸短促,有轻微水饮停留的,应当通过小便祛除停留的水饮,用苓桂术甘汤主治,肾气丸也可以主治。

【原文】

(十八)

病者脉伏,其人欲自利,利反快,虽利,心下续坚满,此为留饮欲去故也,甘遂半夏汤主之。

甘遂半夏汤方

甘遂(大者,三枚)　半夏(十二枚,以水一升,煮取半升,去滓)　芍药(五枚)　甘草(如指大一枚,炙)

右四味,以水二升,煮取半升,去滓,以蜜半升和药汁,煎取八合,顿服之。

【今译】

病人脉伏,将要腹泻,腹泻后反而感到爽快。虽然腹泻,但心下依然坚硬胀满,这是水饮停留将除而未除的原因,用甘遂半夏汤主治。

Volume 2

【英译】

Line 12. 17

Shortness of breath with mild retention of fluid should be eliminated by [promoting] urination. Linggui Zhugan Decoction (苓 桂 术 甘 汤，poria，cinnamon twig，largehead atractylodes rhizome and licorice decoction) [can be used] to treat it. Shenqi Pill (肾气丸，kidney qi pill) [can also be used] to treat it.

【英译】

Line 12. 18

[If] the patient's pulse is hidden，there will be diarrhea. [After] diarrhea，[the patient will feel] comfortable. Although [there is] diarrhea，[there is] still hardness and fullness below the heart. This is due to fluid retention that should be eliminated [but is still not eliminated]. Gansui Banxia Decoction (甘遂半夏汤，kansui and pinellia decoction) [can be used] to treat it.

Gansui Banxia Decoction （甘 遂 半 夏 汤，kansui and pinellia decoction) [is composed of] 3 pieces of Gansui (甘遂，kansui，Radix Kansui)(large)，12 pieces of Banxia (半夏，pinellia，Rhizoma Pinelliae) (to be boiled in 1 *sheng* of water to get 0. 5 *sheng* and the dregs are removed)，5 pieces of Shaoyao (芍药，peony，Radix Paeoniae) and 1 piece of Gancao (甘草，licorice，Radix Glycyrrhizae Praeparata) as big as the size of a finger (broil).

These four ingredients are decocted in 2 *sheng* of water to get 0. 5 *sheng*. [After] removal of the dregs，0. 5 *sheng* of honey is mixed with the medicinal juice and boiled to get 8 *ge*. [The whole decoction is] taken as one dose.

【原文】

(十九)

脉浮而细滑,伤饮。

【今译】

脉象浮而细滑,是被水饮所伤而致。

【原文】

(二十)

脉弦数,有寒饮,冬夏难治。

【今译】

脉象弦数,又有寒饮停留,冬天和夏天都很难治疗。

【原文】

(二十一)

脉沉而弦者,悬饮内痛。

【今译】

脉沉而弦的,是悬饮所致的内痛。

Volume 2

【英译】

Line 12. 19

Floating，thin and slippery pulse is caused by ［damage of］ fluid retention.

【英译】

Line 12. 20

Taut and rapid pulse with ［retention of］ cold fluid is difficult to treat in winter and summer.

【英译】

Line 12. 21

Sunken and taut pulse ［indicates］ internal pain ［caused by］ propped fluid retention.

【原文】

(二十二)

病悬饮者，十枣汤主之。

十枣汤方

芫花（熬） 甘遂、大戟（各等分）

右三味，捣筛，以水一升五合，先煮肥大枣十枚，取八合，去滓，内药末。强人服一钱匕，羸人服半钱，平旦温服之；不下者，明日更加半钱。得快下后，糜粥自养。

【今译】

悬饮所致治病，宜用十枣汤主治。

【英译】

Line 12.22

Disease [caused by] propped fluid retention [can be] treated by Shizao Decoction (十枣汤, ten jujubes decoction).

Shizao Decoction (十枣汤, ten jujubes decoction) [is composed of] Yuanhua (芫花, genkwa, Flos Genkwa)(simmer), Gansui (甘遂, kansui, Radix Kansui) and Daji (大戟, euphorbia, Radix Euphorbiae seu Knoxiae) of the same amount.

These three ingredients are pounded and sieved to decoct in 1 *sheng* and 5 *ge* of water. Ten pieces of plump Dazao (大枣, jujube, Fructus Ziziphus Jujubae) are boiled first to get 8 *ge*. [After] removal of the dregs, the powder [of the three ingredients] are put into [it to boil]. Strong patients take 1 *qianbi* [each time] and weak patients take half a *qianbi* [each time]. [The decoction is] taken warm at daybreak. [If there is] no purgation, half more *qianbi* [should be taken] the next day. When well purged, [the patient can take] porridge to nourish himself.

【原文】

(二十三)

病溢饮者,当发其汗,大青龙汤主之,小青龙汤亦主之。

大青龙汤方

麻黄(六两,去节) 桂枝(二两,去皮) 甘草(二两,炙) 杏仁(四十个,去皮尖) 生姜(三两,切) 大枣(十二枚) 石膏(如鸡子大,碎)

右七味,以水九升,先煮麻黄,减二升,去上沫,内诸药,煮取三升,去滓。温服一升,取微似汗。汗多者,温粉粉之。

小青龙汤方

麻黄(三两,去节) 芍药(三两) 五味子(半升) 干姜(三两) 甘草(三两,炙) 细辛(三两) 桂枝(三两,去皮) 半夏(半升,洗)

右八味,以水一斗,先煮麻黄,减二升,去上沫,内诸药,煮取三升,去滓,温服一升。

【今译】

患溢饮病的,应当通过发汗治疗,用大青龙汤主治,小青龙汤也可主治。

【英译】

Line 12.23

Spilling fluid retention disease with sweating [after occurrence] can be treated by Da Qinglong Decoction (大青龙汤，major blue loong decoction). Xiao Qinglong Decoction (小青龙汤，minor blue loong decoction) [can] also [be used] to treat it.

Da Qinglong Decoction (大青龙汤，major blue loong decoction) [is composed of] 6 *liang* of Mahuang (麻黄，ephedra, Herba Ephedrae) (remove nodes), 2 *liang* of Guizhi (桂枝，cinnamon twig, Ramulus Cinnamomi) (remove the bark), 2 *liang* of Gancao (甘草，licorice, Radix Glycyrrhizae Praeparata) (broil), 40 pieces of Xingren (杏仁，apricot kernel, Semen Armeniacae Amarum) (remove the bark and tips), 3 *liang* of Shengjiang (生姜，fresh ginger, Rhizoma Zingiberis Recens) (cut), 12 pieces of Dazao (大枣，jujube, Fructus Ziziphus Jujubae) and Shigao (石膏，gypsum, Gypsum Fibrosum) (the size of a chicken egg, pound).

These seven ingredients are decocted in 9 *sheng* of water. Mahuang (麻黄，ephedra, Herba Ephedrae) is boiled first. [After] removal of the foam, the other ingredients are put into it to boil and get 3 *sheng*. The dregs are removed and [the decoction is] taken warm 1 *sheng* [each time]. [After taking the first dose, the patient feels] slightly [warm] like sweating. [If there is] profuse sweating, eliminate it with some warm powder.

Xiao Qinglong Decoction (小青龙汤，minor blue loong decoction) [is composed of] 3 *liang* of Mahuang (麻黄，ephedra, Herba Ephedrae) (remove nodes), 3 *liang* of Shaoyao (芍药，peony, Radix Paeoniae), 0.5 *sheng* of Wuweizi (五味子，schisandra, Fructus Schisandrae), 3 *liang* of Ganjiang (干姜，dried ginger, Rhizoma Zingiberis), 3 *liang* of Gancao (甘草，licorice, Radix Glycyrrhizae Praeparata) (broil), 3 *liang* of Xixin (细辛，asarum, Herba Asari), 3 *liang* of Guizhi (桂枝，cinnamon twig, Ramulus Cinnamomi) (remove the bark) and 0.5 *sheng* of Banxia (半夏，pinellia, Rhizoma Pinelliae) (wash).

These eight ingredients are decocted in 1 *dou* of water. Mahuang (麻黄，ephedra, Herba Ephedrae) is boiled first to reduce 2 *sheng*. [After] removal of the foam, the other ingredients are put into [it] to boil and get 3 *sheng*. The dregs are removed and [the decoction is] taken warm 1 *sheng* [each time].

【原文】

(二十四)

膈间支饮,其人喘满,心下痞坚,面色黧黑,其脉沉紧,得之数十日,医吐下之不愈,木防己汤主之。虚者即愈,实者三日复发。复与不愈者,宜木防己汤去石膏加茯苓芒硝汤主之。

木防己汤方

木防己(三两) 石膏(十二枚,如鸡子大) 桂枝(二两) 人参(四两)

右四味,以水六升,煮取二升,分温再服。

木防己去石膏加茯苓芒硝汤方

木防己、桂枝(各二两) 人参、茯苓(各四两) 芒硝(三合)

右五味,以水六升,煮取二升,去滓,内芒硝,再微煎。分温再服,微利则愈。

【今译】

膈间有支饮,患者气喘胀满,心下硬结痞坚,面色黑而晦黄,脉象沉紧,得病已经数十天了,医生用吐下之法治疗而不愈,可用木防己汤主治。心下虚软的,就可及时治愈,心下结实的三天后又复发。再用木防己汤治疗依然不愈的,宜用木防己汤去石膏加茯苓芒硝汤主治。

【英译】
Line 12.24

Propped fluid retention in the diaphgram [results in] panting, [chest] fullness, lump and hardness below the heart, black facial expression, sunken and tight pulse. Dozens of days [after] occurrence, if the doctor has failed to cure it [by using] vomiting and purging [therapies], Mufangji Decoction (木防己汤, the root of stephania tetrandra decoction) [can be used] to treat it. [If it is] deficiency [below the heart], [it will be] easy to cure. [If it is] excess [below the heart], [it will] recur three days later. If Mufangji Decoction (木防己汤, the root of stephania tetrandra decoction) is already used, [but this disease is still] difficult to cure, Mufangji Decoction (木防己汤, the root of stephania tetrandra decoction) with removal of Shigao (石膏, gypsum, Gypsum Fibrosum) and addition of Fuling (茯苓, poria, Poria) and Mangxiao (芒硝, mirabilite, Mirabilitum) [can be used] to treat it.

Mufangji Decoction (木防己汤, the root of stephania tetrandra decoction) [is composed of] 3 *liang* of Mufangji (木防己, the root of stephania tetrandra, Radix Stephaniae Tetrandrae), 12 pieces of Shigao (石膏, gypsum, Gypsum Fibrosum)(the size of a chicken egg), 2 *liang* of Guizhi (桂枝, cinnamon twig, Ramulus Cinnamomi) and 4 *liang* of Renshen (人参, ginseng, Radix Ginseng).

These four ingredients are decocted in 6 *sheng* of water to get 2 *sheng* [after] boiling. [The decoction is] divided into two [doses] and taken warm.

Mufangji Decoction (木防己汤, the root of stephania tetrandra decoction) with removal of Shigao (石膏, gypsum, Gypsum Fibrosum) and addition of Fuling (茯苓, poria, Poria) and Mangxiao (芒硝, mirabilite, Mirabilitum) [is composed of] 2 *liang* of Mufangji (木防己, the root of stephania tetrandra, Radix Stephaniae Tetrandrae), 2 *liang* of Guizhi (桂枝, cinnamon twig, Ramulus Cinnamomi), 4 *liang* of Renshen (人参, ginseng, Radix Ginseng), 4 *liang* of Fuling (茯苓, poria, Poria) and 3 *ge* of Mangxiao (芒硝, mirabilite, Mirabilitum).

These five ingredients are decocted in 6 *sheng* of water to get 2 *sheng* [after] boiling. The dregs are removed and Mangxiao (芒硝, mirabilite, Mirabilitum) is put into [it] to boil mildly. [The decoction is] divided into two [doses] and taken warm. [If there is] slight diarrhea [after taking the decoction], [the disease will be] cured.

【原文】

(二十五)

心下有支饮,其人苦冒眩,泽泻汤主之。

泽泻汤方

泽泻(五两) 白术(二两)

右二味,以水二升,煮取一升,分温再服。

【今译】

心下有支饮,病人苦于冒眩,用泽泻汤主治。

【原文】

(二十六)

支饮胸满者,厚朴大黄汤主之。

厚朴大黄汤方

厚朴(一尺) 大黄(六两) 枳实(四枚)

右三味,以水五升,煮取二升,分温再服。

【今译】

支饮引起胸部胀满的,用厚朴大黄汤主治。

Volume 2

【英译】

Line 12.25

[When] there is propped fluid retention below the heart, the patient will suffer from dizziness and blurred vision. Zexie Decoction (泽泻汤, alisma decoction) [can be used] to treat it.

Zexie Decoction (泽泻汤, alisma decoction) [is composed of] 5 *liang* of Zexie (泽泻, alisma, Rhizoma Alismatis) and 2 *liang* of Baizhu (白术, rhizome of largehead atractylodes, Rhizoma Atractylodis Macrocephalae).

These two ingredients are decocted in 2 *sheng* of water to get 1 *sheng* [after] boiling. [The decoction is] divided into two [doses] and taken warm.

【英译】

Line 12.26

Propped fluid retention with chest fullness [can be] treated by Houpo Dahuang Decoction (厚朴大黄汤, magnolia bark and rhubarb decoction).

Houpo Dahuang Decoction (厚朴大黄汤, magnolia bark and rhubarb decoction) [is composed of] 1 *chi* of Houpo (厚朴, magnolia bark, Cortex Magnoliae Officinalis), 6 *liang* of Dahuang (大黄, rhubarb, Radix et Rhizoma Rhei) and 4 pieces of Zhishi (枳实, processed unripe bitter orange, Fructus Aurantii Immaturus).

These three ingredients are decocted in 5 *sheng* of water to get 2 *sheng* [after] boiling. [The decoction is] divided into two [doses] and taken warm.

【原文】

（二十七）

支饮不得息，葶苈大枣泻肺汤主之。

【今译】

支饮患者呼吸困难的，用葶苈大枣泻肺汤主治。

【原文】

（二十八）

呕家本渴，渴者为欲解，今反不渴，心下有支饮故也，小半夏汤主之。

小半夏汤方

半夏（一升）　生姜（半斤）

右二味，以水七升，煮取一升半，分温再服。

【今译】

经常呕吐之人，本来应该感到口渴的。口渴是疾病将要解除的象征，如今反而不渴，这是心下有支饮的原因，可用小半夏汤主治。

Volume 2

【英译】

Line 12.27

Propped fluid retention with difficulty in breathing [can be] treated by Tingli Dazao Xiefei Decoction (葶苈大枣泻肺汤, tingli and jujube decoction for draining the lung).

【英译】

Line 12.28

Patients with panting are usually thirsty and thirst indicates resolution of [panting]. [But] now [the patient is] not thirsty because there is propped fluid retention below the heart. Xiao Banxia Decoction (小半夏汤, minor pinellia decoction) [can be used] to treat it.

Xiao Banxia Decoction added with Fuling (茯苓, poria, Poria) (小半夏汤, minor pinellia decoction) [is composed of] 1 *sheng* of Banxia (半夏, pinellia, Rhizoma Pinelliae) and 0.5 *jin* of Shengjiang (生姜, fresh ginger, Rhizoma Zingiberis Recens).

These two ingredients are decocted in 7 *sheng* of water and get 1 *sheng* [after] boiling. [The decoction is] divided into two [doses] and taken warm.

【原文】

(二十九)

腹满,口舌干燥,此肠间有水气,己椒苈黄丸主之。

防己椒目葶苈大黄丸方

防己　椒目　葶苈(熬)　大黄(各一两)

右四味,末之,蜜丸如梧子大。先食饮服一丸,日三服,稍增,口中有津液。渴者,加芒硝半两。

【今译】

腹部胀满,口舌干燥,这是因为肠间有水气,宜用己椒苈黄丸主治。

【原文】

(三十)

卒呕吐,心下痞,膈间有水,眩悸者,小半夏加茯苓汤主之。

小半夏加茯苓汤方

半夏(一升)　生姜(半斤)　茯苓(三两)

右三味,以水七升,煮取一升五合,分温再服。

【今译】

突然呕吐,心下痞满,膈间有水饮,头晕目眩,心下悸动,宜用小半夏加茯苓汤主治。

【英译】

Line 12.29

Abdominal fullness with dry tongue and mouth ［is caused by］ water qi（edema）in the intestines. Fangji Jiaomu Tingli Dahuang Pill（防己椒目葶苈大黄丸，the root of stephania tetrandra，lepidium/descurainiae and rhubarb pill）［can be used］to treat it.

Fangji Jiaomu Tingli Dahuang Pill（防己椒目葶苈大黄丸，the root of stephania tetrandra，lepidium/descurainiae and rhubarb pill）［is composed of］1 *liang* of Fangji（防己，the root of stephania tetrandra，Radix Stephaniae Tetrandrae），1 *liang* of Jiaomu（椒目，zanthoxylum seed，Zanthoxyli Semen），1 *liang* of Tingli（葶苈，lepidium/descurainiae，Semen Lepidii seu Descurainiae）（simmer）and 1 *liang* of *Dahuang*（大黄，rhubarb，Radix et Rhizoma Rhei）.

These four ingredients are pounded into powder and made into pills with honey the size of firmiana seeds. Before eating, one pill ［should be］ taken ［each time］ and three times a day. A little increase ［of the dose will］ induce fluid in the mouth. For thirst, 0.5 *liang* of Mangxiao（芒硝，mirabilite，Mirabilitum）is added.

【英译】

Line 12.30

［The disease characterized by］ fulminant panting and vomiting, lump below the heart, ［retention of］ water in the diaphragm, dizziness and palpitation can be treated by Xiao Banxia Decoction added with Fuling（小半夏加茯苓汤，minor pinellia decoction added with poria）.

Xiao Banxia Decoction added with Fuling（小半夏加茯苓汤，minor pinellia decoction added with poria）［is composed of］1 *sheng* of Banxia（半夏，pinellia，Rhizoma Pinelliae），0.5 *jin* of Shengjiang（生姜，fresh ginger，Rhizoma Zingiberis Recens）and 3 *liang* of Fuling（茯苓，poria，Poria）.

These three ingredients are decocted in 7 *sheng* of water to get 1 *sheng* and 5 *ge* ［after］ boiling. ［The decoction is］ divided into two ［doses］ and taken warm.

【原文】

（三十一）

假令瘦人脐下有悸，吐涎沫而癫眩，此水也，五苓散主之。

五苓散方

泽泻（一两一分）　猪苓（三分，去皮）　茯苓（三分）　白术（三分）

桂枝（二分，去皮）

右五味，为末。白饮服方寸匕，日三服，多饮暖水，汗出愈。

【今译】

如果消瘦的患者脐下悸动，呕吐涎沫，眩晕不堪，这是水饮之症，宜用五苓散主治。

附方

【原文】

《外台》茯苓饮治心胸中有停痰宿水，自吐出水后，心胸间虚，气满不能食，消痰气，令能食。

茯苓　人参　白术（各三两）　枳实（二两）　橘皮（二两半）　生姜（四两）　右六味，水六升，煮取一升八合。分温三服，如人行八九里进之。

【今译】

《外台秘要》中的茯苓饮，用以治疗心胸中痰饮宿水停留，自行吐出水后，心胸间显得空虚，气满不能饮食，只有消除了痰气，才能进食。

Volume 2

【英译】

Line 12.31

If there is palpitation below the umbilicus in an emaciated patient，[there will be] vomiting of drool and foam，and dizziness due to [retention of] water. It can be treated by Wuling Powder（五苓散，powder made of five medicinal herbs）.

Wuling Powder（五苓散，powder made of five medicinal herbs [is composed of] 1 *liang* and 1 *fen* of Zexie（泽泻，alisma，Rhizoma Alismatis），3 *fen* of Zhuling（猪苓，polyporus，Polyporus Umbellatus）（remove the bark），3 *fen* of Fuling（茯苓，poria，Poria），3 *fen* of Baizhu（白术，rhizome of largehead atractylodes，Rhizoma Atractylodis Macrocephalae）and 2 *fen* of Guizhi（桂枝，cinnamon twig，Ramulus Cinnamomi）（remove the bark）.

These five ingredients are pounded into powder. [The patient can] take 1 *fangcunbi* [each time] in water and three times a day. [The patient should] drink more warm water [to induce sweating]. [When there is] sweating，[the disease is going] to heal.

Appended formulas

【英译】

Fuling Decoction（茯苓饮，poria decoction）[from the book entitled] *Waitai Miyao*（《外台秘要》，*The Medical Secrets of an Official Named Wang Tao*）[is used] to treat retention of phlegm and accumulation of water in the heart and chest. [When there is] spontaneous sweating，[retention of] water will be eliminated，the chest and diaphragm will be empty. [If] qi is full，[the patient is] unable to eat. [When] phlegmatic qi is resolved，[the patient is] able to eat.

Fuling Decoction（茯苓饮，poria decoction）[is composed of] 3 *liang* of Fuling（茯苓，poria，Poria），3 *liang* of Renshen（人参，ginseng，Radix Ginseng），3 *liang* of Baizhu（白术，rhizome of largehead atractylodes，Rhizoma Atractylodis Macrocephalae），2 *liang* of Zhishi（枳实，processed unripe bitter orange，Fructus Aurantii Immaturus），2.5 *liang* of Jupi（橘皮，tangerine peel，Pericarpium Citri Reticulatae）and 4 *liang* of Shengjiang（生姜，fresh ginger，Rhizoma Zingiberis Recens）.

These six ingredients are decocted in 6 *sheng* of water to get 1 *sheng* and 8 *ge* [after] boiling. [The decoction is] divided into three [doses] and taken warm. [The patient should wait for the time it takes for him] to walk eight or nine *li*（about 4 or 4.5 kilometers）and then take the second [dose].

【原文】

(三十二)

咳家其脉弦,为有水,十枣汤主之。

【今译】

时常咳嗽的患者,脉象弦,是内有水饮所致,宜用十枣汤主治。

【原文】

(三十三)

夫有支饮家,咳烦,胸中痛者,不卒死,至一百日、一岁,宜十枣汤。

【今译】

有支饮病的患者,咳嗽,烦闷,胸中疼痛,如果不突然死亡,延迟至一百天或一年,宜用十枣汤主治。

【原文】

(三十四)

久咳数岁,其脉弱者可治,实大数者死;其脉虚者必苦冒,其人本有支饮在胸中故也,治属饮家。

【今译】

咳嗽数年,脉象弱的可以治疗,脉象实大而数的,将死亡。脉象虚的,必然遭遇头目昏冒。这是病人本来就有支饮在胸的缘故,应按水饮病进行治疗。

【英译】

Line 12.32

Taut pulse in the patient with frequent cough [indicates that] there is water [retention]. [It can be] treated by Shizao Decoction (十枣汤, ten jujubes decoction).

【英译】

Line 12.33

Patients with propped fluid retention [suffer from] panting, vexation and pain in the chest. [The patients will] not immediately die, but in one hundred days or a year. The appropriate [formula used to treat it is] Shizao Decoction (十枣汤, ten jujubes decoction).

【英译】

Line 12.34

[In a patient, there is] incessant cough for years. [If] the pulse is weak, [it is] curable. [If] the pulse is strong, large and rapid, [it is] fatal. [If] the pulse is weak, [the patient] must suffer from dizziness [because] originally there is propped fluid retention in the chest. The treatment is the same as that for fluid retention.

【原文】

(三十五)

咳逆,倚息不得卧,小青龙汤主之。

【今译】

咳嗽气逆的患者,倚床呼吸,不能平卧,宜用小青龙汤主治。

【原文】

(三十六)

青龙汤下已,多唾口燥,寸脉沉,尺脉微,手足厥逆,气从小腹上冲胸咽,手足痹,其面翕热如醉状,因复下流阴股,小便难,时复冒者,与茯苓桂枝五味子甘草汤,治其气冲。

桂苓五味甘草汤方

茯苓(四两)　桂枝(四两,去皮)　甘草(三两,炙)　五味子(半升)

右四味,以水八升,煮取三升,去滓,分温三服。

【今译】

服用青龙汤攻下之后,患者多唾口燥,寸部脉沉,尺部脉微,手足厥逆,气从小腹上冲到胸部和咽喉,手足麻痹,面部微微发热如醉状,气冲又向下流到两腿内侧,小便困难,时时又有头目昏冒的,宜用茯苓桂枝五味子甘草汤主治,治疗患者的气冲之症。

Volume 2

【英译】

Line 12.35

[The disease, marked by] cough, counterflow [of qi], propped breathing and inability to lie down, [can be treated by] Xiao Qinglong Decoction (小青龙汤, minor blue loong decoction).

【英译】

Line 12.36

[When] Qinglong Decoction (青龙汤, blue loong decoction) [has already been used to promote] purgation, [there are still symptoms and signs of] frequent spitting, dry mouth, sunken cun pulse, faint chi pulse, reversal cold of hands and feet, qi surging up to the chest and throat from the lower abdomen, impediment of hands and feet, feverish facial expression like being drunken. [In addition, qi] flows downward to the inner sides [of legs], [resulting in] difficulty in defecation and repeated dizziness occasionally. Fuling Guizhi Wuweizi Gancao Decoction (茯苓桂枝五味子甘草汤, poria, cinnamon twig, schisandra and licorice decoction) [can be used] to treat qi surging.

Fuling Guizhi Wuweizi Gancao Decoction (茯苓桂枝五味子甘草汤, poria, cinnamon twig, schisandra and licorice decoction) [is composed of] 4 *liang* of Fuling (茯苓, poria, Poria), 4 *liang* of Guizhi (桂枝, cinnamon twig, Ramulus Cinnamomi) (remove the bark), 3 *liang* of Gancao (甘草, licorice, Radix Glycyrrhizae Praeparata) (broil) and 0.5 *sheng* of Wuweizi (五味子, schisandra, Fructus Schisandrae).

These four ingredients are decocted in 8 *sheng* of water to get 3 *sheng* [after] boiling. The dregs are removed and [the decoction is] divided into three [doses] and taken warm.

【原文】

(三十七)

冲气即低，而反更咳，胸满者，用桂苓五味甘草汤去桂加干姜、细辛，以治其咳满。

苓甘五味姜辛汤方

茯苓（四两）　甘草　干姜　细辛（各三两）　五味子（半升）

右五味，以水八升，煮取三升，去滓。温服半升，日三服。

【今译】

冲气已平，患者反而更加咳嗽，胸部胀满，宜用桂苓五味甘草汤去桂枝加干姜、细辛主治，以治疗其咳嗽胸满。

Volume 2

【英译】

Line 12.37

[There are cases where] qi surging is already finished, but [there is] severe cough and chest fullness. Guiling Wuwei Gancao Decoction (桂苓五味甘草汤, cinnamon twig, poria, schisandar and licorice decoction) [can be used] to treat cough and fullness.

Guiling Wuwei Gancao Decoction (桂苓五味甘草汤, cinnamon twig, poria, schisandar and licorice decoction) [is composed of] 4 *liang* of Fuling (茯苓, poria, Poria), 3 *liang* of Gancao (甘草, licorice, Radix Glycyrrhizae Praeparata), 3 *liang* of Ganjiang (干姜, dry ginger, Rhizoma Zingiberis), 3 *liang* of Xixin (细辛, asarum, Herba Asari) and 0. 5 *sheng* of Wuweizi (五味子, schisandra, Fructus Schisandrae).

These five ingredients are decocted in 8 *sheng* of water to get 3 *sheng* [after] boiling. The dregs are removed and [the decoction is] taken warm 0. 5 *sheng* [each time] and three times a day.

【原文】

（三十八）

咳满即止，而更复渴，冲气复发者，以细辛、干姜为热药也。服之当遂渴，而渴反止者，为支饮也。支饮者，法当冒，冒者必呕，呕者复内半夏，以去其水。

桂苓五味甘草去桂加干姜细辛半夏汤方

茯苓（四两）　甘草　细辛　干姜（各二两）　五味子　半夏（各半升）

右六味，以水八升，煮取三升，去滓。温服半升，日三服。

【今译】

咳嗽与胸满已经停止，但患者却又感口渴，冲气再次发生，这是因为细辛和干姜是热性药物，患者服用后就会口渴。如果反而不口渴的，是因为有支饮之症。有支饮之症的，应当头目昏冒，昏冒的人必然呕吐，呕吐的再加半夏，以便除去水饮。

Volume 2

【英译】

Line 12.38

[There are cases where] cough and [chest] fullness have already ceased, but [there is] still thirst and qi surges up again [because] Xixin (细辛, asarum, Herba Asari) and Banxia (半夏, pinellia, Rhizoma Pinelliae) are heat [in property]. [After] taking these [two medicinals], there should be thirst. [If there is] no thirst [after taking these two medicinals], [it] is propped fluid retention [disease]. [In] propped fluid retention [disease], there must be dizziness accompanied by retching. [When there is] retching, Banxia (半夏, pinellia, Rhizoma Pinelliae) is added to eliminate water. [It should be] treated by Linggan Wuwei Gancao Decoction (苓甘五味甘草汤, poria, schisandra and licorice decoction) added with Ganjiang (干姜, dried ginger, Rhizoma Zingiberis), Xixin (细辛, asarum, Herba Asari) and Banxia (半夏, pinellia, Rhizoma Pinelliae).

Linggan Wuwei Gancao Decoction (苓甘五味甘草汤, poria, schisandra and licorice decoction) added with Ganjiang (干姜, dried ginger, Rhizoma Zingiberis), Xixin (细辛, asarum, Herba Asari) and Banxia (半夏, pinellia, Rhizoma Pinelliae) [is composed of] 4 *liang* of Fuling (茯苓, poria, Poria), 2 *liang* of Gancao (甘草, licorice, Radix Glycyrrhizae Praeparata), 2 *liang* of Xixin (细辛, asarum, Herba Asari), 2 *liang* of Ganjiang (干姜, dried ginger, Rhizoma Zingiberis), 0.5 *sheng* of Wuweizi (五味子, schisandra, Fructus Schisandrae) and 0.5 *sheng* of Banxia (半夏, pinellia, Rhizoma Pinelliae).

These four ingredients are decocted in 8 *sheng* of water and get 3 *sheng* [after] boiling. The dregs are removed and [the decoction is] taken warm 0.5 *sheng* [each time] and three times a day.

【原文】

（三十九）

水去呕止，其人形肿者，加杏仁主之。其证应内麻黄，以其人遂痹，故不内之；若逆而内之者，必厥。所以然者，以其人血虚，麻黄发其阳故也。

苓甘五味加姜辛半夏杏仁汤方

茯苓（四两）　甘草（三两）　五味子（半升）　干姜（三两）　细辛（三两）　半夏（半升）　杏仁（半升，去皮尖）

右七味，以水一斗，煮取三升，去滓。温服半升，日三服。

【今译】

水饮消除，呕吐停止，患者身体浮肿的，加杏仁主治。这样的证候本来应该加入麻黄，因患者有麻痹之感，所以不宜加入麻黄。如果违反此法而加入了麻黄，就会产生厥冷。之所以如此，是因为患者血虚，麻黄又能发汗，从而导致阳亡。

【英译】

Line 12.39

[After taking Linggan Wuwei Gancao Decoction (苓甘五味甘草汤, poria, schisandra and licorice decoction) added with Ganjiang (干姜, dried ginger, Rhizoma Zingiberis), Xixin (细辛, asarum, Herba Asari) and Banxia (半夏, pinellia, Rhizoma Pinelliae),] water is eliminated and panting is ceased. [If] the body is swollen, Xingren (杏仁, apricot kernel, Semen Armeniacae Amarum) should be added to treat it. Originally Mahuang (麻黄, ephedra, Herba Ephedrae) should be added [to treat such a disease]. Because the patient feels numb, [Mahuang (麻黄, ephedra, Herba Ephedrae)] should not be added. If [it is] added, reversal cold will be inevitable because [there is] blood deficiency in the patient. [Thus when] Mahuang (麻黄, ephedra, Herba Ephedrae) [is added], [collapse of] yang will be caused.

[Therefore it should be treated by] Linggan Wuwei Decoction (苓甘五味汤, poria and licorice decoction) added with Ganjiang (干姜, dried ginger, Rhizoma Zingiberis), Xixin (细辛, asarum, Herba Asari), Banxia (半夏, pinellia, Rhizoma Pinelliae) and Xingren (杏仁, apricot kernel, Semen Armeniacae Amarum).

This formula [Linggan Wuwei Decoction (苓甘五味汤, poria and licorice decoction) added with Ganjiang (干姜, dried ginger, Rhizoma Zingiberis), Xixin (细辛, asarum, Herba Asari), Banxia (半夏, pinellia, Rhizoma Pinelliae) and Xingren (杏仁, apricot kernel, Semen Armeniacae Amarum)is composed of] 4 *liang* of Fuling (茯苓, poria, Poria), 3 *liang* of Gancao (甘草, licorice, Radix Glycyrrhizae Praeparata), 0.5 *sheng* of Wuweizi (五味子, schisandra, Fructus Schisandrae), 3 *liang* of Ganjiang (干姜, dried ginger, Rhizoma Zingiberis), 3 *liang* of Xixin (细辛, asarum, Herba Asari), 0.5 *sheng* of Banxia (半夏, pinellia, Rhizoma Pinelliae) and 0.5 *sheng* of Xingren (杏仁, apricot kernel, Semen Armeniacae Amarum)(remove the bark and tips).

These seven ingredients are decocted in 1 *dou* of water and get 3 *sheng* [after] boiling. The dregs are removed and [the decoction is] taken warm 0.5 *sheng* [each time] and three times a day.

【原文】

(四十)

若面热如醉,此为胃热上冲,熏其面,加大黄以利之。

茯甘五味加姜辛半杏大黄汤方

茯苓(四两)　甘草(三两)　五味子(半升)　干姜(三两)　细辛(三两)　半夏(半升)　杏仁(半升)　大黄(三两)

右八味,以水一斗,煮取三升,去滓。温服半升,日三服。

【今译】

如果患者面部热得如醉状,这是胃热上冲熏蒸面部所致,应加大黄泄除胃热。

【原文】

(四十一)

先渴后呕,为水停心下,此属饮家,小半夏加茯苓汤主之。

【今译】

先口渴而后呕吐,为水停心下的缘故,属于水饮之症,用小半夏加茯苓汤主治。

【英译】

Line 12.40

If ［the patient's］ face is as feverish as being drunken，［it］ indicates heat surging up from the stomach to fumigate the face. ［It can be treated by］ adding Dahuang（大黄，rhubarb，Radix et Rhizoma Rhei）to resolve it.

［It should be treated by］ Fugan Wuwei Decoction（茯甘五味汤，poria，licorice and schisandra decoction）added with Ganjiang（干姜，dried ginger，Rhizoma Zingiberis），Xixin（细辛，asarum，Herba Asari），Banxia（半夏，pinellia，Rhizoma Pinelliae），Xingren（杏仁，apricot kernel，Semen Armeniacae Amarum）and Dahuang（大黄，rhubarb，Radix et Rhizoma Rhei）.

This formula ［is composed of］ 4 *liang* of Fuling（茯苓，poria，Poria），3 *liang* of Gancao（甘草，licorice，Radix Glycyrrhizae Praeparata），0.5 *sheng* of Wuweizi（五味子，schisandra，Fructus Schisandrae），3 *liang* of Ganjiang（干姜，dried ginger，Rhizoma Zingiberis），3 *liang* of Xixin（细辛，asarum，Herba Asari），0.5 *sheng* of Banxia（半夏，pinellia，Rhizoma Pinelliae），0.5 *sheng* of Xingren（杏仁，apricot kernel，Semen Armeniacae Amarum）and 3 *liang* of Dahuang（大黄，rhubarb，Radix et Rhizoma Rhei）.

These eight ingredients are decocted in 1 *dou* of water to get 3 *sheng* ［after］ boiling. The dregs are removed and ［the decoction is］ taken warm 0.5 *sheng* ［each time］ and three times a day.

【英译】

Line 12.41

Thirst followed with panting indicates retention of water below the heart，pertaining to fluid retention disease. Xiao Banxia Decoction added with Fuling（小半夏加茯苓汤，minor pinellia decoction added with poria）［can be used］ to treat it.

消渴小便不利淋病脉证并治第十三

【原文】

(一)

厥阴之为病,消渴,气上冲心,心中疼热,饥而不欲食,食即吐,下之不肯止。

【今译】

厥阴病的症候表现为,消渴,气上冲于心,心中疼痛灼热,饥饿而不想吃饭,吃饭后即呕吐,用下法治疗常导致腹泻不止。

【原文】

(二)

寸口脉浮而迟,浮即为虚,迟即为劳,虚则卫气不足,劳则荣气竭。趺阳脉浮而数,浮即为气,数即为消谷而大坚,气盛则溲数,溲数即坚,坚数相搏,即为消渴。

【今译】

寸口脉既浮又迟,浮脉属虚,迟脉属劳,虚是卫气不足的表现,劳是营气衰竭的表现。趺阳脉既浮又数,脉浮为胃气盛,脉数为消谷而且大便坚硬,气盛又会导致小便频数,小便频数则加剧大便坚硬,大便坚与脉象数相互影响,形成消渴病。

Chapter 13
Wasting-Thirst, Inhibited Urination and Strangury Disease: Pulses, Syndromes/Patterns and Treatment

【英译】

Line 13. 1

Jueyin disease [is characterized by] wasting-thirst, qi surging up to the heart, pain and heat in the heart, hunger without desire to eat and vomiting right after eating. [Application of] purgation [causes] incessant diarrhea.

【英译】

Line 13. 2

[There are cases where] the pulse in cunkou [region] is floating and slow. Floating [pulse] indicates deficiency while slow [pulse] indicates overstrain. Deficiency indicates insufficiency of defense qi while overstrain indicates exhaustion of nutrient qi. [There are cases where] fuyang pulse is floating and rapid. Floating [pulse] indicates [exuberant stomach] qi while rapid [pulse] indicates rapid digestion and hard stool. Exuberant [stomach] qi causes frequent urination and frequent urination causes hard stool. [Mutual] influence of hard [stool] and rapid [pulse] indicates wasting-thirst.

【原文】

(三)

男子消渴,小便反多,以饮一斗,小便一斗,肾气丸主之。

【今译】

男子患了消渴病,小便反而曾多,如果饮水一斗,小便也是一斗,用肾气丸主治。

【原文】

(四)

脉浮,小便不利,微热,消渴者,宜利小便、发汗,五苓散主之。

【今译】

如果患者脉象浮,小便不利,轻微发热,消渴,宜用利小便与发汗法治疗,可用五苓散主治。

【原文】

(五)

渴欲饮水,水入则吐者,名曰水逆,五苓散主之。

【今译】

如果患者口渴想喝水,喝水后就呕吐的,称为水逆,宜用五苓散主治。

Volume 2

【英译】

Line 13.3

[In] a man with wasting-thirst, urination is frequent, [and if he] drinks 1 *dou* of water, he will discharge 1 *dou* of urine. [It can be] treated by Shenqi Pill (肾气丸, kidney qi pill).

【英译】

Line 13.4

[The disease, characterized by] floating pulse, inhibited urination, faint fever and wasting-thirst should [be treated by] promoting urination and sweating. Wuling Powder (五苓散, powder made of five medicinal herbs) [is the appropriate formula for] treating it.

【英译】

Line 13.5

[There are cases where the patient feels] thirsty and wants to drink water. [But after] drinking water, [he begins] to vomit. This is [a case of] water reversal, which [can be] treated by Wuling Powder (五苓散, powder made of five medicinal herbs).

【原文】

（六）

渴欲饮水不止者，文蛤散主之。

文蛤散方

文蛤（五两）

右一味，杵为散，以沸汤五合，和服方寸匕。

【今译】

患者口渴想喝水而口渴不止的，宜用文蛤散主治。

【原文】

（七）

淋之为病，小便如粟状，小腹弦急，痛引脐中。

【今译】

淋病的症候表现为，小便中有如小米一样的硬物，小腹拘急疼痛，牵引脐中。

【英译】

Line 13.6

Thirst that cannot be resolved by drinking water [should be] treated by Wenge Powder（文蛤散，meretrix clam shell powder）.

Wenge Powder （文蛤散，meretrix clam shell powder）[is composed of] 5 *liang* of Wenge（文蛤，meretrix clam shell，Concha Meretricis）.

This ingredient is pounded into powder and boiled into 5 *ge* [of decoction]. [Each time] 1 *fangcunbi* [of the decoction is] taken.

【英译】

Line 13.7

[The manifestations of] strangury [include particles in] urine like millets，spasm of lower abdomen and pain stretching to the umbilicus.

【原文】

(八)

趺阳脉数,胃中有热,即消谷引食,大便必坚,小便即数。

【今译】

趺阳部位脉象数,胃中有邪热,因而大量水谷消耗,饮食不断,大便必然坚硬,小便频数。

【原文】

(九)

淋家不可发汗,发汗则必便血。

【今译】

对于淋病患者,不可以通过发汗治疗,发汗就会引起便血。

Volume 2

【英译】

Line 13.8

［If］ the pulse in fuyang ［region］ is rapid and there is ［pathogenic］ heat in the stomach, causing rapid digestion, constant intake of food, there must be hard stool and frequent urination.

【英译】

Line 13.9

Strangury cannot ［be treated by］ diaphoresis and diaphoresis will cause bloody urine.

【原文】

（十）

小便不利者，有水气，其人若渴，栝蒌瞿麦丸主之。

栝蒌瞿麦丸方

栝蒌根（二两）　茯苓　薯蓣（各三两）　附子（一枚，炮）　瞿麦（一两）

右五味，末之，炼蜜丸梧子大。饮服三丸，日三服，不知，增至七八丸，以小便利，腹中温为知。

【今译】

小便不利是因水气停止所致，患者如果口渴，用栝蒌瞿麦丸主治。

【英译】

Line 13. 10

Inhibited urination [is caused by retention of] water qi. If the patient feels thirsty，Gualou Qumai Pill（栝蒌瞿麦丸，trichosanthes root and dianthus pill）[can be used] to treat it.

Gualou Qumai Pill （栝 蒌 瞿 麦 丸，trichosanthes root and dianthus pill）[is composed of] 2 *liang* of Gualougen（栝蒌根，trichosanthes root，Radix Trichosanthis），3 *liang* of Fuling（茯苓，poria，Poria），3 *liang* of Shuyu （薯 蓣，dioscorea，Rhizoma Dioscoreae），1 piece of Fuzi（附子，aconite，Radix Aconiti Lateralis Preparata）（fry heavily）and 1 *liang* of Qumai（瞿麦，dianthus，Herba Dianthi）.

These five ingredients are pounded into powder and mixed with Lianmi（炼蜜，processed honey，Mel Praeparatum）to produce pills the size of firmiana seeds. 3 pills are taken in water [each time] and three times a day. [If there is] no effect，[the dosage] can increase to seven or eight pills. Promotion of urination and warmth in the abdomen indicate effect.

【原文】

（十一）

小便不利，蒲灰散主之，滑石白鱼散、茯苓戎盐汤并主之。

蒲灰散方

蒲灰（七分）　滑石（三分）

右二味，杵为散，饮服方寸匕，日三服。

滑石白鱼散方

滑石（二分）　乱发（二分，烧）　白鱼（二分）

右三味，杵为散。饮服方寸匕，日三服。

茯苓戎盐汤方

茯苓（半斤）　白术（二两）　戎盐（弹丸大，一枚）

右三味，先将茯苓、白术煎成，入戎盐，再煎，分温三服。

【今译】

小便不利，宜用蒲灰散主治，或用滑石白鱼散、茯苓戎盐汤主治。

Volume 2

【英译】

Line 13. 11

Inhibited urination can be treated by Puhui Powder（蒲灰散，charred dandelion powder），or by Huashi Baiyu Powder（滑石白鱼散，talcum and silverfish powder）and Fuling Rongyan Decoction（茯苓戎盐汤，poria and halite decoction）.

Puhui Powder（蒲灰散，charred dandelion powder）［is composed of］7 *fen* of Puhui（蒲灰，charred dandelion，Herba Taraxaci Carbonisata）and 3 *fen* of Huashi（滑石，talcum，Talcum）.

These two ingredients are pounded into powder. ［The powder is］taken 1 *fangcunbi* ［each time］and three times a day.

Huashi Baiyu Powder （滑石白鱼散，talcum and silverfish powder）［is composed of］2 *fen* of Huashi（滑石，talcum，Talcum），2 *fen* of Luanfa（乱发，human hair，Crinis Carbonisatus）（burn）and 2 *fen* of Baiyu（白鱼，silverfish，Lepisma）.

These three ingredients are pounded into powder. ［The powder is］taken 1 *fangcunbi* ［each time］and three times a day.

Fuling Rongyan Decoction （茯苓戎盐汤，poria and halite decoction）［is composed of］0. 5 *sheng* of Fuling（茯苓，poria，Poria），2 *liang* of Baizhu（白术，rhizome of largehead atractylodes，Rhizoma Atractylodis Macrocephalae）and 1 piece of Rongyan（戎盐，halite，Halitum）（the size of a pillet）.

Among these three ingredients, Fuling（茯苓，poria，Poria）and Baizhu（白术，rhizome of largehead atractylodes，Rhizoma Atractylodis Macrocephalae）are boiled first, then mixed with Rongyan（戎盐，halite，Halitum）and boiled again. ［The decoction is］divided into three ［doses］and taken warm.

【原文】

(十二)

渴欲饮水,口干舌燥者,白虎加人参汤主之。

【今译】

患者口渴想喝水,口干舌燥,用白虎加人参汤主治。

【原文】

(十三)

脉浮发热,渴欲饮水,小便不利者,猪苓汤主之。

猪苓汤方

猪苓(去皮)　茯苓　阿胶　滑石　泽泻(各一两)

右五味,以水四升,先煮四味,取二升,去滓,内胶烊消。温服七合,日三服。

【今译】

脉象浮而发热,口渴想喝水,小便不利的,用猪苓汤主治。

【英译】

Line 13. 12

[The disease with] thirst, desire to drink water, dryness of the mouth and tongue can be treated by Baihu Decoction (白虎汤, white tiger decoction) added with Renshen (人参, ginseng, Radix Ginseng).

【英译】

Line 13. 13

[The disease marked by] floating pulse, fever, thirst with desire to drink water and inhibited urination can be treated by Zhuling Decoction (猪苓汤, polyporus decoction).

Zhuling Decoction (猪苓汤, polyporus decoction) [is composed of] 1 *liang* of Zhuling (猪苓, polyporus, Polyporus Umbellatus) (remove the bark), 1 *liang* of Fuling (茯苓, poria, Poria), 1 *liang* of Ejiao (阿胶, ass-hide glue, Colla Corii Asini), 1 *liang* of Huashi (滑石, talcum, Talcum) and 1 *liang* of Zexie (泽泻, alisma, Rhizoma Alismatis).

These five ingredients are decocted in 4 *sheng* of water. Four ingredients are boiled first to get 2 *sheng*. The dregs are removed and Ejiao (阿胶, ass-hide glue, Colla Corii Asini) is put into [it] to melt. [The decoction is] taken warm 7 *ge* [each time] and three times a day.

水气病脉证并治第十四

【原文】

（一）

师曰：病有风水，有皮水，有正水，有石水，有黄汗。风水，其脉自浮，外证骨节疼痛，恶风；皮水，其脉亦浮，外证胕肿，按之没指，不恶风，其腹如鼓，不渴，当发其汗；正水，其脉沉迟，外证自喘；石水，其脉自沉，外证腹满不喘；黄汗，其脉沉迟，身发热，胸满，四肢头面肿，久不愈，必致痈脓。

【今译】

老师说：水气病有风水、皮水、正水、石水、黄汗等多种。风水病，脉象自浮，外表证有骨节疼痛、恶风等症状；皮水病，脉象也浮，外表证为皮肤浮肿，按之凹陷不起，不恶风，腹胀如鼓，口不渴，应当用发汗的方法治疗；正水病，脉象沉迟，外表证为气喘；石水病，脉象自沉，外表证为腹部胀满，但无气喘；黄汗病，脉象沉迟，身体发热，胸部胀满，四肢、头部和面部浮肿，久治不愈，必然导致痈疮脓肿的发生。

Volume 2

Chapter 14
Water Qi Disease:
Pulses, Syndromes/Patterns and Treatment

【英译】

Line 14. 1

The master said: [Water qi (edema)] diseases include wind water, skin water, regular water, stone water and yellow sweating. [In] wind water [disease], the pulse is spontaneously floating and the external syndrome/pattern [is marked by] pain of joints and aversion to wind; [in] skin water [disease], the pulse is also floating and the external syndrome/pattern [is marked by] skin swelling that engulfs the fingers [when] pressed, aversion to wind, abdominal distension like a drum and no thirst, [which] should [be treated by] inducing sweating; [in] regular water [disease], the pulse is sunken and slow and the external syndrome/pattern is spontaneous panting; [in] stone water [disease], the pulse is spontaneously sunken and the external syndrome [is marked by] abdominal fullness and no panting; [in] yellow sweating [disease], the pulse is sunken and slow, [there are symptoms and signs of] fever over the body, chest fullness, dropsy of the four limbs, head and face, inability to cure after a long time, inevitably resulting in abscess and suppuration.

【原文】

（二）

脉浮而洪，浮则为风，洪则为气，风气相搏。风强则为隐疹，身体为痒，痒为泄风，久为痂癞；气强则为水，难以俯仰。风气相击，身体洪肿，汗出乃愈。恶风则虚，此为风水；不恶风者，小便通利，上焦有寒，其口多涎，此为黄汗。

【今译】

患者脉象浮而洪，脉浮是外感风邪，脉洪为水气涌盛，风邪与水气相搏。风邪盛则引发隐疹，使患者身体瘙痒，痒为排泄风邪的象征，因而称为泄风，若长期不愈，则会变化为痂癞；水气盛则为水气病，患者身体浮肿，难以俯仰。风邪与水气相击，使患者身体严重浮肿，通过发汗法可将其治愈。恶风为阳虚的表现，为风水病；不恶风的，小便通利，这是上焦有寒的表现，患者口中多涎，这是黄汗病的表现。

【英译】

Line 14.2

[There are cases where] the pulse [of the patient] is floating and surging. Floating [pulse] indicates [pathogenic] wind and surging [pulse] indicates [exuberant water] qi. [Pathogenic] wind and [exuberant water] qi coexist. [If pathogenic] wind is strong, [it will cause] urticaria and [make] the body itch [which] indicates discharge of wind. [If it is not resolved] for a long time, [it will cause] leprosy or scab. [If water] qi is strong, [it] indicates [exuberant] water, [making the body] difficult to raise and bend. [When pathogenic] wind and [exuberant water] qi contend with each other, [it will cause] severe generalized swelling [which can be] cured by diaphoresis. Aversion to cold indicates deficiency [of yang qi], [Which is] wind water [disease]. No aversion to wind, normal urination, cold in the upper energizer and copious drool from the mouth [are the manifestations of] yellow sweating [disease].

【原文】

（三）

寸口脉沉滑者,中有水气,面目肿大,有热,名曰风水。视人之目窠上微拥,如蚕新卧起状,其颈脉动,时时咳,按其手足上,陷而不起者,风水。

【今译】

寸口脉象沉滑的患者,体内有水气,面目肿大,身体有热,这种病称为风水。诊断时可看到患者眼胞微肿,就像刚刚起床一样,颈脉搏动,时时咳嗽,按压其手足,皮肤凹陷而不起,这都是风水病的表现。

Volume 2

【英译】

Line 14.3

[The disease, marked by] sunken and slippery pulse, [retention of] water qi inside and fever, is called wind water [disease]. [In diagnosis, one can] observe slight swelling of eyelids like just getting up from the bed, beating of cervical pulse, frequent cough and depression of hands and feet that cannot spring back when pressed, [which are the manifestations of] wind water [disease].

【原文】

(四)

太阳病,脉浮而紧,法当骨节疼痛,反不疼,身体反重而酸,其人不渴,汗出即愈,此为风水。恶寒者,此为极虚,发汗得之。渴而不恶寒者,此为皮水。身肿而冷,状如周痹,胸中窒,不能食,反聚痛,暮躁不得眠,此为黄汗,痛在骨节。咳而喘,不渴者,此为脾胀,其状如肿,发汗即愈。然诸病此者,渴而下利,小便数者,皆不可发汗。

【今译】

太阳病,脉象浮而紧,应当也有骨节疼痛,如今反而不疼,身体反而沉重而酸楚,患者口不渴,使其出汗就能痊愈,这也是风水病。如果患者出汗后恶寒的,这是因为阳气虚弱而发汗所致。如果患者口渴但却不恶寒的,这是皮水病。如果患者身体肿胀而发冷,其症状为周痹,胸中窒塞,不能饮食,疼痛反而集中,傍晚时烦躁而不得眠,这是黄汗病,疼痛集中在骨节部位。如果患者咳嗽而喘,不口渴的,这是脾胀病,其症状为浮肿,可通过发汗法治愈。然而在各种水气病中,如果患者口渴而又腹泻,小便频数,都不可通过发汗治愈。

【英译】

Line 14.4

[In] taiyang disease, the pulse is floating and tight. Originally there is pain of joints, but now there is no pain [of joints], the body is heavy and aching, the patient is not thirsty and [it can be] cured by diaphoresis. This is called wind water [disease]. Aversion to cold indicates deficiency due to sweating. [If there is] thirst but no aversion to cold, this is skin water [disease]. [The case, marked by] swelling and cold of the body like generalized impediment, congestion of the chest, inability to eat, focused pain, vexation and inability to sleep at night, is yellow sweating [disease], and the focused pain is in the joints. [The case marked by] cough, panting and no thirst is spleen distension [disease] with the symptom of dropsy. [It can be] cured by diaphoresis. [In] different [water qi] diseases, [if there are] thirst, diarrhea and frequent urination, no diaphoresis should be used for treatment.

【原文】

（五）

里水者，一身面目黄肿，其脉沉，小便不利，故令病水。假如小便自利，此亡津液，故令渴也。越婢加术汤主之。

【今译】

患皮水病的人，全身及面目黄肿，脉象也沉，小便不利，所以使其患有皮水病。假如患者小便通利，这就是津液的亡失，就会导致津液耗竭，使患者口渴。用越婢加术汤主治。

【原文】

（六）

跌阳脉当伏，今反紧，本自有寒，疝瘕腹中痛，医反下之，下之即胸满短气。

【今译】

跌阳部位的脉象应当是沉伏的，如今反而是紧的，这是素有寒邪所致，使病人患有疝瘕腹痛等症，医生反而用攻下法治之，使患者产生胸满短气的证变。

Volume 2

【英译】

Line 14.5

Internal water (skin water disease) [is characterized by] yellow swelling of the whole body, face and eyes, sunken pulse and inhibited urination, and therefore [resulting in skin] water disease. If urination is normal, it is the loss of fluid and humor, that is why [the patient is] thirsty. [It can be] treated by Yuebi Decoction (越婢汤, decoction for effusing the spleen) added with Baizhu (白术, rhizoma of largehead atractylodes, Rhizoma Atractylodis Macrocephalate).

【英译】

Line 14.6

The pulse in the fuyang [region] should be hidden, but now it is tight due to original [retention of] cold [that causes] hernia, mass and pain in the abdomen. [If] a doctor [treats it with] purgation, chest fullness and shortness of breath [will be caused].

【原文】

（七）

跗阳脉当伏，今反数，本自有热，消谷，小便数，今反不利，此欲作水。

【今译】

跗阳部位脉象应当沉伏，如今反而为数，这是患者素有积热的原因，患者常有消谷善饥、小便频数的症状，如今反而小便不利，就会因此而形成水气病。

【原文】

（八）

寸口脉浮而迟，浮脉则热，迟脉则潜，热潜相搏，名目沉。跗阳脉浮而数，浮脉即热，数脉即止，热止相搏，名曰伏。沉伏相搏，名曰水。沉则脉络虚，伏则小便难，虚难相搏，水走皮肤，即为水矣。

【今译】

寸口部的脉象浮而迟，浮脉为热邪浮行于外，迟脉为热邪潜藏于内，浮行于外的热邪与潜藏于内的热邪相搏，称为沉。跗阳部的脉象浮而数，浮脉为胃气热盛，数脉为小便止而不利，热盛的胃气与止而不利的小便相搏，称为伏。沉潜的热邪与留伏的水邪相搏，称为水。热邪的沉潜使得脉络亏虚，留伏的水邪使得小便困难，脉络亏虚与小便困难相搏，水热之邪泛滥于皮肤，因而形成水气病。

Volume 2

【英译】

Line 14.7

The pulse in fuyang [region] should be hidden, but now it is rapid due to original [accumulation of] heat. [That is why there is usually] rapid digestion and frequent urination [in patients], but now [there is] diarrhea, indicating that water [qi disease] will occur.

【英译】

Line 14.8

[There are cases where] the pulse in cunkou [region] is floating and slow. Floating pulse indicates heat [floating in the external] and slow pulse indicates submersion [of pathogenic heat in the internal]. [When] heat [floating in the external] and submersion [of pathogenic heat in the internal] contend with each other, it is called sinking. [There are cases where] the pulse in fuyang [region] is floating and rapid. Floating pulse indicates [exuberant] heat [in stomach qi] and rapid pulse indicates inhibition [of urination]. [When exuberant] heat [in stomach qi] and inhibition [of urination] contend with each other, it is called hiding. [When] sinking and hiding contend with each other, it is called water. Sinking means deficiency of the meridians and collaterals and hiding means difficulty in urination. [When] deficiency [of meridians and collaterals] and difficulty [in urination] contend with each other, water will run into the skin, causing water [qi disease].

【原文】

(九)

寸口脉弦而紧,弦则卫气不行,即恶寒,水不沾流,走于肠间。

少阴脉紧而沉,紧则为痛,沉则为水,小便即难。

【今译】

寸口部脉弦而紧,脉弦是卫气不行的表现,患者因此恶寒,因水液不能排流,流注于肠道之间。

如果少阴部位的脉紧而沉,脉紧是疼痛的表现,脉沉表明有水气,导致小便困难。

【原文】

(十)

脉得诸沉,当责有水,身体肿重。水病脉出者死。

【今译】

如果患者脉象沉,是水气滞留的表现,使患者身体浮肿沉重。水气病患者的脉象由沉伏而暴出,导致患者死亡。

【英译】

Line 14.9

[There are cases where] the pulse in cunkou [region] is taut and tight. Taut [pulse] indicates failure of defense qi to move, and therefore causing aversion to cold, difficulty in discharging water and water flowing into the intestines.

[There are cases where] the pulse in shaoyin [region] is tight and sunken. Tight [pulse] indicates pain and sunken [pulse] indicates water, resulting in difficulty in urination.

【英译】

Line 14.10

Sunken pulse indicates retention of water [that causes] swelling and heaviness of the body. The pulse [of the patient with] water [qi] disease [is originally sunken, but now it suddenly] bursts out, [inevitably resulting in] death.

【原文】

（十一）

夫水病人，目下有卧蚕，面目鲜泽，脉伏，其人消渴。病水腹大，小便不利，其脉沉绝者，有水，可下之。

【今译】

患水气病的人，下眼胞浮肿，好像有蚕卧于其下，面部和眼胞因浮肿而光亮润泽，脉象沉伏，患者有消渴症候。如果因水气病而腹部肿大，小便不利，脉象沉绝，说明有水积蓄，可用攻下法治疗。

【原文】

（十二）

问曰：病下利后，渴饮水，小便不利，腹满因肿者，何也？答曰：此法当病水，若小便自利及汗出者，自当愈。

【今译】

问：患腹泻之后，患者口渴饮水，小便不利，腹部胀满，阴部也出现水肿。这是什么原因呢？

答：这种情况应当形成水气病，如果小便自利且能出汗的，应当能自愈。

【英译】

Line 14. 11

[In] the patient with water [qi] disease, the lower eyelids are swollen like silkworm lying behind, the face and eyes are bright and fresh [because of dropsy], the pulse is hidden and there is wasting-thirst. In water [qi] disease, [if] the abdomen is swollen seriously, urination is inhibited, the pulse is sunken and expiring, [indicating accumulation of] water [which] can [be treated by] purgation.

【英译】

Line 14. 12

Question: [There are cases where] after diarrhea, [there are symptoms and signs of] thirst, desire to drink water, inhibited urination, abdominal fullness and genital swelling. What is the reason?

Answer: Such pathological conditions will develop into water [qi] disease. If urination is normalized and sweating is induced, [it will] heal spontaneously.

【原文】

(十三)

心水者,其身重而少气,不得卧,烦而躁,其人阴肿。

【今译】

心脏病而导致水肿的,患者身体沉重,呼吸短促,无法平卧,烦躁不安,患者的前阴部也会有水肿。

【原文】

(十四)

肝水者,其腹大,不能自转侧,胁下腹痛,时时津液微生,小便续通。

【今译】

患肝水的病人,腹部肿胀,不能自行转侧,胁下和腹部疼痛,口中津液时时微生,小便也时通而时不通。

【原文】

(十五)

肺水者,其身肿,小便难,时时鸭溏。

【今译】

患肺水的病人,身体肿胀,小便困难,时时大便糖稀如鸭溏。

【英译】

Line 14. 13

[In] heart water (edema) [due to heart disease], [there are symptoms and signs of] heaviness of the body, shortness of breath, inability to lie down, vexation and swelling of the genitals.

【英译】

Line 14. 14

[The manifestations of] liver water [include] enlarged abdomen, inability to turn sides [of the body] freely, abdominal pain below the rib-side, frequent slight fluid [in the mouth] and intermittently inhibited and disinhibited urination.

【英译】

Line 14. 15

[The manifestations of] lung water [include] generalized swelling, difficulty in urination and intermittent sloppy stool.

【原文】

（十六）

脾水者，其腹大，四肢苦重，津液不生，但苦少气，小便难。

【今译】

患脾水的病人，腹部重大，四肢沉重，津液不生，但却时常少气，小便困难。

【原文】

（十七）

肾水者，其腹大，脐肿腰痛，不得溺，阴下湿如牛鼻上汗，其足逆冷，面反瘦。

【今译】

患肾水的病人，腹部肿大，脐部肿胀，腰部疼痛，不得小便，会阴部潮湿得像牛鼻上出汗一样，足部逆冷，面部反而消瘦。

【原文】

（十八）

师曰：诸有水者，腰以下肿，当利小便；腰以上肿，当发汗乃愈。

【今译】

老师说：凡是水肿病，腰以下浮肿，应当以利小便为主治疗；腰以上浮肿的，应当通过发汗治愈。

Volume 2

【英译】

Line 14. 16

[The manifestations of] spleen water [include] enlarged abdomen, heaviness of the four limbs, failure to engender fluid and humor, severe shortness of breath and difficulty in urination.

【英译】

Line 14. 17

[The manifestations of] kidney water [include] enlarged abdomen, swelling of the umbilicus, pain of the waist, inability to urinate, dampness in the genitals as sweat over the nose of an ox, reversal cold of feet and emaciation of the face.

【英译】

Line 14. 18

The master said: [In] all [cases of] water [disease], [there is] swelling below the waist [and it] should [be treated by] promoting urination. [If there is] swelling above the waist, [it] should be cured by diaphoresis.

【原文】

(十九)

师曰：寸口脉沉而迟，沉则为水，迟则为寒，寒水相搏。趺阳脉伏，水谷不化，脾气衰则鹜溏，胃气衰则身肿。少阳脉卑，少阴脉细，男子则小便不利，妇人则经水不通。经为血，血不利则为水，名曰血分。

【今译】

老师说：寸口部脉象沉而迟，沉脉主水，迟脉主寒，寒水相搏。趺阳部的脉象伏，表示脾胃阳气不足，无法消化水谷，由于脾气衰使得大便糖稀如鸭溏，由于胃气衰使得身体浮肿。少阳部的脉象沉弱，少阴部的脉象细小，男子则小便不利，女人则经水不通。月经来自于血，血不利则化而为水，称为血分水气病。

【原文】

(二十)

问曰：病有血分水分，何也？

师曰：经水前断，后病水，名曰血分，此病难治；先病水，后经水断，名曰水分，此病易治。何以故？去水，其经自下。

【今译】

问：妇女水肿病有血分和水分的区分，是什么原因呢？

老师说：如果患者月经先停，后患水肿，称为血分，这种病难治。如果患者先患水肿，其后月经停止，称为水分，这种病易治。为什么是这样的呢？因为祛除了水，月经就自然而下。

Volume 2

【英译】

Line 14. 19

The master said: [There are cases where] the pulse in cunkou [region] is sunken and slow. Sunken [pulse] indicates water while slow [pulse] indicates cold, cold and water contend with each other. [If] the pulse in fuyang [region] is hidden, it indicates indigestion [due to insufficiency of yang qi in the spleen and stomach]. Debilitation of spleen qi results in sloppy stool while debilitation of stomach qi results in generalized swelling. [If] Shaoyang pulse is sunken and weak while shaoyin pulse is thin and small, it indicates inhibited urination in men and dysmenorrhea in women. Menstruation originates from the blood. [If] the blood does not circulate freely, [it will] transform into water, known as [water qi blood in] the blood aspect.

【英译】

Line 14. 20

Question: Diseases [in women are either related to] blood aspect [or] water aspect. What is the reason?

The master said: [If] menstruation stops first and then water [disease] occurs, it is called blood aspect [disease], [which is] very difficult to cure. [If] water disease occurs first and then menstruation stops, it is called water aspect [disease], [which is] easy to cure. Why is it so? [Because when] water is eliminated, menstruation will descend spontaneously.

【原文】

（二十一）

问曰：病者苦水，面目身体四肢皆肿，小便不利，脉之，不言水，反言胸中痛，气上冲咽，状如炙肉，当微咳喘。审如师言，其脉何类？

师曰：寸口沉而紧，沉为水，紧为寒，沉紧相搏，结在关元，始时尚微，年盛不觉。阳衰之后，营卫相干，阳损阴盛，结寒微动，肾气上冲，喉咽塞噎，胁下急痛。医以为留饮而大下之，气击不去，其病不除。后重吐之，胃家虚烦，咽燥欲饮水，小便不利，水谷不化，面目手足浮肿。又以葶苈丸下水，当时如小差，食饮过度，肿复如前，胸胁苦痛，象若奔豚，其水扬溢，则浮咳喘逆。当先平降冲气令止，乃治咳，咳止，其喘自差。先治新病，病当在后。

【今译】

问：患水气病的患者，面目身体四肢都浮肿，小便不利，但为患者切脉诊断的时候，老师却不谈水，反而说患者胸中痛，气上冲咽喉，好像有灼热的肉块堵塞一样，而且还应有微微咳喘。如果病情的确像老师说的那样，那么其脉象又是哪一类呢？

老师说：患者寸口脉沉而紧，沉为有水，紧为有寒，沉紧相搏，常结聚在下焦的关元之处，汗水开始凝聚时，患者年壮气盛，感觉不大。但年龄增大，阳气衰微之后，营气和卫气不和，阳气就会日衰，阴气就会渐盛，聚结肚脐之下的寒水开始微动，肾气上冲，使得患者咽喉阻塞不通，胁下急痛。医生以为留饮胁痛而用峻下之法治疗，如此治疗不仅使气

Volume 2

【英译】

Line 14.21

Question: [When] the patient suffers from water [qi disease], [there are symptoms and signs of] swelling of face, eyes, body and four limbs as well as inhibited urination. [But when diagnosing the patient by taking] pulse, [the master] did not talk about water, just mentioned chest pain, qi surging up into the throat like fried muscles [stagnated in the throat] and slight cough and panting. [If it is just as what the master] mentioned in diagnosis, what category of pulse is it?

The master said: [There are cases where] the pulse in the cunkou [region] is sunken and tight. Sunken [pulse] indicates water and tight [pulse] indicates cold. [When] the sunken [pulse] and tight [pulse] coexist, [they often] bind in Guanyuan (CV 4). Initially [it] is mild and [the patient] does not feel [it because he is] strong. [When] yang [qi] is weakened, nutrient [qi] and defense [qi] interfere with each other, [leading to] decline of yang [qi] and exuberance of yin [qi], making binding cold [below the umbilicus begin] to activate and kidney qi [begin] to surge up, [causing] blockage of the throat and acute pain below the rib-side. [When] feeling [that it is caused by] retention of fluid, the doctor [uses] purgation [to deal with it]. [As a result,] qi [continues] to surge up and will not cease, and the disease is difficult to cure. Afterwards [the doctor uses the therapy for] greatly [inducing] vomiting, [resulting in] deficiency of stomach [qi], vexation, dryness of the throat, desire to drink water, inhibited urination, indigestion of food and swelling of face, eyes, hands and feet. [The

上冲而不降,病也无法根治。其后又重用吐法治疗咽喉梗塞,使得胃气虚弱,烦闷不堪,患者咽喉干燥想饮水,小便不利,水谷不化,面目手足出现浮肿。医生又用葶苈丸攻下水,当时好像浮肿有所缓解,但由于食饮过度,水肿又复发得像以前一样,胸胁部剧烈疼痛,其病情就像奔豚一样。由于水气向上扬溢,所以出现浮肿、咳嗽、气喘和上逆。此时应当先平降冲气,使其停止,再治疗咳嗽,咳嗽停止后,喘息就会自愈。应当先治新病,新病治好后再治水气病。

doctor then] uses Tingli Pill (葶苈丸, lepidium/descurainiae pill) to purge water, seeming to have alleviated [the disease]. [Because of] overtaking of food, [the patient suffers from] swelling as serious as before, pain in the chest and rib-side, pathological condition similar to running piglet and spreading of water, causing dropsy, cough, panting and reversal [counterflow of qi]. [It] should [be treated] by attacking surging qi to cease it. [Then measures should be taken] to treat cough. [When] cough is ceased, panting will stop spontaneously. [In dealing with such a disease, the treatment should] first focus on the new disease and then on the old disease.

【原文】

(二十二)

风水,脉浮身重,汗出恶风者,防己黄芪汤主之。腹痛加芍药。

防己黄芪汤方

防己(一两) 黄芪(一两一分) 白术(三分) 甘草(半两,炙)

右剉,每服五钱匕,生姜四片,枣一枚,水盏半,煎取八分,去滓。温服,良久再服。

【今译】

风水病,脉象浮,身体重,汗出而恶风,宜用防己黄芪汤主治。若有腹痛,可加芍药。

【原文】

(二十三)

风水恶风,一身悉肿,脉浮不渴,续自汗出,无大热,越婢汤主之。

越婢汤方

麻黄(六两) 石膏(半斤) 生姜(三两) 大枣(十五枚) 甘草(二两)

右五味,以水六升,先煮麻黄,去上沫,内诸药,煮取三升,分温三服。恶风者,加附子一枚,炮;风水加术四两。

【今译】

风水病,有恶风、全身浮肿、脉象浮、口不渴、断断续续出汗、无高热的症状,用越婢汤主治。

【英译】

Line 14.22

Wind water [disease, marked by] floating pulse, heaviness of the body, sweating and aversion to wind, [can be] treated by Fangji Huangqi Decoction (防己黄芪汤, the root of stephania tetrandra and astragalus decoction). For abdominal pain, Shaoyao (芍药, peony, Radix Paeoniae) is added.

Fangji Huangqi Decoction (防己黄芪汤, the root of stephania tetrandra and astragalus decoction) [is composed of] 1 *liang* of Fangji (防己, the root of stephania tetrandra, Radix Stephaniae Tetrandrae), 1 *liang* and 1 *fen* of Huangqi (黄芪, astragalus, Radix Astragali), 3 *fen* of Baizhu (白术, rhizome of largehead atractylodes, Rhizoma Atractylodis Macrocephalae) and 0.5 *liang* of Gancao (甘草, licorice, Radix Glycyrrhizae Praeparata) (broil).

These ingredients are grated, 5 *qianbi* for each, 4 pieces of Shengjiang (生姜, fresh ginger, Rhizoma Zingiberis Recens) and 1 piece of Dazao (大枣, jujube, Fructus Ziziphus Jujubae) are decocted in half a cup of water to get 8 *fen* [after] boiling. The dregs are removed and [the decoction is] taken warm and taken again after a longer period of time.

【英译】

Line 14.23

Wind water [disease, marked by] aversion to wind, generalized swelling, floating pulse, thirst, incessant sweating and no great fever, [can be] treated by Yuebi Decoction (越婢汤, decoction for effusing the spleen).

Yuebi Decoction (越婢汤, decoction for effusing the spleen) [is composed of] 6 *liang* of Mahuang (麻黄, ephedra, Herba Ephedrae), 0.5 *jin* of Shigao (石膏, gypsum, Gypsum Fibrosum), 3 *liang* of Shengjiang (生姜, fresh ginger, Rhizoma Zingiberis Recens), 15 pieces of Dazao (大枣, jujube, Fructus Ziziphus Jujubae) and 2 *liang* of Gancao (甘草, licorice, Radix Glycyrrhizae Praeparata).

These five ingredients are decocted in 6 *sheng* of water. Mahuang (麻黄, ephedra, Herba Ephedrae) is boiled first. [After] removal of the dregs, the other ingredients are put into [it] to boil and get 3 *sheng*. [The decoction is] divided into three [doses] and taken warm. For aversion to cold, 1 piece of Fuzi (附子, aconite, Radix Aconiti Lateralis Preparata) (fry heavily) is added. For wind water [disease], 4 *liang* of Baizhu (白术, rhizome of largehead atractylodes, Rhizoma Atractylodis Macrocephalae) is added.

【原文】

(二十四)

皮水为病,四肢肿,水气在皮肤中,四肢聂聂动者,防己茯苓汤主之。

防己茯苓汤方

防己(三两) 黄芪(三两) 桂枝(三两) 茯苓(六两) 甘草(二两)

右五味,以水六升,煮取二升,分温三服。

【今译】

皮水病,四肢肿胀,水气滞留在皮肤中,四肢轻微跳动,用防己茯苓汤主治。

【原文】

(二十五)

里水,越婢加术汤主之,甘草麻黄汤亦主之。

越婢加术汤方

甘草麻黄汤方

甘草(二两) 麻黄(四两)

右二味,以水五升,先煮麻黄,去上沫,内甘草,煮取三升。温服一升,重复汗出,不汗,再服,慎风寒。

【今译】

里水病,宜用越婢加术汤主治,也可用甘草麻黄汤主治。

Volume 2

【英译】

Line 14.24

Skin water disease, [marked by] swelling of the four limbs, [retention of] water qi in the skin and quivering of the four limbs, [can be] treated by Fangji Fuling Decoction (防己茯苓汤, the root of stephania tetrandra and poria decoction).

Fangji Fuling Decoction (防己茯苓汤, the root of stephania tetrandra and poria decoction) [is composed of] 3 *liang* of Fangji (防己, the root of stephania tetrandra, Radix Stephaniae Tetrandrae), 3 *liang* of Huangqi (黄芪, astragalus, Radix Astragali), 3 *liang* of Guizhi (桂枝, cinnamon twig, Ramulus Cinnamomi), 6 *liang* of Fuling (茯苓, poria, Poria) and 2 *liang* of Gancao (甘草, licorice, Radix Glycyrrhizae Praeparata).

These five ingredients are decocted in 6 *sheng* of water to get 2 *sheng* [after] boiling. [The decoction is] divided into three [doses] and taken warm.

【英译】

Line 14.25

Internal water [disease can be] treated by Yuebi Decoction (越婢汤, decoction for effusing the spleen) added with Baizhu (白术, rhizome of largehead atractylodes, Rhizoma Atractylodis Macrocephalae). [It can] also [be] treated by Gancao Mahuang Decoction (甘草麻黄汤, licorice and ephedra deciction).

Gancao Mahuang Decoction (甘草麻黄汤, licorice and ephedra decoction) [is composed of] 2 *liang* of Gancao (甘草, licorice, Radix Glycyrrhizae Praeparata) and 4 *liang* of Mahuang (麻黄, ephedra, Herba Ephedrae).

These two ingredients are decocted in 5 *sheng* of water. Mahuang (麻黄, ephedra, Herba Ephedrae) is boiled first. [After] removal of the foam, Gancao (甘草, licorice, Radix Glycyrrhizae Praeparata) is put into [it] to boil and get 3 *sheng*. [The decoction is] taken warm 1 *sheng* [each time] to induce sweating. [If there is] no sweating, one more [dose should be] taken. Cares [should be taken to avoid attack of] wind and cold.

【原文】

(二十六)

水之为病,其脉沉小,属少阴;浮者为风;无水,虚胀者,为气。水,发其汗即已。脉沉者,宜麻黄附子汤;浮者,宜杏子汤。

麻黄附子汤方

麻黄(三两) 甘草(二两) 附子(一枚,炮)

右三味,以水七升,先煮麻黄,去上沫,内诸药,煮取二升半。温服八分,日三服。

杏子汤方

【今译】

水气病,脉象沉小,属少阴证;脉象浮的,为风水证;没有水肿,但有虚胀的,为气虚证。有水肿证的,通过发汗即可治愈。脉象沉的,宜用麻黄附子汤主治;脉象浮的,宜用杏子汤主治。

【原文】

(二十七)

厥而皮水者,蒲灰散主之。方见消渴中。

【今译】

皮水病出现手足厥冷的,可用蒲灰散主治。

【英译】

Line 14.26

[In] water disease, [if] the pulse is sunken and small, [it] belongs to shaoyin [syndrome/pattern]; [if the pulse is] floating, [it] indicates wind [syndrome/pattern]; [if there is] no water [disease], [it indicates] deficiency and distension due to qi [deficiency]. Water [disease can be] cured by diaphoresis. For sunken pulse, Mahuang Fuzi Decoction (麻黄附子汤, ephedra and aconite decoction) is the appropriate [formula for treating it]. For floating [pulse], Xingzi Decoction (杏子汤, apricot kernel decoction) is the appropriate [formula for treating it].

Mahuang Fuzi Decoction (麻黄附子汤, ephedra and aconite decoction): Already described above.

Mahuang Fuzi Decoction (麻黄附子汤, ephedra and aconite decoction) [is composed of] 3 *liang* of Mahuang (麻黄, ephedra, Herba Ephedrae), 2 *liang* of Gancao (甘草, licorice, Radix Glycyrrhizae Praeparata) and 1 piece of Fuzi (附子, aconite, Radix Aconiti Lateralis Preparata)(fry heavily).

These three ingredients are decocted in 7 *sheng* of water. Mahuang (麻黄, ephedra, Herba Ephedrae) is boiled first. [After] removal of the foam, the other ingredients are put into [it] to boil and get 2.5 *sheng*. [The decoction is] taken warm 8 *fen* [each time] and three times a day.

Xingzi Decoction (杏子汤, apricot kernel decoction)[: This decoction is already described above].

【英译】

Line 14.27

For impediment with skin water [disease], Puhui Powder (蒲灰散, charred dandelion powder) [can be used] to treat it.

Puhui Powder (蒲灰散, charred dandelion powder) is already described in wasting-thirst [disease].

【原文】

（二十八）

问曰：黄汗之为病，身体肿，发热汗出而渴，状如风水，汗沾衣，色正黄如柏汁，脉自沉，何从得之？师曰：以汗出入水中浴，水从汗孔入得之，宜芪芍桂酒汤主之。

黄芪芍药桂枝苦酒汤方

黄芪（五两）　芍药（三两）　桂枝（三两）

右三味，以苦酒一升，水七升，相和，煮取三升。温服一升，当心烦，服至六七日乃解。若心烦不止者，以苦酒阻故也。

【今译】

问：黄汗发病，身体浮肿，发热，出汗，口渴，病状像风水一样，汗液沾湿内衣，颜色显得正黄，就像柏汁一样，脉象自沉，这种病是怎么得的呢？

老师说：这是因为刚出汗就下水洗澡，使得水从汗孔进入肌肤，因而得黄汗病，宜用芪芍桂酒汤主治。

Volume 2

【英译】

Line 14.28

Question：Yellow sweating disease ［is characterized by］ generalized swelling, fever, sweating and thirst, ［the manifestations of which］ look like ［those of］ wind water ［disease］. ［In the patient,］ the clothes are wet ［because of sweating］, the color is just as yellow as the leaves of pine tree and the pulse is spontaneously sunken. What is the cause?

The master said：［This is due to the fact that the patient］ jumps into water for bathing ［when］ there is still sweating. ［As a result,］ water enters the body from the sweat pores. Huangqi Shaoyao Guizhi Kujiu Decoction（黄芪芍药桂枝苦酒汤, astragalus, peony, cinnamon twig and rice vinegar decoction） is the appropriate ［formula for］ treating it.

Huangqi Shaoyao Guizhi Kujiu Decoction（黄芪芍药桂枝苦酒汤, astragalus, peony, cinnamon twig and rice vinegar decoction） ［is composed of］ 5 *liang* of Huangqi（黄芪, astragalus, Radix Astragali）, 3 *liang* of Shaoyao（芍药, peony, Radix Paeoniae） and 3 *liang* of Guizhi（桂枝, cinnamon twig, Ramulus Cinnamomi）.

These three ingredients are decocted in 1 *sheng* of rice vinegar and 7 *sheng* of water to get 3 *sheng* ［after］ boiling. ［The decoction is］ taken warm 1 *sheng* ［each time］. ［If there is］ vexation, ［it will be］ resolved after taking ［the decoction］ for six or seven days. If vexation is incessant, it is due to blockage of rice vinegar.

【原文】

（二十九）

黄汗之病，两胫自冷。假令发热，此属历节。食已汗出，又身常暮盗汗出者，此劳气也。若汗出已，反发热者，久久其身必甲错；发热不止者，必生恶疮。

若身重，汗出已辄轻者，久久必身瞤。瞤即胸中痛，又从腰以上必汗出，下无汗，腰髋弛痛，如有物在皮中状，剧者不能食，身疼重，烦躁，小便不利，此为黄汗。桂枝加黄芪汤主之。

桂枝加黄芪汤方

桂枝、芍药（各三两）　甘草（二两）　生姜（三两）　大枣（十二枚）黄芪（二两）

右六味，以水八升，煮取三升。温服一升，须臾饮热稀粥一升余，以助药力，温服取微汗；若不汗，更取。

【今译】

黄汗之病，两小腿常感寒冷。假如发热，这就属于历节病。饭后汗出，或夜晚入睡身体有盗汗出，这就属于虚劳病。如果汗出后反而发热的，时间一长肌肤就会干燥生屑；发热不止的，必然生恶疮。

如果患者身体沉重，汗出后就会有所缓解。但时间一长患者肌肉就会颤动。肌肉颤动就会引起胸中疼痛。同时患者腰以上还会出汗，但腰以下则无汗，腰髋部弛缓无力，身体疼痛，就像东西积聚在皮肤中一样。病情严重的患者不能进食，其身体疼痛沉重，烦躁不安，小便不利，这就是黄汗病，宜用桂枝加黄芪汤主治。

【英译】

Line 14.29

[In] yellow sweating disease, [there is] spontaneous cold in the two shanks. If there is fever, it pertains to acute swelling of joints. [If] there is sweating after taking food and [if] there is always night sweating, it is consumptive qi [disease]. If there is fever after sweating, squamous dry skin will be present. [If] fever is incessant, there must be malignant sores. If the body is heavy, [it will be] alleviated after sweating. [If it] continues for a long time, the body will eventually twitch. [When the body is] twitching, [there will be] pain in the chest, sweating above the waist, no sweating below [the waist], limpness and pain in the waist and hip, a sensation as if there were something retained in the skin. [If the disease is] acute, [there will be] inability to eat, generalized pain and heaviness, vexation and inhibited urination, [which are the manifestations of] yellow sweating [disease]. Guizhi Decoction (桂枝汤, cinnamon twig decoction) added with Huangqi (黄芪, astragalus, Radix Astragali) [can be used] to treat it.

Guizhi Decoction (桂枝汤, cinnamon twig decoction) added with Huangqi (黄芪, astragalus, Radix Astragali) [is composed of] 3 *liang* of Guizhi (桂枝, cinnamon twig, Ramulus Cinnamomi), 3 *liang* of Shaoyao (芍药, peony, Radix Paeoniae), 2 *liang* of Gancao (甘草, licorice, Radix Glycyrrhizae Praeparata), 3 *liang* of Shengjiang (生姜, fresh ginger, Rhizoma Zingiberis Recens), 12 pieces of Dazao (大枣, jujube, Fructus Ziziphus Jujubae) and 2 *liang* of Huangqi (黄芪, astragalus, Radix Astragali).

These six ingredients are decocted in 8 *sheng* of water to get 3 *sheng* [after] boiling. [The decoction is] taken warm 1 *sheng* [each time]. [After taking the dose] for a while, 1 *sheng* of hot thin porridge should be taken to strengthen the effect of the decoction. Taking warm [decoction] will induce slight sweating. If there is no sweating, one more [dose should be] taken.

【原文】

（三十）

师曰：寸口脉迟而涩，迟则为寒，涩为血不足。趺阳脉微而迟，微则为气，迟则为寒。寒气不足，则手足逆冷；手足逆冷，则营卫不利；营卫不利，则腹满肠鸣相逐，气转膀胱，荣卫俱劳。阳气不通即身冷，阴气不通即骨疼；阳前通则恶寒，阴前通则痹不仁；阴阳相得，其气乃行，大气一转，其气乃散；实则失气，虚则遗尿，名曰气分。

【今译】

老师说：寸口脉象迟而涩，脉象迟则为有寒，脉象涩为血不足。趺阳脉象微而迟，脉象微则为气虚，脉象迟则为有寒。寒气不足，则手足逆冷；手足逆冷，说明营气和卫气运行不利；营气与卫气运行不利，就会导致腹中胀满，肠鸣，气水相逐，使寒气冲入膀胱。如果营气和卫气俱衰，阳气不通就使身体寒冷，阴气不通就会导致骨节疼痛。如果营气和卫气失调，阳气先通就会恶寒，阴气先通就会使肌肤麻木不仁。只有阴阳调和了，气才能正常运行，大气一转，水气就会消散。如果病情属于实证，患者常有矢气的表现。如果病情属于虚证，就会常见小便失禁，称为气分病。

【英译】

Line 14.30

The master said: [There are cases where] the pulse in the cunkou [region] is slow and rough. Slow [pulse] indicates cold and rough [pulse] indicates insufficiency of blood. [There are cases where] the pulse in the fuyang [region] is faint and slow. Faint [pulse] indicates qi [deficiency] and slow [pulse] indicates cold. [When there is] cold and insufficiency of [qi and blood], there will be reversal cold of hands and feet. [When there is] reversal cold of hands and feet, nutrient [qi] and defense [qi] cannot flow smoothly. [When] nutrient [qi] and defense [qi] cannot flow smoothly, [it will cause] abdominal fullness, borborygmus and repelling [between water and qi], [leading to] transmission of [cold] qi into the bladder and debilitation of both nutrient [qi] and defense [qi]. [When] yang qi is obstructed, there will be generalized cold; [when] yin qi is obstructed, there will be pain of joints. [When] yang [qi] begins to flow first, there will be aversion to cold; [when] yin [qi] begins to flow first, there will be impediment and numbness [of skin]. [Only when] yin and yang cooperate with each other, qi is able to move. [Only when] great qi begins to rotate can [pathogenic] qi be dissipated. [When the disease is] excess [in nature], there will be flatus; [when the disease is] deficiency [in nature], there will be enuresis. [Such a pathological condition is] called qi aspect [disease].

【原文】

（三十一）

气分，心下坚大如盘，边如旋杯，水饮所作，桂枝去芍药加麻辛附子汤主之。

桂枝去芍药加麻黄细辛附子汤方

桂枝（三两）　生姜（三两）　甘草（二两）　大枣（十二枚）　麻黄、细辛（各二两）　附子（一枚，炮）

右七味，以水七升，煮麻黄，去上沫，内诸药，煮取二升。分温三服，当汗出，如虫行皮中，即愈。

【今译】

气分病，患者心下坚硬，按之状如盘大，边沿就像旋转的杯子一样，这是水饮凝聚所导致的后果，宜用桂枝去芍药加麻辛附子汤主治。

【英译】

Line 14.31

Qi aspect [disease is characterized by] hardness below the heart like a plate, the edges of which felt like a rotating cup. [It is] caused by retention of water and [can be] treated by Guizhi Decoction (桂枝汤, cinnamon twig decoction) with removal of Shaoyao (芍药, peony, Radix Paeoniae) and addition of Mahuang (麻黄, ephedra, Herba Ephedrae), Xixin (细辛, asarum, Herba Asari) and Fuzi (附子, aconite, Radix Aconiti Lateralis Preparata).

Guizhi Decoction (桂枝汤, cinnamon twig decoction) with removal of Shaoyao (芍药, peony, Radix Paeoniae) and addition of Mahuang (麻黄, ephedra, Herba Ephedrae), Xixin (细辛, asarum, Herba Asari) and Fuzi (附子, aconite, Radix Aconiti Lateralis Preparata) [is composed of] 3 *liang* of Guizhi (桂枝, cinnamon twig, Ramulus Cinnamomi), 3 *liang* of Shengjiang (生姜, fresh ginger, Rhizoma Zingiberis Recens), 2 *liang* of Gancao (甘草, licorice, Radix Glycyrrhizae Praeparata), 12 pieces of Dazao (大枣, jujube, Fructus Ziziphus Jujubae), 2 *liang* of Mahuang (麻黄, ephedra, Herba Ephedrae), 2 *liang* of Xixin (细辛, asarum, Herba Asari) and 1 piece of Fuzi (附子, aconite, Radix Aconiti Lateralis Preparata)(fry heavily).

These seven ingredients are decocted in 7 *sheng* of water. Mahuang (麻黄, ephedra, Herba Ephedrae) is boiled first. [After] removal of the foam, all the other ingredients are put into it to boil and get 2 *sheng*. [The decoction is] divided into three [doses] and taken warm. When there is sweating like worms running beneath the skin, [the disease is] about to cure.

【原文】

(三十二)

心下坚大如盘,边如旋盘,水饮所作,枳术汤主之。

枳术汤方

枳实(七枚) 白术(二两)

右二味,以水五升,煮取三升。分温三服,腹中软,即当散也。

【今译】

患者心下坚硬,坚硬之处大如盘,其边如旋盘,为水饮凝聚所致,宜用枳术汤主治。

附方

【原文】

《外台》防己黄芪汤治风水,脉浮为在表,其人或头汗出,表无他病,病者但下重,从腰以上为和,腰以下当肿及阴,难以屈伸。

【今译】

防己黄芪汤源自《外台》主治风水,脉象浮说明疾患在表,患者或者头部出汗,体表没有其他疾病,患者体下沉重,从腰以上正常,腰以下则肿胀,牵引至阴部,使小腿难以屈伸。

【英译】

Line 14.32

[If there is] hardness as large as a dish and the edge appears like a winding dish, [it is] caused by retention of fluid. Zhizhu Decoction (枳术汤, processed unripe bitter orange and largehead atractylodes rhizome decoction) [can be used] to treat it.

Zhizhu Decoction (枳术汤, processed unripe bitter orange and largehead atractylodes rhizome decoction) [is composed of] 7 pieces of Zhishi (枳实, processed unripe bitter orange, Fructus Aurantii Immaturus) and 2 *liang* of Baizhu (白术, rhizome of largehead atractylodes, Rhizoma Atractylodis Macrocephalae).

These two ingredients are decocted in 5 *sheng* of water to get 3 *sheng* [after] boiling. [The decoction is] divided into three [doses] and taken warm. [If] there is stagnation in the abdomen, [it will] disperse [after taking the decoction].

Appended formula

【英译】

Fangji Huangqi Decoction (防己黄芪汤, the root of stephania tetrandra and astragalus decoction) [is from the book entitled] *Waitai Miyao* (《外台秘要》, *The Medical Secrets of an Official Named Wang Tao*).

Fangji Huangqi Decoction (防己黄芪汤, the root of stephania tetrandra and astragalus decoction) is used to treat wind water [disease], [in which] there is floating pulse in the external, or sweating over the head and no other external diseases, the lower part [of the body] is heavy, the part above the waist is normal, and there is swelling below the waist stretching to the genitals, [making the legs] difficult to bend and stretch.

黄疸病脉证并治第十五

【原文】

(一)

寸口脉浮而缓,浮则为风,缓则为痹。痹非中风。四肢苦烦,脾色必黄,瘀热以行。

【今译】

寸口部位脉象浮而缓,脉象浮为风邪,脉象缓为湿邪痹阻。此处之痹不是中风。四肢苦烦不舒,皮肤必然发黄,这是脾的瘀热行于肌表所致。

Volume 2

Chapter 15
Jaundice Disease:
Pulses, Syndromes/Patterns and Treatment

【英译】

Line 15.1

The pulse in the cunkou [region] is floating and moderate. Floating [pulse] indicates wind and moderate [pulse] indicates impediment. Impediment is not wind stroke. [If the patient suffers from] vexation in the four limbs, the skin must be yellow [due to] movement of stagnated heat [from the spleen to the external].

【原文】

（二）

趺阳脉紧而数，数则为热，热则消谷，紧则为寒，食即为满。尺脉浮为伤肾，趺阳脉紧为伤脾。风寒相搏，食谷即眩，谷气不消，胃中苦浊，浊气下流，小便不通，阴被其寒，热流膀胱，身体尽黄，名曰谷疸。

额上黑，微汗出，手足中热，薄暮即发，膀胱急，小便通利，名曰女劳疸，腹如水状不治。

心中懊侬而热，不能食，时欲吐，名曰酒疸。

【今译】

趺阳脉象紧而数，脉象数为胃有热，胃有热会引起消食善饥；脉象紧为胃有寒气，食后即感到胸部胀满。尺脉浮为肾虚有热而伤肾，趺阳脉紧为寒伤脾。风寒相搏，食后即有眩晕之感，食物不得消化，胃中有苦浊之气，浊气下流，就会引起小便不通。太阴脾受寒湿所困，胃中湿热就会流向膀胱，导致身体发黄，这种病情叫做谷疸。

患者额上发黑，微微汗出，手足的中心发热，黄昏时即发作，膀胱拘急，小便通利，这种病情叫做女劳疸，如果其腹部像有水一样的症状，就无法治疗。

如果患者心中懊恼不舒，有闷热之感，不能饮食，时时欲吐，这种病情叫做酒疸。

【英译】

Line 15.2

The pulse in the fuyang [region] is tight and rapid. Rapid [pulse] indicates heat and heat indicates digestion of food. Tight [pulse] indicates cold and [there will be] fullness after taking food. [When] pulse in the chi [region] is floating, [it] indicates damage of the kidney; [when] the pulse in the fuyang [region] is tight, [it] indicates damage of the spleen. [When] wind and cold contend with each other, [it will cause] dizziness [after] taking food, indigestion of food, bitter turbid [qi] in the stomach, downward flow of turbid qi, inhibited urination, yin covered by cold, heat flowing into the bladder and generalized yellowing, known as cereal jaundice.

[If there are symptoms and signs of] black forehead, slight sweating, feverish hands and feet, occurrence at dusk, tension of the bladder and spontaneous smooth urination, [it is] called female overstrain jaundice. [If] the abdomen appears like water [retention], [it is] incurable.

[If there are symptoms and signs of] anguish and heat in the heart, inability to eat food and frequent nausea, [it is] called wine jaundice.

【原文】

(三)

阳明病,脉迟者,食难用饱,饱则发烦头眩,小便必难,此欲作谷疸。虽下之,腹满如故,所以然者,脉迟故也。

【今译】

阳明病,脉象迟,饮食难以吃饱,饱食后烦闷、头晕、小便困难,这是谷疸即将发作之势。虽然用攻下法治疗,但腹部依然胀满如故,之所以如此,是因为脉迟的缘故。

【原文】

(四)

夫病酒黄疸,必小便不利,其候心中热,足下热,是其证也。

【今译】

患酒黄疸之病的患者,必然有小便不利、心中热、足下热等症状,这就是该证的表现。

【英译】

Line 15.3

Yangming disease [is characterized by] slow pulse, difficulty in taking enough food, vexation and dizziness [after taking] enough food, and difficulty in urination. [Such manifestations indicate that it is] about to develop into cereal jaundice. Although [treated by] purgation, abdominal fullness is still as before because the pulse is slow.

【英译】

Line 15.4

[In] yellow wine jaundice, there must be [symptoms and signs of] inhibited urination, heat in the heart and heat below the feet. [These] are just [the manifestations of] this syndrome/pattern.

【原文】

（五）

酒黄疸者，或无热，靖言了，腹满欲吐，鼻燥。其脉浮者，先吐之；沉弦者，先下之。

【今译】

患酒黄疸的患者，或者无热，神情安静，语言正常，但腹部胀满欲吐，鼻腔干燥。如果脉象浮，可先用吐法治疗；如果脉象沉弦的，可先用下法治疗。

【原文】

（六）

酒疸，心中热，欲呕者，吐之愈。

【今译】

酒疸病患者，心中有热，想呕吐的，可用吐法治疗，吐后即痊愈。

【英译】

Line 15.5

[In] yellow wine jaundice, maybe there is no heat, [the patient is quiet] and speaks normally, but the nose is dry. [If] the pulse is floating, [the therapy for promoting] vomiting [should be used] first; [if the pulse is] sunken and taut, purgation [should be used] first.

【英译】

Line 15.6

[In] wine jaundice, [if there is] heat in the heart and [the patient] wants to vomit, [it can be treated by the therapy for promoting vomiting]. [After] vomiting, [the disease will be] cured.

【原文】

（七）

酒疸下之，久久为黑疸，目青面黑，心中如噉蒜齑状，大便正黑，皮肤爪之不仁，其脉浮弱，虽黑微黄，故知之。

【今译】

酒疸病经下法治疗后，时间一长就转变为黑疸，目青面黑，心中像吃了姜、蒜和韭菜一样的灼热之感，大便正黑，皮肤甲错，但搔而不痒，脉象浮弱，皮肤虽然黑但也显得有些微黄，这就是黑疸病按酒疸下法误治所致。

【原文】

（八）

师曰：病黄疸，发热烦喘，胸满口燥者，以病发时，火劫其汗，两热所得。然黄家所得，从湿得之。一身尽发热而黄，肚热，热在里，当下之。

【今译】

老师说：患黄疸病，证见发热、烦躁、喘息、胸中胀满、口干舌燥的，这是疾病发作时用火攻法发汗，导致热邪与火邪相搏所致。但患者发黄是因湿邪所致。患者全身发热，肤色发黄，腹中有热，热邪在里，应当用攻下法治疗。

Volume 2

【英译】

Line 15.7

[In] wine jaundice, [after treatment with] purgation, [it will eventually transform into] black jaundice after a certain period [of endurance] with blue eyes, black facial expression, scorching sensation in the heart like having taken ginger, garlic and Chinese chives, black stool, squamous and numb skin, floating and weak pulse. Although [the skin is] black, [it is also] slightly yellow. This is the result [of wrong treatment of it with the purgation method used to treat wine jaundice].

【英译】

Line 15.8

The master said: Jaundice [is marked by] fever, vexation, panting, chest fullness and dryness of the mouth. [If] fire attacking [therapy is used to induce] sweating [when] the disease [has just] occurred, [it will cause pathogenic] heat and [pathogenic] fire. But [yellowing of the patient's skin] results from [pathogenic] dampness. [If there is] generalized fever and yellowing with heat in the abdomen and the internal, [it] should [be treated by] purgation.

【原文】

(九)

脉沉,渴欲饮水,小便不利者,皆发黄。

【今译】

脉象沉,口渴欲饮水,小便不利的,肌肤皆会发黄。

【原文】

(十)

腹满,舌痿黄,燥不得睡,属黄家。

【今译】

腹部胀满,肌肤痿黄,烦燥不得安睡的,属于发黄病证。

【原文】

(十一)

黄疸之病,当以十八日为期,治之十日以上瘥,反极为难治。

【今译】

黄疸病,应当以十八日为治疗瘥愈的期限,治疗之十日以上就应该瘥愈,如果病情反而加剧的,就是难治之症。

Volume 2

【英译】

Line 15.9

[If there are symptoms and signs of] sunken pulse, thirst with desire to drink water, and inhibited urination, there is certainly generalized yellowing.

【英译】

Line 15.10

[If there are symptoms and signs of] abdominal distension and fullness, withered yellow body, vexation and inability to sleep well, [it] belongs to jaundice.

【英译】

Line 15.11

Jaundice usually lasts for eighteen days. [After being] treated for over ten days, [it should be] cured. [If it becomes] more serious, [it is] difficult to treat.

金匮要略英译

【原文】

(十二)

疸而渴者,其疸难治;疸而不渴者,其疸可治。发于阴部,其人必呕;阳部,其人振寒而发热也。

【今译】

黄疸病有口渴之症的,就难以治愈;黄疸病而不渴的,就比较可治。病发于内部的,患者必然有呕吐症状;病发于外部的,患者就会有寒战和发热的症状。

【原文】

(十三)

谷疸之为病,寒热不食,食即头眩,心胸不安,久久发黄,为谷疸,茵陈蒿汤主之。

茵陈蒿(六两)　栀子(十四枚)　大黄(二两)

右三味,以水一斗,先煮茵陈,减六升,内二味,煮取三升,去滓。分温三服,小便当利,尿如皂角汁状,色正赤,一宿腹减,黄从小便去也。

【今译】

谷疸病的常见症状为,恶寒、发热、不能进食、食后头晕、心胸不安,持续时间长了就会发黄,成为谷疸,宜用茵陈蒿汤主治。

【英译】

Line 15. 12

Jaundice with thirst is diffcult to treat; jaundice without thirst is curable. [If it is] located in the internal, the patient must vomit; [if it is located] in the external, the patient will quiver with fever.

【英译】

Line 15. 13

Cereal jaundice [is usually characterized by] aversion to cold, fever, inability to eat, dizziness after eating, disquiet in the heart and chest. [If lasting for] a long time, [it will cause] generalized yellowing and become cereal jaundice. [It can be] treated by Yinchenhao Decoction (茵陈蒿汤, virgate wormwood decoction).

Yinchenhao Decoction (茵 陈 蒿 汤, virgate wormwood decoction) [is composed of] 6 *liang* of Yinchenhao (茵陈蒿, virgate wormwood, Artemisiae Scopariae Herba), 14 pieces of Zhizi (栀子, gardenia, Fructus Gardeniae) and 2 *liang* of Dahuang (大黄, rhubarb, Radix et Rhizoma Rhei).

These three ingredients are decocted in 1 *dou* of water. Yinchenhao (茵陈蒿, virgate wormwood, Artemisiae Scopariae Herba) is boiled first to reduce 6 *sheng*. [Then] the other two ingredients are put into [it] to boil and get 3 *sheng*. The dregs are removed and [the decoction is] divided into three [doses] and taken warm. Urination should be normalized [after taking the first dose] and the urine appears like gleditsia juice, quite normal in color. The abdomen will be relieved overnight and yellowing will be eliminated through urination [after taking the decoction].

【原文】

(十四)

黄家日晡所发热,而反恶寒,此为女劳得之。膀胱急,少腹满,身尽黄,额上黑,足下热,因作黑疸。其腹胀如水状,大便必黑,时溏,此女劳之病,非水也。腹满者难治,硝石矾石散主之。

硝石矾石散方

硝石　矾石(烧,等分)

右二味,为散。以大麦粥汁和服方寸匕,日三服,病随大小便去,小便正黄,大便正黑,是候也。

【今译】

素有发黄症的患者,经常在午后3至7时发热。此时如果反而出现恶寒症状,这就属于女劳疸。膀胱拘急,少腹胀满,全身发黄,额上发黑,足下发热,就会发展成为黑疸。腹部胀满如有水聚之状,大便必然发黑,时时有溏泄,这是由于女劳之病所致,而不是有水聚。腹部胀满的难治,宜用硝石矾石散主治。

Volume 2

【英译】

Line 15. 14

［There is usually］ fever ［in the patient with］ jaundice in the time from 3 o'clock to 7 o'clock in the afternoon. ［If there is no fever］ but aversion to cold, this is a woman consumptive ［disease］. ［If there are symptoms and signs of］ tension of bladder, lower abdominal fullness, generalized yellowing, black forehead and heat in the soles of feet, ［it］ will develop into black jaundice. ［If there are symptoms and signs of］ abdominal distension like ［retention of］ water, black stool and frequent sloppy stool, it is a woman consumptive ［disease］, not ［retention of］ water. ［If］ the abdomen is full, ［it is］ difficult to treat. ［The appropriate formula］ for treating it is Xiaoshi Fanshi Powder (硝石矾石散, niter and alum powder).

Xiaoshi Fanshi Powder (硝石矾石散, niter and alum powder) ［is composed of］ Xiaoshi (硝石, niter, Nitrum) (burn) and Fanshi (矾石, alum, Alumen) (burn) of the same amount.

These two ingredients are pounded into powder and mixed with barley juice. ［The powder is］ taken 1 *fangcunbi* ［each time］ and three times a day. The disease will be eliminated through defecation and urination, indication ［of which are］ pure yellow urine and pure black stool.

【原文】

(十五)

酒黄疸,心中懊憹或热痛,栀子大黄汤主之。

栀子大黄汤方

栀子(十四枚)　大黄(一两)　枳实(五枚)　豉(一升)

右四味,以水六升,煮取二升,分温三服。

【今译】

酒黄疸病患者,心中懊恼烦闷,或灼热而痛,宜用栀子大黄汤主治。

【原文】

(十六)

诸病黄家,但利其小便。假令脉浮,当以汗解之,宜桂枝加黄芪汤主之。

【今译】

患发黄病的患者,只须通利小便,就能治愈。如果脉象浮,应当用发汗法治疗,宜用桂枝加黄芪汤主治。

【英译】

Line 15. 15

[In] wine jaundice, [there is] discomfort and vexation in the heart, or heat and pain. The appropriate [formula for] treating it is Zhizi Dahuang Decoction (栀子大黄汤, gardenia and rhubarb decoction).

Zhizi Dahuang Decoction (栀子大黄汤, gardenia and rhubarb decoction) [is composed of] 14 pieces of Zhizi (栀子, gardenia, Fructus Gardeniae), 1 *liang* of Dahuang (大黄, rhubarb, Radix et Rhizoma Rhei), 5 pieces of Zhishi (枳实, processed unripe bitter orange, Fructus Aurantii Immaturus) and 1 *sheng* of Chi (豉, fermented soybean, Sojae Semen Fermentatum).

These four ingredients are decocted in 6 *sheng* of water to get 2 *sheng* [after] boiling. [The decoction is] divided into three [doses] and taken warm.

【英译】

Line 15. 16

[In] patients with jaundice, just normalization of urination [can cure the disease]. If the pulse is floating, [it can be] resolved by diaphoresis. The appropriate [formula for] treating it is Guizhi Decoction (桂枝汤, cinnamon twig decoction) added with Huangqi (黄芪, astragalus, Radix Astragali).

【原文】

(十七)

诸黄,猪膏发煎主之。

猪膏发煎方

猪膏(半斤) 乱发(如鸡子大三枚)

右二味,和膏中煎之,发消药成。分再服,病从小便出。

【今译】

各种发黄之症,用猪膏发煎主治。

【原文】

(十八)

黄疸病,茵陈五苓散主之。

茵陈五苓散方

茵陈蒿末(十分) 五苓散(五分)

右二物和,先食饮方寸匕,日三服。

【今译】

黄疸病,用茵陈五苓散主治。

【英译】

Line 15. 17

Various yellowing [diseases] can be treated by Zhugao Fajian Decoction (猪膏发煎方, pork lard and human hair decoction).

Zhugao Fajian Decoction (猪膏发煎方, pork lard and human hair decoction) [is composed of] 0.5 *jin* of Zhugao (猪膏, pork lard, Suis Adeps) and Luanfa (乱发, human hair, Crinis Carbonisatus) (as large as three chicken eggs).

These two ingredients are blended into paste and fried. [When] the hair is dispersed, the ingredients are decocted well. [The decoction is] divided into two [doses] and taken orally. The disease will be eliminated through urination.

【英译】

Line 15. 18

Jaundice [should be] treated by Yinchen Wuling Powder (茵陈五苓散, virgate wormwood and poria decoction).

Yinchen Wuling Powder (茵陈五苓散, virgate wormwood and poria decoction) [is composed of] 10 *fen* of Yinchenhao (茵陈蒿, virgate wormwood, Artemisiae Scopariae Herba) and 5 *fen* of Wuling Powder (五苓散, poria powder).

These two ingredients are mixed. [The powder is] taken 1 *fangcunbi* for the first time and three times a day.

【原文】

（十九）

黄疸腹满，小便不利而赤，自汗出，此为表和里实，当下之，宜大黄硝石汤。

大黄硝石汤方

大黄、黄柏、硝石（各四两）　栀子（十五枚）

右四味，以水六升，煮取二升，去滓，内硝，更煮取一升，顿服。

【今译】

黄疸病患者，腹部胀满，小便不利，颜色发红，有自汗出，这是表无外邪，内有实热之症，应当用下法治疗，用大黄硝石汤主治。

【原文】

（二十）

黄疸病，小便色不变，欲自利，腹满而喘，不可除热，热除必哕。哕者，小半夏汤主之。

【今译】

黄疸病患者，小便颜色不变，想要自利，腹部胀满而喘息，不可用除热法治疗，因为热邪虽然消除了，但却必然引起呃逆。有呃逆症状的，用小半夏汤主治。

【英译】

Line 15. 19

[In] jaundice，[symptoms and signs of] inhibited urination with red color and spontaneous sweating indicate external harmony and internal excess [heat syndrome/pattern]. [It] should [be treated by] purgation. The appropriate [formula for treating it] is Dahuang Xiaoshi Decoction（大黄硝石汤，rhubarb and niter decoction）.

Dahuang Xiaoshi Decoction（大黄硝石汤，rhubarb and niter decoction）[is composed of] 4 *liang* of Dahuang（大黄，rhubarb，Radix et Rhizoma Rhei），4 *liang* of Huangbo（黄柏，phellodendron，Cortex Phellodendri），4 *liang* of Xiaoshi（硝石，niter，Nitrum）and 15 pieces of Zhizi（栀子，gardenia，Fructus Gardeniae）.

These four ingredients are decocted in 6 *sheng* of water to get 2 *sheng* [after] boiling. The dregs are removed and Xiaoshi（硝石，niter，Nitrum）is put into [it] to boil and get 1 *sheng*. [The decoction should be] taken once the whole.

【英译】

Line 15. 20

[In] jaundice，the color of urine is not changed，[the patient] wants to urinate spontaneously，the abdomen is full and there is panting. [To treat such a disease,] heat cannot be eliminated [because] elimination of heat will cause hiccup. [If there is] hiccup，Xiao Banxia Decoction（小半夏汤，minor pinellia decoction）[can be used] to treat it.

【原文】

(二十一)

诸黄,腹痛而呕者,宜柴胡汤。

【今译】

各种发黄之病中,有腹痛而呕吐的,宜用柴胡汤主治。

【原文】

(二十二)

男子黄,小便自利,当与虚劳小建中汤。

【今译】

男子肌肤发黄,但小便却通利的,应当用治疗虚劳症的小建中汤主治。

附方

【原文】

瓜蒂汤,治诸黄。

《千金》麻黄醇酒汤,治黄疸。

麻黄(三两)

右一味,以美清酒五升,煮取二升半,顿服尽。冬月用酒,春月用水煮之。

【今译】

瓜蒂汤用以治疗各种黄证。

麻黄醇酒汤源自《千金方》,主治黄疸。

Volume 2

【英译】

Line 15.21

[In] various yellowing [diseases], [if there is] abdominal pain and nausea，Chaihu Decoction（柴胡汤，bupleurum decoction）is the appropriate [formula for] treating it.

【英译】

Line 15.22

Male [patients with] yellow [skin] and spontaneous urination [can be] treated by Xiao Jianzhong Decoction（小建中汤，minor decoction for strengthening the middle）.

Appended formula

【英译】

Guadi Decoction（瓜蒂汤，melon stalk decoction）：For treating various yellowing [diseases].

Mahuang Chunjiu Decoction（麻黄醇酒汤，ephedra and pure wine decoction）[from the book entitled] *Qianjin*（《千金方》，*Thousand Golden Formulas*）：For treating jaundice.

Mahuang Chunjiu Decoction（麻黄醇酒汤，ephedra and pure wine decoction）is just composed of 3 *liang* of single Mahuang（麻黄，ephedra，Herba Ephedrae）.

This ingredient is decocted in 5 *sheng* of pure clear wine to get 2.5 *sheng* [after] boiling. [The decoction is] taken once the whole. In winter，[this ingredient is boiled] in wine；in spring，[this ingredient is] decocted in water.

惊悸吐血下血胸满瘀血病脉证治第十六

【原文】

（一）

寸口脉动而弱,动即为惊,弱则为悸。

【今译】

寸口部脉象动而弱,动是惊动的表现,弱是悸动的体现。

【原文】

（二）

师曰:尺脉浮,目睛晕黄,衄未止;晕黄去,目睛慧了,知衄今止。

【今译】

老师说:尺部脉象浮,目睛周围有晕黄现象,说明衄血没有停止;目睛的晕黄消退了,视力就清晰了,说明衄血已停止。

Volume 2

Chapter 16
Fright, Palpitation, Blood vomiting, Bleeding, Chest Fullness and Blood Stasis Disease: Pulses, Syndromes/Patterns and Treatment

【英译】

Line 16. 1

The pulse in the cunkou [region] is quivering and weak. Quivering [pulse] indicates fright and weak [pulse] indicates palpitation.

【英译】

Line 16. 2

The master said: The pulse in the chi [region] is floating and the eyes are yellow [around the pupils], [indicating that] nosebleed does not cease. [When] yellowing [around the pupils of the eyes] has dispersed, [it indicates that] nosebleed has ceased.

【原文】

（三）

又曰：从春至夏，衄者，太阳；从秋至冬，衄者，阳明。

【今译】

老师又说：从春季到夏季，有衄血的，属于太阳；从秋季到冬季，有衄血的，属于阳明。

【原文】

（四）

衄家不可汗，汗出必额上陷，脉紧急，直视不能眴，不得眠。

【今译】

衄血患者不可用汗法治疗，误用汗法必然导致额上凹陷，脉象紧急，眼睛直视不能转动，不得睡眠。

【原文】

（五）

病人面无色，无寒热，脉沉弦者，衄；浮弱，手按之绝者，下血；烦咳者，必吐血。

【今译】

病人面部苍白无色，不恶寒也不发热，脉象沉弦的，有衄血；脉象浮弱，用手按则无所显现的，为下血；烦躁咳嗽的，必然吐血。

Volume 2

【英译】

Line 16.3

The master said again: [If there is] nosebleed from spring to summer, [it belongs to] taiyang; [if there is] nosebleed from autumn to winter, [it belongs to] yangming.

【英译】

Line 16.4

The patient with nosebleed cannot [be treated by] diaphoresis. [If there is] sweating, [there must be] depression in the forehead, tight and urgent pulse, eyes staring straight and unable to move, and inability to lie down.

【英译】

Line 16.5

[The manifestations of] no facial expression, no aversion to cold, no fever, sunken and taut pulse [indicate] nosebleed. [The pulse is] floating and weak, [but there is] no beating when pressed, [indicating] bleeding. [If there is] vexation and cough, blood vomiting is inevitable.

【原文】

(六)

夫吐血,咳逆上气,其脉数而有热,不得卧者,死。

【今译】

吐血,伴有咳嗽,喘逆上气,脉象数而有热,不能平卧的,为死证。

【原文】

(七)

夫酒客咳者,必致吐血,此因极饮过度所致也。

【今译】

嗜酒之人,若咳嗽,必然导致吐血,这是饮酒过度所致。

【原文】

(八)

寸口脉弦而大,弦则为减,大则为芤,减则为寒,芤则为虚,寒虚相击,此名曰革,妇人则半产漏下,男子则亡血。

【今译】

寸口部脉象弦而大,脉象弦表示减缓,脉象大则为浮软,减缓表示有寒,浮软表示为虚,寒虚相击,称为革。在这种情况下,妇女流产而又漏下,男子则失血。

Volume 2

【英译】

Line 16.6

Blood vomiting, [accompanied by] cough, panting, upward counterflow of qi, rapid pulse, fever and inability to lie down, is fatal.

【英译】

Line 16.7

[If there is] cough in a person addicted to wine, [accompanied by] blood vomiting due to overdrinking of wine, [it is] fatal.

【英译】

Line 16.8

The pulse in the cunkou [region] is taut and large. Taut [pulse] indicates reduction and large [pulse] indicates floating-softness. Reduction means cold, floating-softness means deficiency. [When] cold and deficiency contend with each other, it is called tympanic. [In] women, [it indicates] abortion and vaginal bleeding; [in] men, [it indicates] bleeding.

【原文】

(九)

亡血不可发其表,汗出即寒栗而振。

【今译】

失血的患者,不可用发汗法解表,汗出后会引起寒战怕冷。

【原文】

(十)

病人胸满,唇痿舌青,口燥,但欲嗽水,不欲咽,无寒热,脉微大来迟,腹不满,其人言我满,为有瘀血。

【今译】

病人胸部胀满,嘴唇色痿,舌色青,口干燥,但只想嗽水,不想下咽,无恶寒,不发热,脉象微大而迟,腹部无胀满现象,但患者自感腹部胀满,这是体内有瘀血的表现。

【原文】

(十一)

病者如热状,烦满,口干燥而渴,其脉反无热,此为阴伏,是瘀血也,当下之。

【今译】

病人似乎有发热状况,烦躁,胸满,口中干燥而渴,切脉反而感受不到热,这是深伏于血分的郁热瘀血,应当用攻下法治疗。

Volume 2

【英译】

Line 16. 9

[To treat patients with] bleeding, diaphoresis cannot [be used because] sweating causes quivering and shivering.

【英译】

Line 16. 10

[In] the patient, [there are symptoms and signs of] chest fullness, withered lips, bluish tongue, dryness of the mouth, desire to gargle, no aversion to cold, no fever, faint, large and slow pulse. There is no abdominal fullness, [but] the patient feels fullness in the abdomen [because] there is blood stasis [in the internal].

【英译】

Line 16. 11

The patient seems to have fever, [accompanied by] vexation, chest fullness and dryness of the mouth with thirst. [When] the pulse [is taken], no heat [can be felt because] there is blood stasis [and stagnated heat in the blood aspect]. [To treat such a disease,] purgation should [be used].

【原文】

(十二)

火邪者,桂枝去芍药加蜀漆牡蛎龙骨救逆汤主之。

桂枝救逆汤方

桂枝(三两,去皮)　甘草(二两,炙)　生姜(三两)　牡蛎(五两,熬)　龙骨(四两)　大枣(十二枚)　蜀漆(三两,洗去腥)

右为末,以水一斗二升,先煮蜀漆,减二升,内诸药,煮取三升,去滓,温服一升。

【今译】

有火邪致惊的,用桂枝去芍药加蜀漆牡蛎龙骨救逆汤主治。

【原文】

(十三)

心下悸者,半夏麻黄丸主之。

半夏麻黄丸方

半夏　麻黄(等分)

右二味,末之,炼蜜和丸小豆大,饮服三丸,日三服。

【今译】

心下悸动的,用半夏麻黄丸主治。

【英译】

Line 16. 12

[Disease with] pathogenic fire [that causes fright should be] treated by Guizhi Jiuni Decoction（桂枝救逆汤，cinnamon twig decoction for resolving counterflow）with removal of Shaoyao（芍药，peony，Radix Paeoniae）and addition of Shuqi（蜀漆，dichroa，Ramulus et Folium Dichroae），Muli（牡蛎，oyster shell，Concha Ostreae）and Longgu（龙骨，Loong bone，Os Loong）.

Guizhi Jiuni Decoction（桂枝救逆汤，cinnamon twig decoction for resolving counterflow）[is composed of] 3 *liang* of Guizhi（桂枝，cinnamon twig，Ramulus Cinnamomi）（remove the bark），2 *liang* of Gancao（甘草，licorice，Radix Glycyrrhizae Praeparata）（broil），3 *liang* of Shengjiang（生姜，fresh ginger，Rhizoma Zingiberis Recens），5 *liang* of Muli（牡蛎，oyster shell，Concha Ostreae）（boil），4 *liang* of Longgu（龙骨，Loong bone，Os Loong），12 pieces of Dazao（大枣，jujube，Fructus Ziziphus Jujubae）and 3 *liang* of Shuqi（蜀漆，dichroa，Ramulus et Folium Dichroae）（remove fishy smell through washing）.

These ingredients are pounded into powder and decocted in 1 *dou* and 2 *sheng* water. Shuqi（蜀漆，dichroa，Ramulus et Folium Dichroae）is boiled first to reduce 2 *sheng*. [Then] all the other ingredients are put into [it] to boil and get 3 *sheng*. The dregs are removed and [the decoction is] taken warm 1 *sheng* [each time].

【英译】

Line 16. 13

[The disease with] palpitation below the heart [can be] treated by Banxia Mahuang Pill（半夏麻黄丸，pinellia and ephedra pill）.

Banxia Mahuang Pill（半夏麻黄丸，pinellia and ephedra pill）[is composed of] Banxia（半夏，pinellia，Rhizoma Pinelliae）and Mahuang（麻黄，ephedra，Herba Ephedrae）of the same amount.

These two ingredients are pounded into powder and mixed with Lianmi（炼蜜，processed honey，Mel Praeparatum）to form pills the size of small beans. [Each time] 3 pills are taken with water and three times a day.

【原文】

（十四）

吐血不止者,柏叶汤主之。

柏叶汤方

柏叶　干姜(各三两)　艾(三把)

右三味,以水五升,取马通汁一升,合煮,取一升,分温再服。

【今译】

吐血不止的患者,用柏叶汤主治。

【原文】

（十五）

下血,先便后血,此远血也,黄土汤主之。

黄土汤方

甘草　干地黄　白术　附子(炮)　阿胶　黄芩(各三两)　灶中黄土(半斤)

右七味,以水八升,煮取三升,分温二服。

【今译】

有便血症状的,先大便而后出血,这叫作远血,用黄土汤主治。

Volume 2

【英译】

Line 16.14

[To treat] incessant blood vomiting, Baiye Decoction (柏叶汤, arborvitae leaf decoction) should [be used].

Baiye Decoction (柏叶汤, arborvitae leaf decoction) [is composed of] 3 *liang* of Baiye (柏叶, arborvitae leaf, Cacumen Platycladi), 3 *liang* of Ganjiang (干姜, dried ginger, Rhizoma Zingiberis) and 3 handfuls of Ai (艾, mugwort, Folium Artemisiae Argyi).

These three ingredients are decocted in 5 *sheng* of water and mixed with 1 *sheng* of liquid extracted from horse dung to boil and get 1 *sheng*. [The decoction is] divided into two [doses] and taken warm.

【英译】

Line 16.15

[In the patient with] blood in the stool, [if] stool [is discharged] first and then the blood [is discharged], it is called distal bleeding and should be treated by Huangtu Decoction (黄土汤, oven earth decoction).

Huangtu Decoction (黄土汤, oven earth decoction) [is composed of] 3 *liang* of Gancao (甘草, licorice, Radix Glycyrrhizae Praeparata), 3 *liang* of Gandihuang (干地黄, dried rehmannia, Radix Rehmanniae), 3 *liang* of Baizhu (白术, rhizome of largehead atractylodes, Rhizoma Atractylodis Macrocephalae), 3 *liang* of Fuzi (附子, aconite, Radix Aconiti Lateralis Preparata) (fry heavily), 3 *liang* of Ejiao (阿胶, ass-hide glue, Colla Corii Asini), 3 *liang* of Huangqin (黄芩, scutellaria, Radix Scutellariae) and 0.5 *jin* of Huangtu (黄土, oven earth, Terra Flava Usta).

These seven ingredients are decocted in 8 *sheng* of water to get 3 *sheng* [after] boiling. [The decoction is] divided into two [doses] and taken warm.

【原文】

（十六）

下血，先血后便，此近血也，赤小豆当归散主之。

【今译】

有便血症状的，先出血后大便，这叫作近血，用赤小豆当归散主治。

【原文】

（十七）

心气不足，吐血，衄血，泻心汤主之。

泻心汤方

大黄（二两）　黄连　黄芩（各一两）

右三味，以水三升，煮取一升，顿服之。

【今译】

患者心气不足，烦躁不安，吐血，衄血，用泻心汤主治。

【英译】

Line 16. 16

［In the patient with］ bleeding，［if］ the blood ［is discharged］ first and then the stool ［is discharged］, it is called proximal bleeding and should be treated by Chixiaodou Danggui Powder（赤小豆当归散，rice bean and Chinese angelica decoction）.

【英译】

Line 16. 17

The patient with insufficiency of heart qi，blood vomiting and nosebleed ［should be］ treated by Xiexin Decoction（泻心汤，decoction for draining the heart）.

Xiexin Decoction（泻心汤，decoction for draining the heart）［is composed of］ 2 *liang* of Dahuang（大黄，rhubarb，Radix et Rhizoma Rhei），1 *liang* of Huanglian（黄连，coptis，Rhizoma Coptidis）and 1 *liang* of Huangqin（黄芩，scutellaria，Radix Scutellariae）.

These three ingredients are decocted in 3 *sheng* of water to get 1 *sheng* ［after］ boiling. ［The decoction is］ taken once the whole.

呕吐哕下利病脉证治第十七

【原文】

(一)

夫呕家有痈脓,不可治呕,脓尽自愈。

【今译】

　　经常呕吐的患者,有痈脓溃疡,不可用止呕吐之法治疗,等待脓血排尽后就能自愈。

【原文】

(二)

　　先呕却渴者,此为欲解;先渴却呕者,为水停心下,此属饮家。呕家本渴,今反不渴者,以心下有支饮故也,此属支饮。

【今译】

　　患者先呕吐后口渴,说明呕吐欲解;患者先口渴后呕吐,为水饮停留在心下,称为水饮病。呕吐的患者本来应该口渴,如今反不口渴,是心下有水饮停留的缘故,属于支饮病。

Chapter 17
Retching, Vomiting, Hiccup and Diarrhea Disease:
Pulses, Syndromes/Patterns and Treatment

【英译】

Line 17. 1

The patient with frequent retching [suffers from] abscess with pus. [It] cannot be treated [by the therapy for] stopping retching. [When] pus has disappeared completely, [the disease will] spontaneously heal.

【英译】

Line 17.2

[When the patient] vomits first and then [feels] thirsty, it indicates [that vomiting is] about to resolve. [When the patient feels] thirsty first and then vomits, [it is caused by] retention of water below the heart, pertaining to water retention disease. The patient with vomiting should be thirsty, but now there is no thirst because there is propping retention of water below the heart. [That is why] it belongs to propping retention of water.

【原文】

(三)

问曰：病人脉数，数为热，当消谷引食，而反吐者，何也？师曰：以发其汗，令阳微，膈气虚，脉乃数。数为客热，不能消谷，胃中虚冷故也。

脉弦者，虚也，胃气无余，朝食暮吐，变为胃反。寒在于上，医反下之，今脉反弦，故名曰虚。

【今译】

问：病人脉象数，脉象数为有热，应当消谷善饥，如今反而呕吐，是什么原因呢？

老师说：因为发汗，使阳气衰微，宗气虚弱，所以脉象数。脉象数说明有虚热，所以不能消谷，这是引起胃中虚冷的原因。

脉象弦，属虚，说明胃气不足，早上吃的饭，晚上就吐出，变化为胃反病。因为寒邪在上部，医生反而用攻下法治疗，所以现在脉象就反而变弦了，因此称为虚。

【原文】

(四)

寸口脉微而数，微则无气，无气则荣虚，荣虚则血不足，血不足则胸中冷。

【今译】

寸口脉象微而数，脉象微说明阳气虚衰。如果阳气虚衰，营气也虚。如果营气虚，则血分不足。如果血分不足，则胸中寒冷。

【英译】

Line 17.3

Question: The patient's pulse is rapid and rapid [pulse] indicates heat. [Hence] there should be swift digestion with frequent hunger. But [now there is] vomiting. What is the reason?

The master said: Because sweating [is promoted], [making] yang faint, qi in the diaphragm deficient and the pulse rapid. Rapid [pulse] indicates [deficient pathogenic] heat [that] cannot promote digestion due to deficiency-cold in the stomach.

The pulse is taut, [indicating] deficiency and insufficiency of stomach qi. [As a result, the food] taken in the morning will be vomited in the evening, changing into stomach regurgitation. Cold is in the upper, [but] the doctor [has treated the patient with] purgation. [That is why] the pulse becomes taut. [Hence it is] called deficiency.

【英译】

Line 17.4

The pulse in the cunkou [region] is faint and rapid. Faint [pulse] indicates no qi (collapse of yang qi); no qi indicates deficiency of nutrient [qi]; deficiency of nutrient [qi] indicates insufficiency of the blood; insufficiency of the blood indicates cold in the chest.

【原文】

（五）

趺阳脉浮而涩，浮则为虚，涩则伤脾，脾伤则不磨，朝食暮吐，暮食朝吐，宿谷不化，名曰胃反。脉紧而涩，其病难治。

【今译】

趺阳部脉象浮而涩，脉象浮为胃虚，脉象涩为伤脾，脾伤则无法运化水谷，早上用餐，晚上吐出，晚上用餐，早上吐出，饮食停留于胃，不能消化，称为胃反。如果趺阳部脉象紧而涩，这种病就难治。

【原文】

（六）

病人欲吐者，不可下之。

【今译】

病人想呕吐，不可用攻下法治疗。

【原文】

（七）

哕而腹满，视其前后，知何部不利，利之即愈。

【今译】

患者呃逆而腹部胀满的，要了解患者大小便的情况，了解哪部不利，通过通大便或利小便就可以治愈病患。

Volume 2

【英译】

Line 17.5

The pulse in the fuyang [region] is floating and rough. Floating [pulse] indicates deficiency and rough [pulse] indicates damage of the spleen. [When] the spleen is damaged, [food] cannot be digested. [As a result,] food taken in the morning is vomited in the evening and food taken in the evening is vomited in the morning [because of] inability to digest food. [Hence it is] called stomach regurgitation. [If] the pulse is tight and rough, the disease is difficult to treat.

【英译】

Line 17.6

[When] the patient is about to vomit, purgation cannot [be used].

【英译】

Line 17.7

[In patients with] hiccup and abdominal fullness, observation of the posterior and anterior (defecation and urination) [will enable one] to know which is inhibited. Disinhibition [of urination and defecation] will cure [the patient].

【原文】

（八）

呕而胸满者，茱萸汤主之。

茱萸汤方

吴茱萸（一升）　人参（三两）　生姜（六两）　大枣（十二枚）

右四味，以水五升，煮取三升。温服七合，日三服。

【今译】

呕吐而胸部胀满的，用茱萸汤主治。

【原文】

（九）

干呕，吐涎沫，头痛者，茱萸汤主之。

【今译】

患者干呕，吐涎沫，头痛的，用茱萸汤主治。

【原文】

（十）

呕而肠鸣，心下痞者，半夏泻心汤主之。

半夏泻心汤方

半夏（半升，洗）　黄芩、干姜、人参（各三两）　黄连（一两）　大枣（十二枚）　甘草（三两，炙）

右七味，以水一斗，煮取六升，去滓，再煮取三升。温服一升，日三服。

【今译】

呕吐而肠鸣，心下痞满的，用半夏泻心汤主治。

【英译】

Line 17.8

Retching and chest fullness can be treated by Zhuyu Decoction (茱萸汤，evodia decoction).

Zhuyu Decoction (茱萸汤，evodia decoction) [is composed of] 1 *sheng* of Wuzhuyu (吴茱萸，evodia，Fructus Evodiae)，3 *liang* of Renshen (人参，ginseng，Radix Ginseng)，6 *liang* of Shengjiang (生姜，fresh ginger，Rhizoma Zingiberis Recens) and 12 pieces of Dazao (大枣，jujube，Fructus Ziziphus Jujubae).

These four ingredients are decocted in 5 *sheng* of water to get 3 *sheng* [after] boiling. [The decoction is] taken warm 7 *ge* [each time] and three times a day.

【英译】

Line 17.9

[To treat] dry retching, vomiting of drool and headache, Zhuyu Decoction (茱萸汤，evodia decoction) can be used.

【英译】

Line 17.10

[To treat] retching, borborygmus and lump below the heart, Banxia Xiexin Decoction (半夏泻心汤，pinellia decoction for draining the heart) can be used.

Banxia Xiexin Decoction (半夏泻心汤，pinellia decoction for draining the heart) [is composed of] 0.5 *sheng* of Banxia (半夏，pinellia，Rhizoma Pinelliae)(wash)，3 *liang* of Huangqin (黄芩，scutellaria，Radix Scutellariae)，3 *liang* of Ganjiang (干姜，dried ginger，Rhizoma Zingiberis)，3 *liang* of Renshen (人参，ginseng，Radix Ginseng)，1 *liang* of Huanglian (黄连，coptis，Rhizoma Coptidis)，12 pieces of Dazao (大枣，jujube，Fructus Ziziphus Jujubae) and 3 *liang* of Gancao (甘草，licorice，Radix Glycyrrhizae Praeparata)(broil).

These seven ingredients are decocted in 1 *dou* of water to get 6 *sheng* [after] boiling. The dregs are removed and [the ingredients are] boiled again to get 3 *sheng*. [The decoction is] taken warm 1 *sheng* [each time] and three times a day.

【原文】

(十一)

干呕而利者,黄芩加半夏生姜汤主之。

黄芩加半夏生姜汤方

黄芩(三两) 甘草(二两,炙) 芍药(二两) 半夏(半升) 生姜(三两) 大枣(二十枚)

右六味,以水一斗,煮取三升,去滓。温服一升,日再、夜一服。

【今译】

患者干呕而下利的,用黄芩加半夏生姜汤主治。

【原文】

(十二)

诸呕吐,谷不得下者,小半夏汤主之。

【今译】

凡是呕吐而饮食不能消化和排泄的,用小半夏汤主治。

【英译】

Line 17.11

[To treat] dry retching and diarrhea，Huangqin Decoction（黄芩，scutellaria decoction） added with Banxia （半夏，pinellia，Rhizoma Pinelliae） and Shengjiang（生姜，fresh ginger，Rhizoma Zingiberis Recens） should be used.

Huangqin Decoction （黄芩，scutellaria decoction） added with Banxia（半夏，pinellia，Rhizoma Pinelliae） and Shengjiang（生姜，fresh ginger，Rhizoma Zingiberis Recens） [is composed of] 3 *liang* of Huangqin （黄芩，scutellaria，Radix Scutellariae）, 2 *liang* of Gancao（甘草，licorice，Radix Glycyrrhizae Praeparata）（broil）, 2 *liang* of Shaoyao（芍药，peony，Radix Paeoniae）, 0.5 *sheng* of Banxia（半夏，pinellia，Rhizoma Pinelliae）, 3 *liang* of Shengjiang （生姜，fresh ginger，Rhizoma Zingiberis Recens） and 20 pieces of Dazao（大枣，jujube，Fructus Ziziphus Jujubae）.

These six ingredients are decocted in 1 *dou* of water to get 3 *sheng*. The dregs are removed and [the decoction is] taken warm 1 *sheng* [each time], twice in the daytime and once at night.

【英译】

Line 17.12

[To treat] all kinds of retching，vomiting，inability to swallow food and defecate Xiao Banxia Decoction（小半夏汤，minor pinellia decoction） should be used.

【原文】

(十三)

呕吐而病在膈上,后思水者,解,急与之。思水者,猪苓散主之。

猪苓散方

猪苓、茯苓、白术(各等分)

右三味,杵为散。饮服方寸匕,日三服。

【今译】

呕吐而病在膈上的,呕吐之后想喝水的,疾病有消解的倾向,应急时给患者水喝。想喝水的,用猪苓散主治。

【原文】

(十四)

呕而脉弱,小便复利,身有微热,见厥者难治,四逆汤主之。

四逆汤方

附子(一枚,生用) 干姜(一两半) 甘草(二两,炙)

右三味,以水三升,煮取一升二合,去滓,分温再服。强人可大附子一枚,干姜三两。

【今译】

呕吐而脉象弱,小便反而通利,身上有微热,四肢逆冷的,则难以治愈,用四逆汤主治。

【英译】

Line 17. 13

［When］the disease is ［located］ above the diaphragm，［there is］ retching and vomiting. ［If there is］ desire to drink water after ［retching and vomiting］，［the disease is about］ to resolve and ［water should be］ immediately given to ［the patient］. ［When the patient］ wants to drink water，Zhuling Powder（猪苓散，polyporus powder）should be used.

Zhuling Powder（猪苓散，polyporus powder）［is composed of］ Zhuling（猪苓，polyporus，Polyporus Umbellatus），Fuling（茯苓，poria，Poria）and Baizhu（白术，rhizome of largehead atractylodes，Rhizoma Atractylodis Macrocephalae）of the same amount.

These three ingredients are pounded into powder. ［Each time］ 1 *fangcunbi* is taken with water and three times a day.

【英译】

Line 17. 14

Retching，［accompanied by］ weak pulse，normal urination，slight fever and reversal ［cold of the four limbs］，is difficult to treat. Sini Decoction（四逆汤，decoction for resolving four kinds of adverseness）［can be used］ to treat it.

Sini Decoction（四逆汤，decoction for resolving four kinds of adverseness）［is composed of］ 1 piece of Fuzi（附子，aconite，Radix Aconiti Lateralis Preparata）（raw），1. 5 *liang* of Ganjiang（干姜，dried ginger，Rhizoma Zingiberis）and 2 *liang* of Gancao（甘草，licorice，Radix Glycyrrhizae Praeparata）（broil）.

These three ingredients are decocted in 3 *sheng* of water to get 1 *sheng* and 2 *ge*. The dregs are removed and ［the decoction is］ divided into two ［doses］ and taken warm. ［For］ strong patients，1 piece of large Fuzi（附子，aconite，Radix Aconiti Lateralis Preparata）and 3 *liang* of Ganjiang（干姜，dried ginger，Rhizoma Zingiberis）［can be used］.

【原文】

(十五)

呕而发热者,小柴胡汤主之。

小柴胡汤方

柴胡(半斤)　黄芩(三两)　人参(三两)　甘草(三两)　半夏(半斤)　生姜(三两)　大枣(十二枚)

右七味,以水一斗二升,煮取六升,去滓,再煎取三升。温服一升,日三服。

【今译】

呕吐而发热的,宜用小柴胡汤主治。

【原文】

(十六)

胃反呕吐者,大半夏汤主之。

大半夏汤方

半夏(二升,洗完用)　人参(三两)　白蜜(一升)

右三味,以水一斗二升,和蜜扬之二百四十遍,煮药取二升半。温服一升,余分再服。

【今译】

胃反而呕吐的,用大半夏汤主治。

Volume 2

【英译】

Line 17. 15

[To treat] retching and fever，Xiao Chaihu Decoction（小柴胡汤，minor bupleurum decoction）can be used.

Xiao Chaihu Decoction （ 小 柴 胡 汤， minor bupleurum decoction）[is composed of] 0. 5 *jin* of Chaihu（柴胡，bupleurum，Radix Bupleuri），3 *liang* of Huangqin（黄芩，scutellaria，Radix Scutellariae），3 *liang* of Renshen（人参，ginseng，Radix Ginseng），3 *liang* of Gancao（甘草，licorice，Radix Glycyrrhizae Praeparata），0. 5 *jin* of Banxia（半夏，pinellia，Rhizoma Pinelliae），3 *liang* of Shengjiang（生姜，fresh ginger，Rhizoma Zingiberis Recens）and 12 pieces of Dazao（大枣，jujube，Fructus Ziziphus Jujubae）.

These seven ingredients are decocted in 1 *dou* and 2 *sheng* of water to get 6 *sheng* [after] boiling. The dregs are removed and [the ingredients are] boiled again to get 3 *sheng*. [The decoction is] taken warm 1 *sheng* [each time] and three times a day.

【英译】

Line 17. 16

[To treat] stomach regurgitation with retching and vomiting，Da Banxia Decoction（大半夏汤，major pinellia decoction）can be used.

Da Banxia Decoction（大半夏汤，major pinellia decoction）[is composed of] 2 *sheng* of Banxia （半夏，pinellia，Rhizoma Pinelliae）（wash），3 *liang* of Renshen（人参，ginseng，Radix Ginseng）and 1 *sheng* of Baimi（白蜜，white honey，Mel）.

These three ingredients are blended in 1 *dou* and 2 *sheng* of water. [After] splashing for 240 times，[the ingredients are] boiled to get 2. 5 *sheng*. [The decoction is] taken warm 1 *sheng* [each time] and the rest is divided into two [doses].

【原文】

（十七）

食已即吐者，大黄甘草汤主之。

大黄甘草汤方

大黄（四两） 甘草（一两）

右二味，以水三升，煮取一升，分温再服。

【今译】

用餐之后即呕吐的，用大黄甘草汤主治。

【原文】

（十八）

胃反，吐而渴欲饮水者，茯苓泽泻汤主之。

茯苓泽泻汤方

茯苓（半斤） 泽泻（四两） 甘草（二两） 桂枝（二两） 白术（三两） 生姜（四两）

右六味，以水一斗，煮取三升，内泽泻，再煮取二升半。温服八合，日三服。

【今译】

胃反而呕吐，口渴想喝水的，宜用茯苓泽泻汤主治。

【英译】

Line 17. 17

［To treat］ vomiting right after taking food，Dahuang Gancao Decoction (大黄甘草汤，rhubarb and licorice decoction) can be used.

Dahuang Gancao Decoction（大黄甘草汤，rhubarb and licorice decoction)［is composed of］4 *liang* of Dahuang（大黄，rhubarb，Radix et Rhizoma Rhei) and 1 *liang* of Gancao（甘草，licorice，Radix Glycyrrhizae Praeparata).

These two ingredients are decocted in 3 *sheng* of water to get 1 *sheng* ［after］boiling.［The decoction is］divided into two［doses］and taken warm.

【英译】

Line 17. 18

［To treat］stomach regurgitation with vomiting，thirst and desire to drink water，Fuling Zexie Decoction (茯苓泽泻汤，poria and alisma decoction) should be used.

Fuling Zexie Decoction（茯苓泽泻汤，poria and alisma decoction)［is composed of］0.5 *jin* of Fuling（茯苓，poria，Poria)，4 *liang* of Zexie（泽泻，alisma，Rhizoma Alismatis)，2 *liang* of Gancao（甘草，licorice，Radix Glycyrrhizae Praeparata)，2 *liang* of Guizhi（桂枝，cinnamon twig，Ramulus Cinnamomi)，3 *liang* of Baizhu（白术，rhizome of largehead atractylodes，Rhizoma Atractylodis Macrocephalae) and 4 *liang* of Shengjiang（生姜，fresh ginger，Rhizoma Zingiberis Recens).

These six ingredients are decocted in 1 *dou* of water to get 3 *sheng*［after］boiling.［Then］Zexie（泽泻，alisma，Rhizoma Alismatis) is added and boiled again to get 2. 5 *sheng*.［The decoction is］taken warm 8 *ge*［each time］and three times a day.

【原文】

(十九)

吐后渴欲得水而贪饮者,文蛤汤主之,兼主微风脉紧头痛。

文蛤汤方

文蛤(五两) 麻黄、甘草、生姜(各三两) 石膏(五两) 杏仁(五十枚) 大枣(十二枚)

右七味,以水六升,煮取二升。温服一升,汗出即愈。

【今译】

呕吐后口渴,想得水而且贪饮水的,宜用文蛤汤主治,兼治微受风邪侵袭,脉紧而头痛。

【原文】

(二十)

干呕吐逆,吐涎沫,半夏干姜散主之。

半夏干姜散方

半夏、干姜(各等分)

右二味,杵为散,取方寸匕,浆水一升半,煎取七合,顿服之。

【今译】

患者干呕,胃气上逆,吐涎沫,用半夏干姜散主治。

【英译】

Line 17. 19

[To treat] thirst with desire to drink water and drinking rapaciously after vomiting, Wenge Decoction (文蛤汤, meretrix clam shell decoction) should be used. [This decoction can] also treat tight pulse and headache [due to invasion of] mild wind.

Wenge Decoction (文蛤汤, meretrix clam shell decoction) [is composed of] 5 *liang* of Wenge (文蛤, meretrix clam shell, Concha Meretricis), 3 *liang* of Mahuang (麻黄, ephedra, Herba Ephedrae), 3 *liang* of Gancao (甘草, licorice, Radix Glycyrrhizae Praeparata), 3 *liang* of Shengjiang (生姜, fresh ginger, Rhizoma Zingiberis Recens), 5 *liang* of Shigao (石膏, gypsum, Gypsum Fibrosum), 50 pieces of Xingren (杏仁, apricot kernel, Semen Armeniacae Amarum) and 12 pieces of Dazao (大枣, jujube, Fructus Ziziphus Jujubae).

These seven ingredients are decocted in 6 *sheng* of water to get 2 *sheng* [after] boiling. [The decoction is] taken warm 1 *sheng* [each time]. [When there is] sweating, [it will be] cured.

【英译】

Line 17. 20

[To treat] dry retching, vomiting, counterflow [of stomach qi] and vomiting of drool and foam, Banxia Ganjiang Powder (半夏干姜散, pinellia and dried ginger powder) should be used.

Banxia Ganjiang Powder (半夏干姜散, pinellia and dried ginger powder) [is composed of] Banxia (半夏, pinellia, Rhizoma Pinelliae) and Ganjiang (干姜, dried ginger, Rhizoma Zingiberis) of the same amount.

These two ingredients are pounded into powder. And 1 *fangcunbi* is mixed with 1.5 *sheng* of water and boiled to get 7 *ge*. [It is] taken once the whole.

【原文】

（二十一）

病人胸中似喘不喘，似呕不呕，似哕不哕，彻心中愦愦然无奈者，生姜半夏汤主之。

生姜半夏汤方

半夏（半斤）　生姜汁（一升）

右二味，以水三升，煮半夏，取二升，内生姜汁，煮取一升半，小冷，分四服。日三、夜一服，止，停后服。

【今译】

病人胸中好像气喘，但实际上没有气喘，好像呕吐，但实际上没有呕吐，好像哕逆，但实际上没有哕逆。但患者心中烦闷懊恼得无可奈何，用生姜半夏汤主治。

【原文】

（二十二）

干呕，哕，若手足厥者，橘皮汤主之。

橘皮汤方

橘皮（四两）　生姜（半斤）

右二味，以水七升，煮取三升。温服一升，下咽即愈。

【今译】

患者干呕，哕逆，如果手足厥冷的，用橘皮汤主治。

【英译】

Line 17. 21

[In the patient], there seems to have panting in the chest but actually there is no panting, there seems to have retching but actually there is no retching but there seems to have hiccup but actually there is no hiccup. [But the patient feels] unbearably vexing and depressed in the heart. Shengjiang Banxia Decoction (生姜半夏汤, fresh ginger and pinellia decoction) [can be used] to treat it.

Shengjiang Banxia Decoction (生姜半夏汤, fresh ginger and pinellia decoction) [is composed of] 0. 5 *jin* of Banxia (半夏, pinellia, Rhizoma Pinelliae) and 1 *sheng* of Shengjiangzhi (生姜汁, fresh ginger juice, Rhizoma Zingiberis Recens).

These two ingredients are decocted in 3 *sheng* of water. Banxia (半夏, pinellia, Rhizoma Pinelliae) is boiled first to get 2 *sheng*. [Then] Shengjiangzhi (生姜汁, fresh ginger juice, Rhizoma Zingiberis Recens) is added to boil and get 1. 5 *sheng*. [After] cooling, [it is] divided into four [doses] and taken three in the daytime and one at night. Stop taking [the decoction when all the symptoms have] disappeared.

【英译】

Line 17. 22

[To treat] dry retching and hiccup, if there is reversal [cold of] hands and feet, Jupi Decoction (橘皮汤, tangerine peel decoction) should be used.

Jupi Decoction (橘皮汤, tangerine peel decoction) [is composed of] 4 *liang* of Jupi (橘皮, tangerine peel, Pericarpium Citri Reticulatae) and 0. 5 *jin* of Shengjiang (生姜, fresh ginger, Rhizoma Zingiberis Recens).

These two ingredients are decocted in 7 *sheng* of water to get 3 *sheng*. [The decoction is] taken warm 1 *sheng* [each time]. [When the patient is able to] swallow, [the disease is] about to cure.

【原文】

（二十三）

哕逆者,橘皮竹茹汤主之。

橘皮竹茹汤方

橘皮（二升）　竹茹（二升）　大枣（三十个）　生姜（半斤）　甘草（五两）　人参（一两）

右六味,以水一斗,煮取三升。温服一升,日三服。

【今译】

呃逆证患者,用橘皮竹茹汤主治。

【原文】

（二十四）

夫六腑气绝于外者,手足寒,上气脚缩;五脏气绝于内者,利不禁,下甚者,手足不仁。

【今译】

如果六腑气机衰竭于外,就会引发手足寒冷,气机上逆,下肢挛缩。如果五脏气机衰竭绝于内,下利难以制止,下利严重的,手足就会麻木不仁。

【英译】

Line 17.23

［To treat］hiccup，Jupi Zhuru Decoction （橘皮竹茹汤，tangerine peel and bamboo shavings decoction）should be used.

Jupi Zhuru Decoction（橘皮竹茹汤，tangerine peel and bamboo shavings decoction）［is composed of］2 *sheng* of Jupi （橘皮，tangerine peel，Pericarpium Citri Reticulatae），2 *sheng* of Zhuru （竹茹，bamboo shavings，Caulis Bambusae in Taenia），30 pieces of Dazao （大枣，jujube，Fructus Ziziphus Jujubae），0.5 *jin* of Shengjiang （生姜，fresh ginger，Rhizoma Zingiberis Recens），5 *liang* of Gancao （甘草，licorice，Radix Glycyrrhizae Praeparata） and 1 *liang* of Renshen（人参，ginseng，Radix Ginseng）.

These six ingredients are decocted in 1 *dou* of water to get 3 *sheng*.［The decoction is］taken warm 1 *sheng* ［each time］and three times a day.

【英译】

Line 17.24

Exhaustion of qi from the six fu-organs in the external ［is marked by］ cold of hands and feet，upward flow of qi and contraction of feet；exhaustion of qi from the five zang-organs in the internal ［is marked by］diarrhea difficult to cease and numbness of hands and feet if more serious.

【原文】

(二十五)

下利,脉沉弦者,下重;脉大者,为未止;脉微弱数者,为欲自止,虽发热不死。

【今译】

患下利的,脉象沉弦,里急后重;脉象大的,是下利没有停止;脉象微弱数的,说明下利将要自止,虽有发热症状,但不会导致死亡。

【原文】

(二十六)

下利,手足厥冷,无脉者,灸之不温。若脉不还,反微喘者,死。少阴负趺阳者,为顺也。

【今译】

患者下利,手足厥冷,诊不到脉象,使用灸法治疗后患者四肢依然不温。如果脉象也没有恢复,反而出现微喘症状,就会导致死亡。如果少阴脉小于趺阳脉,则为顺证。

【英译】

Line 17. 25

Diarrhea with sunken and taut pulse [indicates] tenesmus. Large pulse indicates [that diarrhea is] not ceased; faint, weak and rapid pulse indicates [that diarrhea is] about to cease. Although there is fever, [it is] not fatal.

【英译】

Line 17. 26

[In patients with] diarrhea, [there are symptoms and signs of] reversal cold of hands and feet and insensible pulse. Moxibustion is unable to warm [the limbs]. If the pulse is still insensible, and there appears slight panting, [it is] fatal. [If] shaoyin [pulse] is smaller than fuyang [pulse], it is favorable.

【原文】

(二十七)

下利,有微热而渴,脉弱者,今自愈。

【今译】

患者下利,有微热而口渴,脉象弱的,就将自愈。

【原文】

(二十八)

下利,脉数,有微热汗出,今自愈;设脉紧,为未解。

【今译】

患者下利,脉象数,有微热和汗出的,将自愈;如果脉象紧,说明其病未愈。

【原文】

(二十九)

下利,脉数而渴者,今自愈。设不差,必清脓血,以有热故也。

【今译】

患者下利,脉象数而口渴的,将自愈。如果病没有痊愈,大便必有脓血,因为有热所致。

Volume 2

【英译】

Line 17.27

[In patients with] diarrhea, [if there are manifestations of] slight heat, thirst and weak pulse, [it is] about to heal.

【英译】

Line 17.28

[In patients with] diarrhea, [if there are manifestations of] rapid pulse, slight heat and sweating, [it is] about to heal. If the pulse is tight, [it indicates that the disease is] not resolved.

【英译】

Line 17.29

[In patients with] diarrhea, [if there is] rapid pulse and thirst, [it is] about to heal. If [it is] not cured, there must be [stool with] pus and blood due to [accumulation of] heat.

【原文】

(三十)

下利,脉反弦,发热身汗者,自愈。

【今译】

患者下利,脉象反而弦,发热,身上出汗,病将自愈。

【原文】

(三十一)

下利气者,当利其小便。

【今译】

患者下利而矢气的,应当通过利小便的方法治疗。

【原文】

(三十二)

下利,寸脉反浮数,尺中自涩者,必清脓血。

【今译】

患者下利,寸脉反而浮数,尺中脉象自涩的,大便必有脓血。

Volume 2

【英译】

Line 17.30

[In patients with] diarrhea, [if there are manifestations of] taut pulse, fever and sweating, [it is] about to heal.

【英译】

Line 17.31

Diarrhea with [discharge of] flatus should [be treated by] promoting urination.

【英译】

Line 17.32

[In] diarrhea with floating and rapid pulse in the cun [region] and rough pulse in the chi [region], there must be [stool with] pus and blood.

【原文】

(三十三)

下利清谷,不可攻其表,汗出必胀满。

【今译】

患者下利清谷,不可用解表法强行发表,误发汗必然引起腹中胀满。

【原文】

(三十四)

下利,脉沉而迟,其人面少赤,身有微热,下利清谷者,必郁冒,汗出而解,病人必微热。所以然者,其面戴阳,下虚故也。

【今译】

患者下利,脉沉而迟,面色微有红赤,身上有微热,下利清谷的,必然郁闷头冒,如果发汗病情就能缓解,病人必有微热。之所以如此,是因为患者面部戴阳,下元虚冷所致。

Volume 2

【英译】

Line 17.33

[Patients suffering from] diarrhea with undigested food cannot [be treated by] attacking the external [because promoting] sweating will [cause abdominal] distension and fullness.

【英译】

Line 17.34

[In patients with] diarrhea [marked by] sunken and slow pulse, slightly reddish face, slight fever and watery defecation with undigested food, there must be depression and dizziness. [If there is] sweating, [it will be] resolved and the patient must have slight fever. The reason is that there is daiyang (red face as if decorated with rouge due to up-floating of yang) and deficiency in the lower [part of the body].

【原文】

(三十五)

下利后,脉绝,手足厥冷,晬时脉还,手足温者生,脉不还者死。

【今译】

下利之后,脉象诊查不到,手足厥冷,一昼夜之后脉象复还,手足温暖的可以治愈,脉象没有复还的,则会导致死亡。

【原文】

(三十六)

下利,腹胀满,身体疼痛者,先温其里,乃攻其表。温里宜四逆汤,攻表宜桂枝汤。

四逆汤方

桂枝汤方

桂枝(三两,去皮)　芍药(三两)　甘草(二两,炙)　生姜(三两)大枣(十二枚)

右五味,哎咀,以水七升,微火煮取三升,去滓。适寒温,服一升。服已须臾,啜稀粥一升,以助药力。温覆令一时许,遍身漐漐微似有汗者益佳,不可令如水淋漓。若一服汗出病差,停后服。

【今译】

患者下利,腹部胀满,身体疼痛的,应先温其里,再通过攻法治疗其表。温里宜用四逆汤,攻表宜用桂枝汤。

【英译】

Line 17.35

After diarrhea, the pulse is insensible, hands and feet are in reversal cold and the pulse returns overnight. [If] the hands and feet are warm, [it is] curable; [if] the pulse fails to return, [it is] fatal.

【英译】

Line 17.36

[Patients with] diarrhea, [accompanied by] abdominal distension and fullness and generalized pain [should be treated by] warming the internal first and then attacking the external. Sini Decoction (四逆汤, decoction for resolving four kinds of adverseness) [can be used] to warm the internal and Guizhi Decoction (桂枝汤, cinnamon twig decoction) [can be used] to attack the external.

Guizhi Decoction (桂枝汤, cinnamon twig decoction) [is composed of] 3 _liang_ of Guizhi (桂枝, cinnamon twig, Ramulus Cinnamomi)(remove the bark), 3 _liang_ of Shaoyao (芍药, peony, Radix Paeoniae), 2 _liang_ of Gancao (甘草, licorice, Radix Glycyrrhizae Praeparata)(broil), 3 _liang_ of Shengjiang (生姜, fresh ginger, Rhizoma Zingiberis Recens) and 12 pieces of Dazao (大枣, jujube, Fructus Ziziphus Jujubae).

These five ingredients are chewed and decocted in 7 _sheng_ of water to get 3 _sheng_ [after] boiling with mild fire. The dregs are removed. To adapt to cold and warm [temperature], 1 _sheng_ [of the decoction is] taken. After a while, 2 _sheng_ of porridge is taken to strengthen the effect of medicine. [Then the patient is] covered [with clothes or quilt] for about two hours [to induce] generalized slight sweating for better [treatment]. But the sweating should not be profuse. If the disease is cured [when there is] sweating after taking just one dose, stop taking the rest [doses].

【原文】

(三十七)

下利,三部脉皆平,按之心下坚者,急下之,宜大承气汤。

【今译】

患者下利,三部脉均属正常,用手按压心下,有坚硬之感,要急用下法治疗,宜用大承气汤主治。

【原文】

(三十八)

下利,脉迟而滑者,实也。利未欲止,急下之,宜大承气汤。

【今译】

患者下利,脉迟而滑的,属于实证。下利没有停止的,应急用下法治疗,宜用大承气汤主治。

【原文】

(三十九)

下利,脉反滑者,当有所去,下乃愈,宜大承气汤。

【今译】

患者下利,脉反而滑的,应当祛除实邪,用下法治疗,就可治愈,宜用大承气汤主治。

【英译】

Line 17.37

[In patients with] diarrhea，the pulses in three regions are normal and there is hardness below the heart when pressed，purgation [should be used] immediately [to treat it]. The appropriate [formula is] Da Chengqi Decoction（大承气汤，major decoction for harmonizing qi）.

【英译】

Line 17.38

Diarrhea with slow and slippery pulse [pertains to] excess [syndrome/pattern]. [If] diarrhea is not ceased，purgation [should be used] immediately. The appropriate [formula for treating it is] Da Chengqi Decoction（大承气汤，major decoction for harmonizing qi）.

【英译】

Line 17.39

[In] diarrhea with slippery pulse，[measures] should [be taken] to eliminate [pathogenic factors]. Purgation can cure [it]. The appropriate [formula for treating it is] Da Chengqi Decoction（大承气汤，major decoction for harmonizing qi）.

【原文】

(四十)

下利已差,至其年月日时复发者,以病不尽故也,当下之,宜大承气汤。

大承气汤方(见痉病中)

【今译】

下利已经治愈,但每年到了下利初发的年月日时,下利又复发,这是因为病邪没有完全祛除的缘故,应当用下法治疗,宜用大承气汤主治。

【原文】

(四十一)

下利,谵语者,有燥屎也,小承气汤主之。

小承气汤方

大黄(四两)　厚朴(二两,炙)　枳实(大者三枚,炙)

右三味,以水四升,煮取一升二合,去滓,分温二服。

【今译】

患者下利,有谵语,有燥屎的,宜用小承气汤主治。

【英译】

Line 17. 40

[Although] diarrhea is already ceased，[it] recurs every year in the time of its initial occurrence because [the disease is] not completely cured. Purgation can cure [it]. The appropriate [formula for treating it is] Da Chengqi Decoction (大承气汤，major decoction for harmonizing qi).

【英译】

Line 17. 41

Diarrhea with delirium and dry stool should be treated by Xiao Chengqi Decoction (小承气汤，minor decoction for harmonizing qi).

Xiao Chengqi Decoction (小承气汤，minor decoction for harmonizing qi) [is composed of] 4 *liang* of Dahuang (大黄，rhubarb，Radix et Rhizoma Rhei)，2 *liang* of Houpo (厚朴，magnolia bark，Cortex Magnoliae Officinalis)(broil) and 3 pieces of big Zhishi (枳实，processed unripe bitter orange，Fructus Aurantii Immaturus)(broil).

These three ingredients are decocted in 4 *sheng* of water to get 1 *sheng* and 2 *ge*. The dregs are removed and [the decoction is] divided into two [doses] and taken warm.

【原文】

(四十二)

下利,便脓血者,桃花汤主之。

桃花汤方

赤石脂(一斤,一半剉,一半筛末)　干姜(一两)　粳米(一升)

右三味,以水七升,煮米令熟,去滓,温七合,内赤石脂末方寸匕。

日三服,若一服愈,余勿服。

【今译】

患者下利,大便有脓血的,宜用桃花汤主治。

【原文】

(四十三)

热利下重者,白头翁汤主之。

白头翁汤方

白头翁(二两)　黄连、黄柏、秦皮(各三两)

右四味,以水七升,煮取二升,去滓。温服一升,不愈更服。

【今译】

湿热下利,里急后重的患者,宜用白头翁汤主治。

【英译】

Line 17.42

Diarrhea [accompanied by] stool with pus and blood [can be] treated by Taohua Decoction (桃花汤，peach blossom decoction).

Taohua Decoction （桃花汤，peach blossom decoction） [is composed of] 1 *jin* of Chishizhi (赤石脂，halloysite，Halloysitum Rubrum)（half is grated and half is sieved），1 *liang* of Ganjiang（干姜，dried ginger，Rhizoma Zingiberis) and 1 *sheng* of Jingmi（粳米，polished round-grained rice，Semen Oryzae Nonglutinosae).

These three ingredients are decocted in 7 *sheng* of water and the rice is cooked well. The dregs are removed and 7 *ge* [is taken] warm added with 1 *fangcunbi* of Chishizhi (赤石脂，halloysite，Halloysitum Rubrum)，three times a day. If [the disease is] cured [after] taking one [dose]，the rest [doses] should not be taken.

【英译】

Line 17.43

Diarrhea with [dampness-] heat and tenesmus should be treated by Baitouweng Decoction (白头翁汤，pulsatilla decoction).

Baitouweng Decoction （白头翁汤，pulsatilla decoction） [is composed of] 2 *liang* of Baitouweng (白头翁，pulsatilla，Radix Pulsatillae)，3 *liang* of Huanglian （黄连，coptis，Rhizoma Coptidis)，3 *liang* of Huangbo （黄柏，phellodendron，Cortex Phellodendri) and 3 *liang* of Qinpi (秦皮，ash，Cortex Fraxini).

These four ingredients are decocted in 7 *sheng* of water to get 2 *sheng* [after] boiling. The dregs are removed and [the decoction is] taken warm 1 *sheng* [each time]. [If it is] not cured，one more [dose] should be taken.

【原文】

(四十四)

下利后更烦,按之心下濡者,为虚烦也,栀子豉汤主之。

栀子豉汤方

豉子(十四枚)　香豉(四合,绵裹)

右二味,以水四升,先煮栀子,得二升半,内豉,煮取一升半,去滓。分二服,温进一服,得吐则止。

【今译】

患者下利后更烦躁的,按压心下感到濡软的,为虚烦之症,宜用栀子豉汤主治。

【原文】

(四十五)

下利清谷,里寒外热,汗出而厥者,通脉四逆汤主之。

通脉四逆汤方

附子(大者一枚,生用)　干姜(三两,强人可四两)　甘草(二两,炙)

右三味,以水三升,煮取一升二合,去滓,分温再服。

【今译】

患者下利清谷,里寒外热,汗出而四肢厥冷的,宜用通脉四逆汤主治。

Volume 2

【英译】

Line 17.44

After diarrhea, [there is] more serious vexation and soft [lump] below the heart when pressed, indicating deficiency-vexation. Zhizi Chi Decoction (栀子豉汤, gardenia and fermented soybean decoction) [can be used] to treat it.

Zhizi Chi Decoction (栀子豉汤, gardenia and fermented soybean decoction) [is composed of] 14 pieces of Zhizi (栀子, gardenia, Fructus Gardeniae) and 4 ge of Xiangchi (香豉, fermented soybean, Sojae Semen Fermentatum)(wrap in the gauze).

These two ingredients are decocted in 4 *sheng* of water. Zhizi (栀子, gardenia, Fructus Gardeniae) is boiled first to get 2 *sheng*. [Then] Chi (豉, fermented soybean, Sojae Semen Fermentatum) is added to boil and get 1.5 *sheng*. The dregs are removed and [the decoction is] divided into two [doses] and taken warm 1 [dose each time]. [When] vomiting is induced, stop [taking the decoction].

【英译】

Line 17.45

Diarrhea with undigested food, [accompanied by] internal cold, external heat, sweating and reversal [cold of limbs], [can be] treated by Tongmai Sini Decoction (通脉四逆汤, decoction for freeing vessels and resolving four kinds of adverseness).

Tongmai Sini Decoction (通脉四逆汤, decoction for freeing vessels and resolving four kinds of adverseness) [is composed of] 1 big piece of Fuzi (附子, aconite, Radix Aconiti Lateralis Preparata) (raw), 3 *liang* of Ganjiang (干姜, dried ginger, Rhizoma Zingiberis)(4 *liang* for strong patients) and 2 *liang* of Gancao (甘草, licorice, Radix Glycyrrhizae Praeparata)(broil).

These three ingredients are decocted in 3 *sheng* of water to get 1 *sheng* and 2 *ge* [after] boiling. The dregs are removed and [the decoction is] divided into two [doses] and taken warm.

【原文】

(四十六)

下利,肺痛,紫参汤主之。

紫参汤方

紫参(半斤) 甘草(三两)

右二味,以水五升,先煮紫参,取二升,内甘草,煮取一升半,分温三服。

【今译】

患者下利,肺部疼痛的,宜用紫参汤主治。

【原文】

(四十七)

气利,诃梨勒散主之。

诃梨勒散方

诃梨勒(十枚,煨)

右一味,为散,粥饮和,顿服。

【今译】

患者下利并伴有矢气的,宜用诃梨勒散主治。

【英译】

Line 17. 46

Diarrhea with lung pain ［should be］ treated by Zishen Decoction（紫参汤，bistort rhizome decoction）.

Zishen Decoction（紫参汤，bistort rhizome decoction）［is composed of］0.5 *jin* of Zishen（紫参，bistort rhizome，Rhizoma Bistortae）and 3 *liang* of Gancao（甘草，licorice，Radix Glycyrrhizae Praeparata）.

These two ingredients are decocted in 5 *sheng* of water. Zishen（紫参，bistort rhizome，Rhizoma Bistortae）is boiled first to get 2 *sheng*.［Then］Gancao（甘草，licorice，Radix Glycyrrhizae Praeparata）is added to boil and get 1.5 *sheng*.［The decoction is］divided into three［doses］and taken warm.

【英译】

Line 17. 47

Diarrhea with flatus［should be］treated by Helile Powder（诃梨勒散，chebule powder）.

Helile Powder（诃梨勒散，chebule powder）［is composed of］10 pieces of Helile（诃梨勒，chebule，Fructus Chebulae）(roast).

This ingredient is pounded into powder and taken with porridge once the whole.

附方

【原文】

《千金翼》小承气汤　治大便不通,哕数,谵语。

《外台》黄芩汤　治干呕下利。

黄芩　人参　干姜(各三两)　桂枝(一两)　大枣(十二枚)　半夏(半升)

右六味,以水七升,煮取三升,温分三服。

【今译】

《千金翼》中的小承气汤：用以治疗大便不通,呃逆频数,有谵语。

《外台秘要》中的黄芩汤：用以治疗干呕下利。

Appended formula

【英译】

Xiao Chengqi Decoction（小承气汤，minor decoction for harmonizing qi）［from the book entitled］ *Qianjin Yifang* (《千金翼方》, *Supplemented Thousand Golden Formulas*)：For treating inhibited defecation, hiccup and frequent delirium.

Huangqin Decoction（黄芩汤，scutellaria decoction）［from the book entitled］ *Waitai Miyao* (《外台秘要》, *The Medical Secrets of an Official Named Wang Tao*)：For treating dry retching and diarrhea.

Huangqin Decoction （黄芩汤，scutellaria decoction）［is composed of］ 3 *liang* of Huangqin（黄芩，scutellaria，Radix Scutellariae），3 *liang* of Renshen（人参，ginseng，Radix Ginseng），3 *liang* of Ganjiang（干姜，dried ginger，Rhizoma Zingiberis），1 *liang* of Guizhi（桂枝，cinnamon twig，Ramulus Cinnamomi），12 pieces of Dazao（大枣，jujube，Fructus Ziziphus Jujubae）and 0.5 *sheng* of Banxia（半夏，pinellia，Rhizoma Pinelliae）.

These six ingredients are decocted in 7 *sheng* of water to get 3 *sheng* ［after］ boiling. ［The decoction is］ divided into three ［doses］ and taken warm.

疮痈肠痈浸淫病脉证并治第十八

【原文】

(一)

诸浮数脉,应当发热,而反洒淅恶寒,若有痛处,当发其痈。

【今译】

凡是脉象浮的,都应发热,如今反而洒洒淅淅的有恶寒症状,如果有疼痛之处,应当发生痈肿。

【原文】

(二)

师曰:诸痈肿,欲知有脓无脓,以手掩肿上,热者为有脓,不热者为无脓。

【今译】

老师说:大凡痈肿,要想知道有脓无脓的情况,用手按压痈肿之上,热的为有脓,不热的为无脓。

Chapter 18
Sores, Abscess, Intestinal Abscess and Dampness Spreading Disease: Pulses, Syndromes/Patterns and Treatment

【英译】

Line 18. 1

[Patients with] floating and rapid pulse should have fever, but now [there is] aversion to cold [as if] soaking [in cold water]. If there is pain, abscess must occur.

【英译】

Line 18. 2

The master said: [In] all [cases of] abscess and swelling, [if one] wants to know whether there is pus, [he can] press the swollen [area] with hand. [If it is] hot, there is pus; [if it is] not hot, there is no pus.

【原文】

（三）

肠痈之为病，其身甲错，腹皮急，按之濡，如肿状，腹无积聚，身无热，脉数，此为腹内有痈脓，薏苡附子败酱散主之。

薏苡附子败酱散方

薏苡仁（十分）　附子（二分）　败酱（五分）

右三味，杵为末，取方寸匕，以水二升，煎减半，顿服。小便当下。

【今译】

患肠痈的病人，肌肤甲错，腹部皮肤急拘，按之感觉濡软，但又有肿胀之相，腹中并无积聚僵硬之处，身上无热，脉象数，这种情况属于腹内有痈脓，用薏苡附子败酱散主治。

【英译】

Line 18.3

Disease with intestinal abscess [is characterized by] squamous skin, tension of abdominal skin, softness like swelling when pressed, no accumulation in the abdomen, no generalized fever and rapid pulse, indicating abscess and pus in the abdomen. Yiyi Fuzi Baijiang Powder (薏苡附子败酱散, coix, aconite and patrinia powder) [can be used] to treat it.

Yiyi Fuzi Baijiang Powder (薏苡附子败酱散, coix, aconite and patrinia powder) [is composed of] 10 *fen* of Yiyiren (薏苡仁, coix, Semen Coicis), 2 *fen* of Fuzi (附子, aconite, Radix Aconiti Lateralis Preparata) and 5 *fen* of Baijiang (败酱, patrinia, Herba Patriniae).

These three ingredients are pounded into powder. 1 *fangcunbi* is put into 2 *sheng* of water to boil and reduce half. [It should be] taken once the whole. [After taking the powder], urine will be discharged.

【原文】

(四)

肠痈者,少腹肿痞,按之即痛,如淋,小便自调,时时发热,自汗出,复恶寒。其脉迟紧者,脓未成,可下之,当有血。脉洪数者,脓已成,不可下也。大黄牡丹汤主之。

大黄牡丹汤方

大黄(四两)　牡丹(一两)　桃仁(五十个)　瓜子(半升)　芒硝(三合)

右五味,以水六升,煮取一升,去滓,内芒硝,再煎沸。顿服之,有脓当下,如无脓,当下血。

【今译】

有肠痈的患者,少腹肿胀痞满,按压时感到疼痛,好像有淋病一样,但小便还是正常的,患者时时发热,汗自出,又有恶寒之感。脉象迟紧,说明脓还未形成,可通过下法治疗,大便时应当有污血随之排出。脉象洪数的,说明脓已形成,就不可用下法治疗。宜用大黄牡丹汤主治。

【原文】

(五)

问曰:寸口脉浮微而涩,法当亡血,若汗出,设不汗者云何? 答曰:若身有疮,被刀斧所伤,亡血故也。

【今译】

问:寸口脉象浮微而涩,应当属于亡血,应当有汗出,如果没有出汗,属于什么原因呢?

答:如果患者身上有疮,应当是因刀斧所伤而失血。

Volume 2

【英译】

Line 18.4

[In] patients with intestinal abscess, there is swelling and lump in the lower abdomen and [there will be] pain like strangury when pressed, [but] urination is normal. [In addition, there are symptoms and signs of] frequent fever, spontaneous sweating and aversion to cold again. [If] the pulse is slow and tight, [it indicates that] pus is not formed yet. [When] purgation is used, there will be blood [in stool]. [If] the pulse is surging and rapid, [it indicates that] pus is already formed, [but] cannot [be treated by] purgation. Dahuang Mudan Decoction (大黄牡丹汤, rhubarb and moutan decoction) [can be used] to treat it.

Dahuang Mudan Decoction (大黄牡丹汤, rhubarb and moutan decoction) [is composed of] 4 *liang* of Dahuang (大黄, rhubarb, Radix et Rhizoma Rhei), 1 *liang* of Mudan (牡丹, moutan, Cortex Moutan Radicis), 50 pieces of Taoren (桃仁, peach kernel, Semen Persicae), 0.5 *sheng* of Guazi (瓜子, wax gourd seed, Semen Benincasae) and 3 *ge* of Mangxiao (芒硝, mirabilite, Mirabilitum).

These five ingredients are decocted in 6 *sheng* of water to get 1 *sheng* [after] boiling. The dregs are removed and Mangxiao (芒硝, mirabilite, Mirabilitum) is added to boil again. [The decoction is] taken once the whole. [If] there is pus, [it] should [be] purged [through defecation]; if there is no pus, there will be blood [in stool].

【英译】

Line 18.5

Question: The pulse in the cunkou [region] is floating, faint and rough. [In such a case] there should be collapse of blood and sweating. But there is [in fact] no sweating. What is the reason?

Answer: If there is wound in the body, [it is] injured by a knife or an axe. That is why [there is] collapse of blood.

【原文】

（六）

病金疮，王不留行散主之。

王不留行散方

王不留行（十分，八月八日采）　蒴藋细叶（十分，七月七日采）　桑东南根（白皮，十分，三月三日采）　甘草（十八分）　川椒（三分，除目及闭口者，去汗）　黄芩（二分）　干姜（二分）　芍药（二分）　厚朴（二分）

右九味，桑根皮以上三味烧灰存性，勿令灰过，各别杵筛，合治之为散，服方寸匕。小疮即粉之，大疮但服之，产后亦可服。如风寒，桑东根勿取之。前三物皆阴干百日。

排脓散方

枳实（十六枚）　芍药（六分）　桔梗（二分）

右三味，杵为散，取鸡子黄一枚，以药散与鸡黄相等，揉和令相得。饮和服之，日一服。

排脓汤方

甘草（二两）　桔梗（三两）　生姜（一两）　大枣（十枚）

右四味，以水三升，煮取一升。温服五合，日再服。

【英译】

Line 18.6

Disease [caused by] wound [due to injury of] knife should be treated by Wangbuliuxing Powder (王不留行散, vaccaria powder).

Wangbuliuxing Powder (王不留行散, vaccaria powder)

Wangbuliuxing Powder （王不留行散, vaccaria powder）[is composed of] 10 *fen* of Wangbuliuxing (王不留行, vaccaria, Semen Vaccariae)（collected on August eighth）, 10 *fen* of Zhuodiaoxiye (蒴藋细叶, fine elder leaves, Folium Sambucus Chinensis)（collected on July seventh）, 10 *fen* of Sangdongnan'gen (桑东南根, mulberry root bark, Cortex Moutan Radicis)（white bark, collected on the third of Mary）, 18 *fen* of Gancao （甘草, licorice, Radix Glycyrrhizae Praeparata）, 3 *fen* of Chuanjiao (川椒, zanthoxylum, Pericarpium Zanthoxyli Praeparata)（remove the seeds and closed husks）, 2 *fen* of Huangqin (黄芩, scutellaria, Radix Scutellariae), 2 *fen* of Ganjiang (干姜, dried ginger, Rhizoma Zingiberis), 2 *fen* of Shaoyao (芍药, peony, Radix Paeoniae) and 2 *fen* of Houpo (厚朴, magnolia bark, Cortex Magnoliae Officinalis).

Among these nine ingredients, the first three above Sangdongnan'gen （桑东南根, mulberry root bark, Cortex Moutan Radicis) are burnt into ash with properties kept. The ash is sieved and blended into powder, 1 *fangcunbi* is taken [each time]. For mild wound, the powder [can be applied to the affected] region; for severe wound, [the powder is] taken orally. [Women] also can take [the powder] after childbirth. If [there is] wind cold, Sangdongnan'gen (桑东南根, mulberry root bark, Cortex Moutan Radicis) should be removed. [Before application,] the first three ingredients [should be] placed in a shady place to dry for one hundred days.

【今译】

因金刃所伤而引起的病患，宜用王不留行散主治。

Volume 2

Painong Powder（排脓散，powder for expelling pus）

Painong Powder（排脓散，powder for expelling pus）［is composed of］16 pieces of Zhishi（枳实，processed unripe bitter orange，Fructus Aurantii Immaturus），6 *fen* of Shaoyao（芍药，peony，Radix Paeoniae）and 2 *fen* of Jiegeng（桔梗，platycodon grandiflorum，Radix Platycodi）.

These three ingredients are pounded into powder. One Jizihuang（鸡子黄，egg yolk，Galli Vitellus）is blended with an equal amount of powder，mixed thoroughly. ［The powder is］taken with water once a day.

Painong Decoction（排脓汤，decoction for expelling pus）

Painong Decoction（排脓汤，decoction for expelling pus）［is composed of］2 *liang* of Gancao（甘草，licorice，Radix Glycyrrhizae Praeparata），3 *liang* of Jiegeng（桔梗，platycodon grandiflorum，Radix Platycodi），1 *liang* of Shengjiang（生姜，fresh ginger，Rhizoma Zingiberis Recens）and 10 pieces of Dazao（大枣，jujube，Fructus Ziziphus Jujubae）.

These four ingredients are decocted in 3 *sheng* of water to get 1 *sheng* ［after］boiling. ［The decoction is］taken warm 5 *ge* ［each time］and twice a day.

【原文】

（七）

浸淫疮，从口流向四肢者可治，从四肢流来入口者不可治。

【今译】

浸淫疮之病，从口腔流向四肢的，可以治疗，从四肢流向口腔的，难以治疗。

【原文】

（八）

浸淫疮，黄连粉主之。

【今译】

浸淫疮之病，宜用黄连粉主治。

【英译】

Line 18.7

Excessive wet sore (acute eczema) flowing from the mouth to the four limbs is curable, [but] flowing from the four limbs to the mouth is incurable.

【英译】

Line 18.8

For excessive wet sore (acute eczema), Huanglian Powder (黄连粉, coptis powder) [is the appropriate formula for] treating it.

趺蹶手指臂肿转筋阴狐疝蛔虫病脉证治第十九

【原文】

（一）

师曰：病趺蹶，其人但能前，不能却，刺腨入二寸，此太阳经伤也。

【今译】

老师说：患趺蹶病的人，只能向前行走，不能往后退，治疗时可针刺小腿肚上的穴位，刺入二寸。这种病是太阳经伤所致。

【原文】

（二）

病人常以手指臂肿动，此人身体瞤瞤者，藜芦甘草汤主之。

藜芦甘草汤方：方未见。

【今译】

病人时常出现手指手臂肿胀颤动，其身体肌肉也因牵引而有微微颤动之相，宜用藜芦甘草汤主治。

藜芦甘草汤方：此方未见。

Volume 2

Chapter 19
Fujue (Hobbled Dorsum of Foot), Swelling of Fingers and Arms, Spasm of Sinews, Inguinal Hernia and Roundworm Disease: Pulses, Syndromes/Patterns and Treatment

【英译】

Line 19.1

The master said: [The patient] suffering from fujue (hobbled dorsum of foot) is able to walk forward, [but] not backward. [It can be treated by] inserting [a needle to a depth of] 2 *cun* [into the acupoint located in] the calf. Such [a disease is caused by] damage of taiyang meridian.

【英译】

Line 19.2

The patient frequently suffers from swelling of fingers and arms with twitching of the body. Lilu Gancao Decoction (藜芦甘草汤，veratrum and licorice decoction) [can be used] to treat it.

Lilu Gancao Decoction (藜芦甘草汤，veratrum and licorice decoction) is not found yet.

【原文】

（三）

转筋之为病，其人臂脚直，脉上下行，微弦。转筋入腹者，鸡屎白散主之。

鸡屎白散方

鸡屎白

右一味，为散，取方寸匕，以水六合和，温服。

【今译】

患有转筋之病的人，其上臂或脚强直，脉象上下跳动有力，或略有微弦之感。转筋引起的疼痛牵引到腹部的，宜用鸡屎白散主治。

【原文】

（四）

阴狐疝气者，偏有小大，时时上下，蜘蛛散主之。

蜘蛛散方

蜘蛛（十四枚，熬焦） 桂枝（半两）

右二味，为散，取八分一匕，饮和服，日再服。蜜丸亦可。

【今译】

阴狐疝气之病，阴囊一边小一边大，时上时下，宜用蜘蛛散主治。

Volume 2

【英译】

Line 19.3

[In the patient with] cramping disease, the arms and legs are stiff, the pulse moves up and down [or appears] faint and taut. [When pain caused by] cramping stretches to the abdomen, Jishibai Powder (鸡屎白散, chicken's white excrement powder) [can be used] to treat it.

Jishibai Powder (鸡屎白散, chicken's white excrement powder) [is only composed of] Jishibai (鸡屎白, chicken's white excrement, Album Galli Excrementum).

This ingredient is ground into powder. 1 *fangcunbi* is blended with 6 *ge* of water. [The powder is] taken warm.

【英译】

Line 19.4

[In] fox-like-hernia (hernia like a fox running upward and downward) disease, [the scrotum is] distorted either small or large, either upward or downward. [It should be] treated by Zhizhu Powder (蜘蛛散, spider powder).

Zhizhu Powder (蜘蛛散, spider powder) [is composed of] 14 pieces of Zhizhu (蜘蛛, spider, Aranea)(simmer and scorch)and 0.5 *liang* of Guizhi (桂枝, cinnamon twig, Ramulus Cinnamomi).

These two ingredients are ground into powder and [per dose] is 8 *fen*. [The powder is] mixed with water and taken twice a day. [It] can also [be made into] pills with honey.

【原文】

（五）

问曰：病腹痛有虫，其脉何以别之？师曰：腹中痛，其脉当沉，若弦，反洪大，故有蛔虫。

【今译】

问：病人腹痛且有虫，其脉象如何鉴别呢？

老师说：腹部疼痛，其脉象应当沉，或者弦，如今反而洪大，这就是因为有蛔虫的缘故。

【原文】

（六）

蛔虫之为病，令人吐涎，心痛，发作有时，毒药不止，甘草粉蜜汤主之。

甘草粉蜜汤方

甘草（二两）　粉（一两）　蜜（四两）

右三味，以水三升，先煮甘草，取二升，去滓，内粉、蜜，搅令和，煎如薄粥。温服一升，差即止。

【今译】

蛔虫病，使患者吐涎，心痛，发作有时，用杀虫的毒药无法治愈时，用甘草粉蜜汤主治。

Volume 2

【英译】

Line 19.5

Question: [When a patient] suffers from abdominal pain with worms, how to differentiate the pulse?

The master said: [In a patient with] abdominal pain, the pulse should be sunken or taut, but [now it is] surging and large because there is roundworm [in the abdomen].

【英译】

Line 19.6

The disease caused by roundworms [is marked by] vomiting of drool and pain in the heart occurring intermittently. [It] cannot be stopped [by applying] toxic medicinals [for killing roundworms]. Gancao Fenmi Decoction (甘草粉蜜汤, licorice, processed galenite and honey decoction) [can be used] to treat it.

Gancao Fenmi Decoction (甘草粉蜜汤, licorice, processed galenite and honey decoction) [is composed of] 2 *liang* of Gancao (甘草, licorice, Radix Glycyrrhizae Praeparata), 1 *liang* of Fen (粉, processed galenite, Galenitum Praeparatum) and 4 *liang* of Mi (蜜, honey, Mel).

These three ingredients are decocted in 3 *sheng* of water. Gancao (甘草, licorice, Radix Glycyrrhizae Praeparata) is boiled first to get 2 *sheng*. The dregs are removed, Fen (粉, processed galenite, Galenitum Praeparatum) and Mi (蜜, honey, Mel) are added to blend with each other and boil like thin porridge. [The decoction is] taken warm 1 *sheng* [each time]. [When the disease is] cured, stop [taking the decoction].

【原文】

（七）

蛔厥者，当吐蛔。令病者静而复时烦，此为脏寒，蛔上入膈，故烦。须臾复止，得食而呕，又烦者，蛔闻食臭出，其人当自吐蛔。

【今译】

患蛔厥病的人，应当吐蛔。如今患者虽然心静，但却时时有烦躁之感，这是内脏虚寒所致，蛔虫上扰入胸膈，所以就引起患者烦躁。但烦躁之感很快就会停止，饮食时又出现呕吐和烦躁现象，这是因为蛔虫闻到食味而上扰，所以使患者吐出蛔虫。

【原文】

（八）

蛔厥者，乌梅丸主之。

乌梅丸方

乌梅（三百个）　细辛（六两）　干姜（十两）　黄连（一斤）　当归（四两）　附子（六两，炮）　川椒（四两，去汗）　桂枝（六两）　人参（六两）　黄柏（六两）

右十味，异捣筛，合治之，以苦酒渍乌梅一宿，去核，蒸之五升米下，饭熟，捣成泥，和药令相得，内臼中，与蜜杵二千下，丸如梧子大。先食，饮服十丸，三服，稍加至二十丸。禁生冷滑臭等食。

【今译】

蛔厥病，用乌梅丸主治。

Volume 3

【英译】

Line 19. 7

[The patient suffering from] roundworm reversal [disease] (reversal cold of the four limbs due to acute abdominal pain caused by roundworm disease) should vomit roundworms. Now the patient is quiet, but sometimes is vexing due to cold in the viscera [caused by] roundworms entering the diaphragm. That is why [there is] vexation. After a while, [vexation] stops. [However, when] taking [food], [there is] retching and vexation again [because] roundworms smell food [and move upward]. [That is why] the patient spontaneously vomit roundworms.

【英译】

Line 19. 8

Roundworm reversal [disease] is treated by Wumei Pill (乌梅丸, mume pill).

Wumei Pill (乌梅丸, mume pill) [is composed of] 300 pieces of Wumei (乌梅, mume, Fructus Mume), 6 *liang* of Xixin (细辛, asarum, Herba Asari), 10 *liang* of Ganjiang (干姜, dried ginger, Rhizoma Zingiberis), 1 *jin* of Huanglian (黄连, coptis, Rhizoma Coptidis), 4 *liang* of Danggui (当归, Chinese angelica, Radix Angelicae Sinensis), 6 *liang* of Fuzi (附子, aconite, Radix Aconiti Lateralis Preparata)(fry heavily), 4 *liang* of Chuanjiao (川椒, zanthoxylum, Pericarpium Zanthoxyli Praeparata)(remove sweat), 6 *liang* of Guizhi (桂枝, cinnamon twig, Ramulus Cinnamomi), 6 *liang* of Renshen (人参, ginseng, Radix Ginseng) and 6 *liang* of Huangbo (黄柏, phellodendron, Cortex Phellodendri).

These ten ingredients are ground and sieved to blend with each other. Wumei (乌梅, mume, Fructus Mume) is soaked in vinegar overnight. [After] removal of pits, [it is] steamed in 5 *sheng* of rice. [When] the rice is well cooked, [it is] crushed into paste and blended with other ingredients. [It is] placed in a jar with some honey and pounded for two thousand times to form pills the size of firmiana seeds. Before eating, 10 pills are taken with water and three times a day. [The dosage can be] gradually increased to 20 pills. [It is] forbidden to take cold, slippery and fetid foods.

卷下

妇人妊娠病脉证并治第二十

【原文】

（一）

师曰：妇人得平脉，阴脉小弱，其人渴，不能食，无寒热，名妊娠，桂枝汤主之。于法六十日当有此证，设有医治逆者，却一月加吐下者，则绝之。

【今译】

老师说：通过诊断发现妇女的脉象如常人一样平和，只有阴脉（即尺部之脉）小而弱，口渴，不能饮食，无恶寒发热现象，这就是妊娠，宜用桂枝汤主治。按常规，怀孕六十日内应当有这种情况的出现，如果医治不当，迁延一月未解，呕吐下利加剧，应采取措施予以解除。

Volume 3

Chapter 20
Women's Pregnancy Disease:
Pulses, Syndromes/Patterns and Treatment

【英译】

Line 20. 1

The master said: [Diagnosis shows that] a woman's pulse is normal, [but] the yin pulse (the pulse in the chi region) is small and weak, [accompanied by] thirst, inability to eat, no aversion to cold and no heat. [Such a condition is] known as pregnancy [and can be] treated by Guizhi Decoction (桂枝汤, cinnamon twig decoction). There is such a syndrome/pattern sixty days [after pregnancy]. If [it is] not well treated and continues for one month, [there will be] vomiting and diarrhea. [Measures should be taken] to eliminate it.

【原文】

（二）

妇人宿有症病，经断未及三月，而得漏下不止，胎动在脐上者，为症痼害。妊娠六月动者，前三月经水利时，胎也。下血者，后断三月衃也。所以血不止者，其症不去故也。当下其症，桂枝茯苓丸主之。

桂枝茯苓丸方

桂枝　茯苓　牡丹（去心）　桃仁（去皮尖，熬）　芍药（各等分）

右五味，末之，炼蜜和丸，如兔屎大。每日食前服一丸，不知，加至三丸。

【今译】

妇人素有此种症积之病，月经停止未及三月，又下血淋漓不止，好像脐上有胎动，这是症积之病危害所致。妊娠六个月时有胎动，怀孕前三月月经正常，属于怀胎。停经时月经失调，时有下血，停经后三个月又下衃血。所以下血不止的，是症病没有除去的缘故。应当采取措施攻下症病，用桂枝茯苓丸主治。

Volume 3

【英译】

Line 20.2

Woman always suffers from accumulation disease（blood stasis accumulating in the abdomen and binding into lump）. Less than three months ［after interruption of］ menstruation, vaginal bleeding is incessant and a sensation ［felt］ above the umbilicus like fetus stirring. ［This is caused by］ damage of accumulation and lump. ［After］ six months of pregnancy, ［there is］ movement of fetus. In the previous three months before pregnancy, menstruation is normal and pregnancy is ready. ［After menstruation has ceased, there is］ vaginal bleeding occasionally. Three months later ［there is］ coagulated blood due to failure to eliminate accumulation ［of blood stasis］. Such a disease ［should be］ treated by Guizhi Fuling Pill（桂枝茯苓丸, cinnamon twig and poria pill）.

Guizhi Fuling Pill（桂枝茯苓丸, cinnamon twig and poria pill）［is composed of］ Guizhi（桂枝, cinnamon twig, Ramulus Cinnamomi）, Fuling（茯苓, poria, Poria）, Mudan（牡丹, moutan, Cortex Moutan Radicis）（remove the center）, Taoren（桃仁, peach kernel, Semen Persicae）（remove the bark and tips, simmer）and Shaoyao（芍药, peony, Radix Paeoniae）of the same amount.

These five ingredients are ground into powder and blended with Lianmi（炼蜜, processed honey, Mel Praeparatum）to form pills, the size of rabbit droppings. Every day before eating, 1 pill is taken. ［If there is］ no effect, ［the dosage can be］ increased to 3 pills ［per dose］.

【原文】

(三)

妇人怀娠六七月,脉弦发热,其胎愈胀,腹痛恶寒者,少腹如扇。所以然者,子脏开故也,当以附子汤温其脏。

方未见。

【今译】

妇人怀娠六七个月,脉象弦而发热,胎气更加膨胀,腹部疼痛恶寒,就像扇冷风入少腹一样。之所以如此,是由于子脏开启的原因,应当以附子汤温暖子脏。

此方未曾见到。

【原文】

(四)

师曰:妇人有漏下者,有半产后因续下血都不绝者,有妊娠下血者。假令妊娠腹中痛,为胞阻,胶艾汤主之。

芎归胶艾汤方

芎䓖　阿胶　甘草(各二两)　艾叶　当归(各三两)　芍药(四两)　干地黄(四两)

右七味,以水五升,清酒三升,合煮,取三升,去滓,内胶,令消尽。温服一升,日三服,不差更作。

【今译】

老师说:妇人有下漏血液的,有因小产后继续下血不止的缘故,有因妊娠而下血的缘。假如妊娠后腹中疼痛,是因为胞阻的缘故,宜用胶艾汤主治。

【英译】

Line 20.3

[In] a woman, six or seven months [after] pregnancy, [there are symptoms and signs of] taut pulse, fetal distension, abdominal pain, aversion to cold and the lower abdomen seeming to be fanned. The reason is that the fetal viscus (uterus) is open. Fuzi Decoction (附子汤, aconite decoction) [can be used] to warm the fetal viscus (uterus).

【英译】

Line 20.4

The master said: [In] a woman there is vaginal spotting [because of] incessant vaginal bleeding after miscarriage. There is same problem after pregnancy. If there is abdominal pain after pregnancy, [it is caused by] uterine obstruction. Jiaoai Decoction (胶艾汤, ass hide glue and mugwort decoction) [can be used] to treat it.

Xionggui Jiaoai Decoction (芎归胶艾汤, xiongqiong, Chinese angelica, ass-hide glue and mugwort decoction) [is composed of] 2 *liang* of Xiongqiong (芎莠, xiongqiong, Rhizoma Chuanxiong), 2 *liang* of Ejiao (阿胶, ass-hide glue, Colla Corii Asini), 2 *liang* of Gancao (甘草, licorice, Radix Glycyrrhizae Praeparata), 3 *liang* of Aiye (艾叶, mugwort, Folium Artemisiae Argyi), 3 *liang* of Danggui (当归, Chinese angelica, Radix Angelicae Sinensis), 4 *liang* of Shaoyao (芍药, peony, Radix Paeoniae) and 4 *liang* of Gandihuang (干地黄, dried rehmannia, Radix Rehmanniae).

These seven ingredients are decocted in 5 *sheng* of water and 3 *sheng* of clear wine to get 3 *sheng* [after] boiling. The dregs are removed and [the decoction is] taken warm 1 *sheng* [each time] and three times a day. [If the disease is] not cured, [the treatment should be] repeated.

【原文】

（五）

妇人怀妊，腹中疞痛，当归芍药散主之。

当归芍药散方

当归（三两）　芍药（一斤）　茯苓（四两）　白术（四两）　泽泻（半斤）　芎䓖（半斤）

右六味，杵为散，取方寸匕，酒和，日三服。

【今译】

妇人怀妊，腹中拘急疼痛，应用当归芍药散主治。

【原文】

（六）

妊娠呕吐不止，干姜人参半夏丸主之。

干姜人参半夏丸方

干姜、人参（各一两）　半夏（二两）

右三味，末之，以生姜汁糊为丸，如梧子大。饮服十丸，日三服。

【今译】

妊娠后呕吐不止的，用干姜人参半夏丸主治。

Volume 3

【英译】

Line 20.5

[In] a pregnant woman, [there is] abdominal tension and pain. Danggui Shaoyao Powder（当归芍药散，Chinese angelica and peony powder）[can be used] to treat it.

Danggui Shaoyao Powder（当归芍药散，Chinese angelica and peony powder）[is composed of] 3 *liang* of Danggui（当归，Chinese angelica，Radix Angelicae Sinensis）, 1 *jin* of Shaoyao（芍药，peony，Radix Paeoniae）, 4 *liang* of Fuling（茯苓，poria，Poria）, 4 *liang* of Baizhu（白术，rhizome of largehead atractylodes, Rhizoma Atractylodis Macrocephalae）, 0.5 *jin* of Zexie（泽泻，alisma，Rhizoma Alismatis）and 0.5 *jin* of Xiongqiong（芎䓖，xiongqiong，Rhizoma Chuanxiong）.

These six ingredients are pounded into powder and 1 *fangcunbi* is taken with wine [each time] and three times a day.

【英译】

Line 20.6

[To treat] incessant retching and vomiting [after] pregnancy, [the appropriate formula is] Ganjiang Renshen Banxia Pill（干姜人参半夏丸，dried ginger，ginseng and pinellia pill）.

Ganjiang Renshen Banxia Pill（干姜人参半夏丸，dried ginger，ginseng and pinellia pill）[is composed of] 1 *liang* of Ganjiang（干姜，dried ginger，Rhizoma Zingiberis）, 1 *liang* of Renshen（人参，ginseng，Radix Ginseng）and 2 *liang* of Banxia（半夏，pinellia，Rhizoma Pinelliae）.

These three ingredients are ground into powder and blended with juice of Shengjiang（生姜，fresh ginger，Rhizoma Zingiberis Recens）to form pills，the size of firmiana seeds. 10 pills are taken with water [each time] and three times a day.

【原文】

(七)

妊娠小便难,饮食如故,归母苦参丸主之。

当归贝母苦参丸方

当归、贝母、苦参(各四两)

右三味,末之,炼蜜丸如小豆大。饮服三丸,加至十丸。

【今译】

妊娠后小便困难,但饮食却正常的,用归母苦参丸主治。

【原文】

(八)

妊娠有水气,身重,小便不利,洒淅恶寒,起即头眩,葵子茯苓散主之。

葵子茯苓散方

葵子(一斤) 茯苓(三两)

右二味,杵为散,饮服方寸匕。日三服,小便利则愈。

【今译】

妊娠后有水气,身体肿胀而沉重,小便不利,洒淅恶寒,站起时头眩,用葵子茯苓散主治。

【英译】

Line 20. 7

[There is] difficulty in urination [after] pregnancy, [but] drinking [water] and taking [food] are normal. [Such a case can be] treated by Danggui Beimu Kushen Pill (当归贝母苦参丸, Chinese angelica, fritillaria and flavescent sophora pill).

Danggui Beimu Kushen Pill (当归贝母苦参丸, Chinese angelica, fritillaria and flavescent sophora pill) [is composed of] 4 *liang* of Danggui (当归, Chinese angelica, Radix Angelicae Sinensis), 4 *liang* of Beimu (贝母, fritillaria, Bulbus Fritillariae Thunbergii) and 4 *liang* of Kushen (苦参, flavescent sophora, Radix Sophorae Flavescentis).

These three ingredients are ground into powder and blended with Lianmi (炼蜜, processed honey, Mel Praeparatum) to form pills the size of big soybeans. 3 pills are taken with water [each time]. [And the dosage can be] increased to 10 pills [per dose].

【英译】

Line 20. 8

There is water qi (edema) [after] pregnancy, [accompanied by] heaviness of the body, inhibited urination, chilly quivering, aversion to cold and dizziness when standing up. [The appropriate formula for] treating it [is] Kuizi Fuling Powder (葵子茯苓散, mallow seed and poria powder).

Kuizi Fuling Powder (葵子茯苓散, mallow seed and poria powder) [is composed of] 1 *jin* of Kuizi (葵子, mallow seed, Semen Malvae) and 3 *liang* of Fuling (茯苓, poria, Poria).

These two ingredients are ground into powder. 1 *fangcunbi* is taken [each time] and three times a day. [When] urination is disinhibited, [the disease will] heal.

【原文】

(九)

妇人妊娠,宜常服当归散主之。

当归散方

当归、黄芩、芍药 芎䓖(各一斤) 白术(半斤)

右五味,杵为散,酒饮服方寸匕,日再服。妊娠常服即易产,胎无疾苦。产后百病悉主之。

【今译】

妇人妊娠之后,即便无病,也宜常服用当归散保健。

【原文】

(十)

妊娠养胎,白术散主之。

白术散方

白术(四分) 芎䓖(四分) 蜀椒(三分,去汗) 牡蛎(二分)

右四味,杵为散,酒服一钱匕,日三服,夜一服。但苦痛,加芍药;心下毒痛,倍加芎䓖;心烦吐痛,不能食饮,加细辛一两、半夏大者二十枚。服之后,更以醋浆水服之。若呕,以醋浆水服之复不解者,小麦汁服之;已后渴者,大麦粥服之。病虽愈,服之勿置。

【今译】

妊娠期间养胎,宜用白术散主治。

Volume 3

【英译】

Line 20.9

[In] a pregnant woman, [even if there is no disease, there is still need to use] Danggui Powder（当归散，Chinese angelica powder）[to prevent any disease].

Danggui Powder（当归散，Chinese angelica powder）[is composed of] 1 *jin* of Danggui（当归，Chinese angelica，Radix Angelicae Sinensis），1 *jin* of Huangqin（黄芩，scutellaria，Radix Scutellariae），1 *jin* of Shaoyao（芍药，peony，Radix Paeoniae），1 *jin* of Xiongqiong（芎䓖，xiongqiong，Rhizoma Chuanxiong）and 0.5 *jin* of Baizhu（白术，rhizome of largehead atractylodes，Rhizoma Atractylodis Macrocephalae）.

These five ingredients are ground into powder. 1 *fangcunbi* is taken with wine [each time] and twice a day. [If this powder is] often taken [after] pregnancy, delivery will be easy, and there will be no suffering and all postpartum diseases will be prevented.

【英译】

Line 20.10

For cultivating fetus [during] pregnancy, [the appropriate formula] is Baizhu Powder（白术散，rhizome of largehead atractylodes powder）.

Baizhu Powder（白术散，rhizome of largehead atractylodes powder）[is composed of] 4 *fen* of Baizhu（白术，rhizome of largehead atractylodes，Rhizoma Atractylodis Macrocephalae），4 *fen* of Xiongqiong（芎䓖，xiongqiong，Rhizoma Chuanxiong），3 *fen* of Shujiao（蜀椒，zanthoxylum，Pericarpium Zanthoxyli）(remove sweat)and 2 *fen* of Muli（牡蛎，oyster shell，Concha Ostreae）.

These four ingredients are ground into powder. 1 *qianbi* is taken with wine [each time], three times a day and once at night. For suffering pain, Shaoyao（芍药，peony，Radix Paeoniae）should be added；for toxic pain below the heart, Xiongqiong（芎䓖，xiongqiong，Rhizoma Chuanxiong）should be doubled；for vexation, vomiting, pain and inability to eat food and drink water, 1 *liang* of Xixin（细辛，asarum，Herba Asari）and 20 big pieces of Banxia（半夏，pinellia，Rhizoma Pinelliae）should be added. After taking [the powder], more vinegar should be taken. If there is retching it cannot be resolved after taking vinegar, juice of Xiaomai（小麦，wheat，Semen Tritici）should be taken. [If there is] thirst after [taking vinegar and juice of wheat], barley porridge [should be] taken. Although the disease is about to cure, there is no need to take all [the ingredients in the formula].

【原文】

（十一）

妇人伤胎，怀身腹满，不得小便，从腰以下重，如有水气状，怀身七月，太阴当养不养，此心气实，当刺泻劳宫及关元，小便微利则愈。

【今译】

妇人怀孕后伤胎，是由于怀孕之后腹部胀满，小便不利，腰以下沉重，犹如有水气病一样。怀孕七个月后，太阴肺经养胎却不能养，这是心气实的缘故，应当用刺法泻劳宫穴及关元穴，小便基本通利后病就可以治愈了。

【英译】

Line 20. 11

A woman has damaged the fetus [after pregnancy due to] abdominal fullness, and has difficulty in urination and heaviness below the waist like the condition of water qi (edema). Seven months [after] pregnancy, taiyin (lung meridian of hand-taiyin) should nourish [the fetus] but has failed due to excess of heart qi. [It can be treated by] needling Laogong (PC 8) and Guanyuan (CV 4). [If] urination is slightly normalized, [the disease is about] to heal.

妇人产后病脉证治第二十一

【原文】

(一)

问曰：新产妇人有三病，一者病痓，二者病郁冒，三者大便难，何谓也？师曰：新产血虚，多汗出，喜中风，故令病痓；亡血复汗，寒多，故令郁冒；亡津液，胃燥，故大便难。

【今译】

问：新产妇有三种疾病，第一种是病痓（即痓病），第二种病是郁冒（即郁闷昏晕），第三种是大便困难。这是什么原因呢？

老师说：由于刚生育时失血，汗出较多，容易中风，所以常患病痓；失血后又出汗，是外感寒邪较多，所以引起郁冒；失血后津液枯竭，胃部干燥，所以大便困难。

Chapter 21
Postpartum Disease:
Pulses, Syndromes/Patterns and Treatment

【英译】

Line 21. 1

Question: [Just after] delivery, women usually suffer from three major diseases, namely tetany, depression and dizziness, and difficulty in defecation. What is the reason?

The master said: [There is] blood deficiency right [after] delivery with copious sweating and frequent wind attack, that is why there is tetany. Sweating [after] collapse of blood [results from] serious cold, that is why there is depression and dizziness. Exhaustion of fluid and humor [after collapse of blood results in] dryness of the stomach, that is why there is difficulty in defecation.

【原文】

（二）

产妇郁冒，其脉微弱，不能食，大便反坚，但头汗出。所以然者，血虚而厥，厥而必冒，冒家欲解，必大汗出。以血虚下厥，孤阳上出，故头汗出。所以产妇喜汗出者，亡阴血虚，阳气独盛，故当汗出，阴阳乃复。大便坚，呕不能食，小柴胡汤主之。

【今译】

产妇有郁闷、眩晕之症，其脉微弱，不能进食，大便反而坚硬，但头部出汗。之所以如此，是因为产后血虚，引起阴虚阳气上逆。阳气上逆必然引起眩晕，眩晕要解除，就必须通过发汗实现。如今因血虚下寒，孤阳盛行于上，所以头部汗出。产妇之所以容易汗出，是因为亡阴血虚，阳气独盛，所以引起汗出，因而使阴阳得以调理。大便坚硬，呕吐而不能进食，用小柴胡汤主治。

【原文】

（三）

病解能食，七八日更发热者，此为胃实，大承气汤主之。

【今译】

郁闷眩晕的病情消解后就能进食，七八日后再次发热的，属于胃实，宜用大承气汤主治。

Volume 3

【英译】

Line 21.2

[Right after] delivery, women [tend to suffer from] depression, dizziness, faint and weak pulse, inability to eat, hard stool and sweating over the head. The reason is that blood deficiency [after delivery] causes counterflow [of yang qi] and counterflow [of yang qi] causes dizziness. [If] the patient wants to resolve dizziness, great sweating must be induced. [But now] blood deficiency [results in] reversal cold [in the lower part of the body and drives] yang to flow alone upwards. That is why [there is] sweating over the head. [Thus right after delivery,] women tend to sweat [because of] yin collapse, blood deficiency and exuberance of yang qi alone. That is why [there is] sweating and balance between yin and yang. For hard stool, retching and inability to eat, Xiao Chaihu Decoction (小柴胡汤, minor bupleurum decoction) [can be used] to treat it.

【英译】

Line 21.3

[After] resolution of the disease, [the patient is] able to eat [but there is] fever again seven or eight days later. This is stomach excess and [can be] treated by Da Chengqi Decoction (大承气汤, major decoction for harmonizing qi).

【原文】

(四)

产后腹中疠痛,当归生姜羊肉汤主之,并治腹中寒疝,虚劳不足。

当归生姜羊肉汤方:方未见。

【今译】

产后腹中拘急疼痛,应当用当归生姜羊肉汤主治,也可以治疗腹中寒疝及虚劳不足之症。

当归生姜羊肉汤方:此方未曾见到。

【原文】

(五)

产后腹痛,烦满不得卧,枳实芍药散主之。

枳实芍药散方

枳实(烧令黑,勿太过) 芍药(等分)

右二味,杵为散。服方寸匕,日三服,并主痈脓,以麦粥下之。

【今译】

产后腹部疼痛,烦躁,腹满,无法躺卧,用枳实芍药散主治。

【英译】

Line 21.4

Abdominal tension and pain after delivery should be treated by Danggui Shengjiang Yangrou Decoction（当归生姜羊肉汤，Chinese angelica, fresh ginger and goat meat decoction）. [It] can also treat cold hernia in the abdomen, deficiency, overstrain and insufficiency.

【英译】

Line 21.5

[The disease marked by] abdominal pain, vexation, [abdominal] fullness and inability to lie down after delivery [can be] treated by Zhishi Shaoyao Powder（枳实芍药散，processed unripe bitter orange and peony powder）.

Zhishi Shaoyao Powder（枳实芍药散，processed unripe bitter orange and peony powder）[is composed of] Zhishi（枳实，processed unripe bitter orange, Fructus Aurantii Immaturus）(burn black, but not excessively) and Shaoyao（芍药，peony, Radix Paeoniae) of the same amount.

These two ingredients are ground into powder. 1 *fangcunbi* is taken [each time] and three times a day. [This powder] also treats abscess and pus and [should be] taken with wheat porridge.

【原文】

（六）

师曰：产妇腹痛，法当以枳实芍药散。假令不愈者，此为腹中有干血着脐下，宜下瘀血汤主之，亦主经水不利。

下瘀血汤方

大黄（二两） 桃仁（二十枚） 蟅虫（二十枚，熬，去足）

右三味，末之，炼蜜和为四丸，以酒一升，煎一丸，取八合。顿服之，新血下如豚肝。

【今译】

老师说：产妇腹部疼痛，按常理应当用枳实芍药散主治。假如没有治愈，这是腹中有瘀血凝聚脐下所致，宜用下瘀血汤主治，也可以主治经水不利。

【原文】

（七）

产后七八日，无太阳证，少腹坚痛，此恶露不尽。不大便，烦躁发热，切脉微实，再倍发热，日晡时烦躁者，不食，食则谵语，至夜即愈，宜大承气汤主之。热在里，结在膀胱也。

【今译】

产后七八日后，无太阳表证，少腹坚硬疼痛，这是恶露不尽所致。如果大便不解，烦躁，发热，切脉时感觉微实，加倍发热，日晡（下午 3 至 7 时）时有烦躁之感，不能进食，进食后则出现谵语，直到夜晚才逐步缓解，宜用大承气汤主治。这是因为热在肠胃，结在下焦所致。

Volume 3

【英译】

Line 21.6

The master said: [To treat] abdominal pain after delivery, usually Zhishi Shaoyao Powder (枳实芍药散, processed unripe bitter orange and peony powder) should be used. If [it has] failed to cure [the disease], it is due to blood stasis in the abdomen binding below the umbilicus. The appropriate [formula for] treating it is Xia Yuxue Decoction (下瘀血汤, decoction for resolving blood stasis). [This decoction] can also treat dysmenorrhea.

Xia Yuxue Decoction (下瘀血汤, decoction for resolving blood stasis) [is composed of] 2 *liang* of Dahuang (大黄, rhubarb, Radix et Rhizoma Rhei), 20 pieces of Taoren (桃仁, peach kernel, Semen Persicae) and 20 pieces of Zhechong (蟅虫, ground beetle, Eupolyphaga seu Steleophaga) (broil, remove the legs).

These three ingredients are ground into powder and blended with Lianmi (炼蜜, processed honey, Mel Praeparatum) to form 4 pills. 1 pill is boiled in 1 *sheng* of wine to get 8 *ge*. [The decoction is] taken once the whole. New blood will be discharged like piglet's liver [after taking the decoction].

【英译】

Line 21.7

Seven or eight days after delivery, there is no taiyang syndrome/pattern, but lower abdominal hardness and pain due to incessant lochia. [If there are symptoms and signs of] constipation, vexation, fever, slightly strong pulse when pressed, doubled fever, vexation from 3 o'clock to 7 o'clock in the afternoon, inability to eat and delirium after eating [that lasts till midnight], the appropriate [formula for] treating it is Da Chengqi Decoction (大承气汤, major decoction for harmonizing qi). [The reason is that] heat is in the internal and binding is in the lower energizer.

【原文】

（八）

产后风,续之数十日不解,头微痛,恶寒,时时有热,心下闷,干呕汗出,虽久,阳旦证续在耳,可与阳旦汤。

【今译】

产后因风邪而患病,延续数十天而不解,头部微痛,恶寒,时时发热,心下郁闷,干呕,汗出,虽然延续日久,阳旦证依然存在,仍可用阳旦汤主治。

【原文】

（九）

产后中风发热,面正赤,喘而头痛,竹叶汤主之。

竹叶汤方

竹叶（一把）　葛根（三两）　防风　桔梗　桂枝　人参　甘草（各一两）　附子（一枚,炮）　大枣（十五枚）　生姜（五两）

右十味,以水一斗,煮取二升半,分温三服,温覆使汗出。颈项强,用大附子一枚,破之如豆大,煎药,扬去沫。呕者,加半夏半升洗。

【今译】

产后中风发热,面色红赤,气喘而头痛,用竹叶汤主治。

【英译】

Line 21.8

Wind attack after delivery continues dozens of days, ［accompanied by］ slight headache, aversion to cold, frequent fever, depression below the heart, dry retching and sweating. Although ［these symptoms and signs continue for］ a long period of time, yangdan（阳旦, yang dawn）syndrome/pattern is still present and Yangdan Decoction（阳旦汤, yang dawn decoction）can still ［be used］ to treat it.

【英译】

Line 21.9

［To treat］ wind attack, fever, redness of the whole face, panting and headache, ［the appropriate formula is］ Zhuye Decoction（竹叶汤, bamboo leaf decoction）.

Zhuye Decoction （竹叶汤, bamboo leaf decoction） ［is composed of］ 1 handful of Zhuye（竹叶, bamboo leaf, Folium Bambusae）, 3 *liang* of Gegen（葛根, pueraria, Radix Puerariae）, 1 *liang* of Fangfeng（防风, saposhnikovia, Radix Saposhnikoviae）, 1 *liang* of Jiegeng（桔梗, platycodon grandiflorum, Radix Platycodi）, 1 *liang* of Guizhi（桂枝, cinnamon twig, Ramulus Cinnamomi）, 1 *liang* of Renshen（人参, ginseng, Radix Ginseng）, 1 *liang* of Gancao（甘草, licorice, Radix Glycyrrhizae Preparata）, 1 piece of Fuzi（附子, aconite, Radix Aconiti Lateralis Preparata）(fry heavily), 15 pieces of Dazao（大枣, jujube, Fructus Ziziphus Jujubae）and 5 *liang* of Shengjiang（生姜, fresh ginger, Rhizoma Zingiberis Recens）.

These ten ingredients are decocted in 1 *dou* of water to get 2.5 *sheng* ［after］ boiling. ［The decoction is］ divided into three ［doses］ and taken warm. ［The patient is］ covered ［with clothes or quilt］ to warm ［the body］. ［To treat］ stiff neck and nape, 1 big piece of Fuzi（附子, aconite, Radix Aconiti Lateralis Preparata）is used. ［It is］ pounded into pieces the size of beans and boiled with the foam removed. ［To treat］ retching, 0.5 *sheng* of Banxia（半夏, pinellia, Rhizoma Pinelliae）is added for washing.

【原文】

（十）

妇人乳中虚，烦乱呕逆，安中益气，竹皮大丸主之。

竹皮大丸方

生竹茹（二分）　石膏（二分）　桂枝（一分）　甘草（七分）　白薇（一分）

右五味，末之，枣肉和丸弹子大。以饮服一丸，日三、夜二服。有热者，倍白薇，烦喘者，加柏实一分。

【今译】

妇女产后哺乳期间，中气虚，心烦意乱，呕吐，呃逆，可用安中益气治疗，用竹皮大丸主治。

【原文】

（十一）

产后下利虚极，白头翁加甘草阿胶汤主之。

白头翁加甘草阿胶汤方

白头翁（二两）　黄连　柏皮　秦皮（各三两）　甘草（二两）　阿胶（二两）

右六味，以水七升，煮取二升半，内胶，令消尽，分温三服。

【今译】

产后下利，气血极虚，宜用白头翁加甘草阿胶汤主治。

【英译】

Line 21. 10

［In］ a woman ［during lactation］, deficiency of middle qi, vexation, retching and counterflow ［of qi can be treated by］ tranquilizing the middle and replenishing qi. ［The appropriate formula for］ treating it is ZhupiDa Pill (竹皮大丸, big bamboo leaf pill).

ZhupiDa Pill (竹皮大丸, big bamboo leaf pill) ［is composed of］ 2 *fen* of Shengzhuru (生竹茹, fresh bamboo shavings, Caulis Bambusae in Taenia), 2 *fen* of Shigao (石膏, gypsum, Gypsum Fibrosum), 1 *fen* of Guizhi (桂枝, cinnamon twig, Ramulus Cinnamomi), 7 *fen* of Gancao (甘草, licorice, Radix Glycyrrhizae Praeparata) and 1 *fen* of Baiwei (白薇, black swallowwort, Radix Cynanchi Atrati).

These five ingredients are ground into powder and blended with jujube pulp to form pills the size of pellets. 1 pill is taken with water ［each time］, three times a day and twice at night. For heat, Baiwei (白薇, black swallowwort, Radix Cynanchi Atrati) is doubled. For vexation and panting, 1 *fen* of Baishi (柏实, arborvitae seed, Semen Biotae) is added.

【英译】

Line 21. 11

Diarrhea and extreme deficiency ［of qi and blood］ after delivery ［should be］ treated by Baitouweng Decoction (白头翁汤, pulsatilla decoction) added with Gancao (甘草, licorice, Radix Glycyrrhizae Praeparata) and Ejiao (阿胶, ass-hide glue, Colla Corii Asini).

Baitouweng Decoction (白头翁汤, pulsatilla decoction) added with Gancao (甘草, licorice, Radix Glycyrrhizae Praeparata) and Ejiao (阿胶, ass-hide glue, Colla Corii Asini) ［is composed of］ 2 *liang* of Baitouweng (白头翁, pulsatilla, Radix Pulsatillae), 3 *liang* of Huanglian (黄连, coptis, Rhizoma Coptidis), 3 *liang* of Baipi (柏皮, arborvitae bark, Cortex Platycladi), 3 *liang* of Qinpi (秦皮, ash, Cortex Fraxini), 2 *liang* of Gancao (甘草, licorice, Radix Glycyrrhizae Praeparata) and 2 *liang* of Ejiao (阿胶, ass-hide glue, Colla Corii Asini).

These six ingredients are decocted in 7 *sheng* of water to get 2.5 *sheng* ［after］ boiling. ［Then］ Ejiao (阿胶, ass-hide glue, Colla Corii Asini) is added to melt completely. ［The decoction is］ divided into three ［doses］ and taken warm.

附方

【原文】

《千金》三物黄芩汤治妇人在草蓐,自发露得风。四肢苦烦热,头痛者,与小柴胡汤。头不痛但烦者,此汤主之。

黄芩(一两) 苦参(二两) 干地黄(四两)

右三昧,以水八升,煮取二升。温服一升,多吐下虫。

【今译】

《千金方》中的三物黄芩汤,治疗妇女分娩时床上不洁、或产后感受风邪所致之病。其四肢烦热,头痛的,可用小柴胡汤治疗。头不痛但却烦热的,也可用此汤主治。

【原文】

《千金》内补当归建中汤治妇人产后虚羸不足,腹中刺痛不止,吸吸少气,或苦少腹中急,摩痛引腰者,不能食饮。产后一月,日得四五剂为善,令人强壮,宜。

当归(四两) 桂枝(三两) 芍药(六两) 生姜(三两) 甘草(二两) 大枣(十二枚)

Volume 3

Appended formula

【英译】

Huangqin Decoction (黄芩汤, scutellaria decoction) [from the book entitled] *Qianjin* (《千金方》, *Thousand Golden Formulas*): For treating women with vexation and heat in the four limbs and headache [due to] unclean bed [during delivery] and wind attack [after delivery], Xiao Chaihu Decoction (小柴胡汤, minor bupleurum decoction) can be used. [If there is] no headache but vexation, this decoction also [can be used] to treat it.

Xiao Chaihu Decoction (小柴胡汤, minor bupleurum decoction) [is composed of] 1 *liang* of Huangqin (黄芩, scutellaria, Radix Scutellariae), 2 *liang* of Kushen (苦参, flavescent sophora, Radix Sophorae Flavescentis) and 4 *liang* of Gandihuang (干地黄, dried rehmannia, Radix Rehmanniae).

These three ingredients are decocted in 8 *sheng* of water to get 2 *sheng* [after] boiling. [The decoction is] taken warm 1 *sheng* [each time]. [This decoction induces] more vomiting to discharge worms.

【英译】

Neibu Danggui Jianzhong Decoction (内补当归建中汤, Chinese angelica decoction for tonifying the internal and strengthening the middle) [from the book entitled] *Qianjin* (《千金方》, *Thousand Golden Formulas*): For treating women [who], after delivery, [suffer from the disease marked by] weakness, emaciation, insufficiency [of qi and blood], incessant sharp pain in the abdomen, strong inhalation with shortness of breath, or tension and pain in the lower abdomen stretching to the waist, and inability to drink and eat. One month after delivery, four to five doses should be taken every day to strengthen the body. [When the body is strengthened, it is] appropriate [for cultivating health].

[Neibu Danggui Jianzhong Decoction (内补当归建中汤, Chinese angelica decoction for tonifying the internal and strengthening the

右六味，以水一斗，煮取三升。分温三服，一日令尽。若大虚，加饴糖六两，汤成，内之于火上暖，令饴消。若去血过多，崩伤内衄不止，加地黄六两、阿胶二两，合八味，汤成，内阿胶。若无当归，以芎䓖代之；若无生姜，以干姜代之。

【今译】

《千金方》内补当归建中汤，用以治疗妇女产后虚弱，消瘦，气血不足，腹中刺痛不已，用力呼吸，但少气，或少腹拘急疼痛，牵引腰部，不能饮食。产后一个月，每天应该服用四五剂，使其身体强壮，就宜于康复。

middle) is composed of] 4 *liang* of Danggui (当归, Chinese angelica, Radix Angelicae Sinensis), 3 *liang* of Guizhi (桂枝, cinnamon twig, Ramulus Cinnamomi), 6 *liang* of Shaoyao (芍药, peony, Radix Paeoniae), 3 *liang* of Shengjiang (生姜, fresh ginger, Rhizoma Zingiberis Recens), 2 *liang* of Gancao (甘草, licorice, Radix Glycyrrhizae Praeparata) and 12 pieces of Dazao (大枣, jujube, Fructus Ziziphus Jujubae).

These six ingredients are decocted in 1 *dou* of water to get 3 *sheng* [after] boiling. [The decoction is] divided into three [doses], taken warm and finished in a day. If [there is] severe deficiency, 6 *liang* of malt sugar should be added to the formed decoction and kept warm over fire to melt the sugar. If bleeding is excessive, it will cause incessant internal bleeding. 6 *liang* of Dihuang (地黄, rehmannia, Radix Rehmanniae), 2 *liang* of Ejiao (阿胶, ass-hide glue, Colla Corii Asini) are added. Altogether there are eight ingredients to perfect the decoction, [in which] Ejiao (阿胶, ass-hide glue, Colla Corii Asini) [is melted]. If there is no Danggui (当归, Chinese angelica, Radix Angelicae Sinensis), Xiongqiong (芎劳, xiongqiong, Rhizoma Chuanxiong) can replace it; if there is no Shengjiang (生姜, fresh ginger, Rhizoma Zingiberis Recens), Ganjiang (干姜, dried ginger, Rhizoma Zingiberis) can replace it.

妇人杂病脉证并治第二十二

【原文】

（一）

妇人中风，七八日续来寒热，发作有时，经水适断，此为热入血室，其血必结，故使如疟状，发作有时，小柴胡汤主之。

【今译】

妇女遭受风邪侵袭，七八日后连续出现寒热现象，发作有一定的时间，月经又恰巧中断，这是热邪乘虚入血室，使血必然凝结，故而寒热往来如疟疾之状，发作有时，用小柴胡汤主治。

【原文】

（二）

妇人伤寒发热，经水适来，昼日明了，暮则谵语，如见鬼状者，此为热入血室，治之无犯胃气及上二焦，必自愈。

【今译】

妇女遭受寒邪入侵而发热，恰逢月经来潮，白天神志清晰，入夜则出现谵语，好像见到了鬼似的，这是热入血室的缘故，治疗时不能用攻下法伤及胃气和二焦，应使其自行痊愈。

Volume 3

Chapter 22
Women's Miscellaneous Disease:
Pulses, Syndromes/Patterns and Treatment

【英译】

Line 22. 1

[In] a woman attacked by wind, [aversion to] cold and heat continues for seven or eight days and occurs at intervals with interruption of menstruation. This is heat entering blood chamber. [In this case] the blood is binding inevitably. That is why [it] appears like malaria with occasional occurrence. Xiao Chaihu Decoction (小柴胡汤, minor bupleurum decoction) [can be used] to treat it.

【英译】

Line 22.2

[In] a woman with cold damage and fever, menstruation has just started. [In] the daytime, [her mind is] clear; [at] night there is delirium as if seeing a ghost. This is heat entering blood chamber. To treat [it], stomach qi and two energizers cannot be damaged. [The patient] will heal spontaneously.

【原文】

(三)

妇人中风,发热恶寒,经水适来,得七八日,热除脉迟,身凉和,胸胁满,如结胸状,谵语者,此为热入血室也,当刺期门,随其实而取之。

【今译】

妇女中风,发热,恶寒,正值月经来潮,患病七八日后,热退,脉迟,身体凉和,胸胁胀满,如结胸之状,有谵语的,这是热入血室所致,治疗时应当针刺期门,血室的瘀血可随泻其实邪而消除。

【原文】

(四)

阳明病,下血谵语者,此为热入血室,但头汗出,当刺期门,随其实而泻之,濈然汗出者愈。

【今译】

阳明病有下血、谵语症状的,这是热入血室所致,但头上有汗出,治疗时应当针刺期门,血室的热邪可随泻其实邪而消除,当患者周身汗出时,疾病就将痊愈。

Volume 3

【英译】

Line 22.3

[In] a woman attacked by wind, [there is] fever and aversion to cold, [during which] menstruation has just started. Seven or eight days [after occurrence], [there are symptoms and signs of] elimination of fever, slow pulse, cool and harmonious body, fullness in the chest and rib-side like chest bind, and delirium. This is heat entering blood chamber. [It] should [be treated by] needling Qimen (LR 14) and [blood stasis will be] eliminated together with purgation of excess.

【英译】

Line 22.4

Yangming disease [is marked by] bleeding and delirium. This is heat entering blood chamber. If there is sweating over the head, [it] should [be treated by] needling Qimen (LR 14) and [blood stasis will be] eliminated together with purgation of excess. [When there is] generalized sweating, [the disease will be] cured.

【原文】

(五)

妇人咽中如有炙脔,半夏厚朴汤主之。

半夏厚朴汤方

半夏(一升)　厚朴(三两)　茯苓(四两)　生姜(五两)　干苏叶(二两)

右五味,以水七升,煮取四升。分温四服,日三、夜一服。

【今译】

妇女咽中好像有烤炙肉块梗阻,宜用半夏厚朴汤主治。

【原文】

(六)

妇人脏躁,喜悲伤欲哭,象如神灵所作,数欠伸,甘麦大枣汤主之。

甘草小麦大枣汤方

甘草(三两)　小麦(一升)　大枣(十枚)

右三味,以水六升,煮取三升,温分三服。亦补脾气。

【今译】

妇女患脏躁病,经常悲伤而想哭,好像受神灵影响一样,频频呵欠,时时伸懒腰,宜用甘麦大枣汤主治。

Volume 3

【英译】

Line 22.5

[When] there is [a sensation of lump] like roasted meat in the throat，Banxia Houpo Decoction（半夏厚朴汤，pinellia and magnolia bark decoction）[can be used] to treat it.

Banxia Houpo Decoction（半夏厚朴汤，pinellia and magnolia bark decoction）[is composed of] 1 *sheng* of Banxia（半夏，pinellia，Rhizoma Pinelliae），3 *liang* of Houpo（厚朴，magnolia bark，Cortex Magnoliae Officinalis），4 *liang* of Fuling（茯苓，poria，Poria），5 *liang* of Shengjiang（生姜，fresh ginger，Rhizoma Zingiberis Recens）and 2 *liang* of Gansuye（干苏叶，dried perilla leaf，Folium Penillae Exsiccatum）.

These five ingredients are decocted in 7 *sheng* of water to get 4 *sheng* [after] boiling. [The decoction is] divided into four [doses] and taken warm，three times a day and once at night.

【英译】

Line 22.6

A woman [suffering from] visceral dryness [disease] tends to sorrow and cry as if being haunted by spirits with frequent yawning and stretching. Gancao Xiaomai Dazao Decoction（甘草小麦大枣汤，licorice，wheat and jujube decoction）[can be used] to treat it.

Gancao Xiaomai Dazao Decoction（甘草小麦大枣汤，licorice，wheat and jujube decoction）[is composed of] 3 *liang* of Gancao（甘草，licorice，Radix Glycyrrhizae Praeparata），1 *sheng* of Xiaomai（小麦，wheat，Semen Tritici）and 10 pieces of Dazao（大枣，jujube，Fructus Ziziphus Jujubae）.

These three ingredients are decocted in 6 *sheng* of water to get 3 *sheng* [after] boiling. [The decoction is] divided into three [doses] and taken warm. [This formula] can also tonify spleen qi.

【原文】

（七）

妇人吐涎沫,医反下之,心下即痞。当先治其吐涎沫,小青龙汤主之;涎沫止,乃治痞,泻心汤主之。

小青龙汤方:见痰饮中。

泻心汤方:见惊悸中。

【今译】

妇女患吐涎沫之症,医生反而用下法治疗,心下因而就出现了痞满。治疗时应当先治其吐涎沫,宜用小青龙汤主治;涎沫停止了,再治疗痞满,宜用泻心汤主治。

【原文】

（八）

妇人之病,因虚、积冷、结气,为诸经水断绝至有历年,血寒积结,胞门寒伤,经络凝坚。

在上呕吐涎唾,久成肺痈,形体损分;在中盘结,绕脐寒疝,或两胁疼痛,与脏相连;或结热中,痛在关元。脉数无疮,肌若鱼鳞,时着男子,非止女身。在下未多,经候不匀。冷阴掣痛,少腹恶寒,或引腰脊,下根气街,气冲急痛,膝胫疼烦,奄忽眩冒,状如厥癫,或有忧惨,悲伤多嗔,此皆带下,非有鬼神。

【英译】

Line 22.7

A woman [suffers from] vomiting of drool and foam. [If] a doctor [uses] purgation [to treat] it, there will be lump below the heart. Vomiting of drool and foam should be treated first and [the appropriate formula is] Xiao Qinglong Decoction (小青龙汤, minor blue long decoction). [Only when vomiting of] drool and foam is ceased can lump be treated, [the appropriate formula is] Xiexin Decoction (泻心汤, decoction for draining the heart).

Xiao Qinglong Decoction (小青龙汤, minor blue long decoction) is mentioned in treatment about phlegm and fluid retention.

Xiexin Decoction (泻心汤, decoction for draining the heart) is mentioned in treatment about palpitation.

【英译】

Line 22.8

Diseases in women are caused by deficiency, cold accumulation and qi binding that lead to interruption of menstruation for years, accumulation and binding of cold in the blood, damage of uterus by cold and stagnation of meridians and collaterals.

In the upper [part of the body, it causes] retching and vomiting of drool and foam, eventually resulting in lung abscess and damage the body. In the middle [part of the body], [invasion of cold into the spleen and liver results in] cold hernia around the umbilicus, or pain in the rib-sides stretching to the viscera, or heat binding in the

久则羸瘦,脉虚多寒。三十六病,千变万端,审脉阴阳,虚实紧弦,行其针药,治危得安,其虽同病,脉各异源,子当辨记,勿谓不然。

【今译】

妇女所患的各种疾病,多因虚损、积冷、结气引起各种月经病变多年,甚至导致经断绝,时间一长,因血分受寒而积结,胞宫遭受寒伤,经络凝坚不通。

在其身体上部,出现呕吐涎唾,时间一长就形成肺痈,导致身体消瘦;在其身体的中部,肝脾受邪之侵袭,导致绕脐寒疝,或两胁疼痛,与肝脏相连;或结热在中,疼痛出现在关元。脉象数,但身体并无疮,肌肤枯燥得像鱼鳞一样,这种情况有时会出现在男子的身上,并非仅仅出现在妇女的身上。在身体的下部,虽然下血并不多,但经候却不匀。阴部寒冷掣痛,少腹恶寒,或牵引到腰脊,疼痛源自气街,发生气冲急痛,又涉及到膝胫,引起疼烦,甚至出现猝然眩晕昏冒,状如昏厥癫狂一样,或者出现忧虑悲痛,悲伤时经常发怒,这都是妇女所患的各种带下杂病,并非因鬼神作祟所致。

久病则身体羸瘦,脉象虚而多寒。妇女常患的三十六种带下之病,变化多端,医生应通过审查脉象之阴阳、虚实、紧弦,用针刺及方药治疗,可转危为安,其病虽然相同,但脉象却各异,应当仔细审辨,不要以为其并不重要。

middle and pain at Guanyuan (CV 4). The pulse is rapid, the skin is like fish scale. [Such a pathological condition] sometimes also appear in men, not only in women. In the lower [part of the body], [bleeding is] less, [but] menstrual cycle is not even. In the genitals [there is] pulling pain; in the lower abdomen, [there is] aversion to cold, or stretching to the waist and spine and originating from Qijie (ST 30), [leading to] surging qi, acute pain, pain and vexation in the knees and shanks, sudden dizziness like syncope and epilepsy, or anxiety and sorrow as well as sadness and anger. All these are menstrual [disorders], not haunting of ghosts and spirits.

After a long period of time there will be emaciation, weak pulse and increased cold. [In women, usually there are] thirty-six diseases, tending to change. By examining yin and yang, deficiency and excess and tightness and tautness of the pulse, [doctors can use] acupuncture and medicinals to treat urgency and secure [health]. Although these diseases are the same [in nature], [the conditions of] pulse vary. Doctors must [carefully] differentiate [varied conditions of pulse] and do not neglect [it].

【原文】

(九)

问曰：妇人年五十所，病下利数十日不止，暮即发热，少腹里急，腹满，手掌烦热，唇口干燥，何也？师曰：此病属带下。何以故？曾经半产，瘀血在少腹不去，何以知之？其证唇口干燥，故知之。当以温经汤主之。

温经汤方

吴茱萸（三两）　当归、芎䓖、芍药（各二两）　人参、桂枝、阿胶　牡丹（去心）　生姜、甘草（各二两）　半夏（半升）　麦门冬（一升，去心）

右十二味，以水一斗，煮取三升，分温三服。亦主妇人少腹寒，久不受胎，兼取崩中去血，或月水来过多，及至期不来。

【今译】

问：妇女已五十岁左右了，前阴下血数十日不止，傍晚发热，少腹里急，腹中胀满，手掌烦热，唇口干燥，这是什么原因呢？

老师说：此病属于带脉以下的病变。是什么原因呢？因为曾经有过小产，瘀血依然停留在少腹没有消除，如何知道的呢？因为证见唇口干燥，所以就可以知道其原因了。应当以温经汤主治。

【英译】

Line 22.9

Question: [In] a woman, already 50 years old, [there is] frequent vaginal bleeding for over ten days, [accompanied by] fever at night, lower abdominal tension, abdominal fullness, vexing fever in the palms and dryness of lips and mouth. What is the reason?

The master said: This disease is located below the conception vessel. Why it is so? [Because there was] abortion before and blood stasis in the lower abdomen. How to know such [a problem]? Dryness of the lips and mouth is the evidence. [It] should be treated by Wenjing Decoction (温经汤, decoction for warming meridians).

Wenjing Decoction (温经汤, decoction for warming meridians) [is composed of] 3 *liang* of Wuzhuyu (吴茱萸, evodia, Fructus Evodiae), 2 *liang* of Danggui (当归, Chinese angelica, Radix Angelicae Sinensis), 2 *liang* of Xiongqiong (芎蔖, xiongqiong, Rhizoma Chuanxiong), 2 *liang* of Shaoyao (芍药, peony, Radix Paeoniae), 2 *liang* of Renshen (人参, ginseng, Radix Ginseng), 2 *liang* of Guizhi (桂枝, cinnamon twig, Ramulus Cinnamomi), 2 *liang* of Ejiao (阿胶, ass-hide glue, Colla Corii Asini), 2 *liang* of Mudan (牡丹, moutan, Cortex Moutan Radicis) (remove the center), 2 *liang* of Shengjiang (生姜, fresh ginger, Rhizoma Zingiberis Recens), 2 *liang* of Gancao (甘草, licorice, Radix Glycyrrhizae Praeparata), 0.5 *sheng* of Banxia (半夏, pinellia, Rhizoma Pinelliae) and 1 *sheng* of Maimendong (麦门冬, ophiopogon, Radix Ophiopogonis)(remove the center).

These twelve ingredients are decocted in 1 *dou* of water to get 3 *sheng* [after] boiling. [The decoction is] divided into three [doses] and taken warm. [This formula] can also treat women with lower abdominal cold and failure to conceive a baby for a long time. Besides, [it is] helpful for eliminating blood from vaginal bleeding, or excessive menstruation and failure of menstruation to occur [at the proper time].

【原文】

（十）

带下经水不利，少腹满痛，经一月再见者，土瓜根散主之。

土瓜根散方：阴㿉肿亦主之。

土瓜根　芍药　桂枝　蟅虫（各三分）

右四味，杵为散。酒服方寸匕，日三服。

【今译】

带脉以下经水不利，少腹胀满疼痛，月经一月出现两次，用土瓜根散主治。

【原文】

（十一）

寸口脉弦而大，弦则为减，大则为芤，减则为寒，芤则为虚，寒虚相搏，此名曰革，妇人则半产漏下，旋覆花汤主之。

旋覆花汤方：见五脏风寒积聚篇。

旋覆花（三两）　葱（十四茎）　新绛（少许）

右三味，以水三升，煮取一升，顿服之。

【今译】

寸口脉象弦而且大，脉象弦为衰减，脉象大为空弱，脉象衰减为寒，脉象空弱为虚，寒虚相搏，称为革脉。在妇女中革脉主患小产或漏下，宜用旋覆花汤主治。

Volume 3

【英译】

Line 22. 10

[The disease marked by] inhibited menstruation below the conception vessel, lower abdominal fullness and pain, and menstruation occurs twice a month [can be] treated by Tuguagen Powder (土瓜根散, cucumber gourd root powder).

Tuguagen Powder (土瓜根散, cucumber gourd root powder): For treating withering and swelling of the genitals.

Tuguagen Powder (土瓜根散, cucumber gourd root powder) [is composed of] 3 *fen* of Tuguagen (土瓜根, cucumber gourd root, Cucumeroidis Trichosanthis), 3 *fen* of Shaoyao (芍药, peony, Radix Paeoniae), 3 *fen* of Guizhi (桂枝, cinnamon twig, Ramulus Cinnamomi) and 3 *fen* of Zhechong (蟅虫, ground beetle, Eupolyphaga seu Steleophaga).

These four ingredients are ground into powder. 1 *fangcunbi* is taken with wine [each time] and three times a day.

【英译】

Line 22. 11

The pulse [of a patient] is taut and large. Taut [pulse] indicates reduction while large [pulse] indicates hollowness. Reduction means cold while hollowness means deficiency. [When] deficiency and cold contend with each other, it is called tympanic [pulse]. [Such a pulse in] a woman indicates miscarriage and vaginal bleeding. The appropriate [formula for] treating it is Xuanfuhua Decoction (旋覆花汤, inula flower decoction).

Xuanfuhua Decoction (旋覆花汤, inula flower decoction) [is composed of] 3 *liang* of Xuanfuhua Decoction (旋覆花, inula flower, Flos Insulae), 14 pieces of Cong (葱, scallion, Herba Alli Fistulosi) and a little of Xinjiang (新绛, fresh madder, Radix Rubiae Recens).

These three ingredients are decocted in 3 *sheng* of water to get 1 *sheng* [after] boiling. [The decoction is] taken once the whole.

【原文】

(十二)

妇人陷经,漏下黑不解,胶姜汤主之。

【今译】

妇女经气下陷,下漏黑血不止,用胶姜汤主治。

【原文】

(十三)

妇人少腹满如敦状,小便微难而不渴,生后者,此为水与血并结在血室也,大黄甘遂汤主之。

大黄甘遂汤方

大黄(四两) 甘遂(二两) 阿胶(二两)

右三味,以水三升,煮取一升。顿服之,其血当下。

【今译】

妇女少腹胀满如隆起之状,小便略微困难,不渴,生病后,这是为水与血俱结在血室,用大黄甘遂汤主治。

【英译】

Line 22. 12

A woman [who suffers from] collapse of meridian qi and vaginal bleeding with black color [that is] difficult to resolve [can be] treated by Jiaojiang Decoction (胶姜, ass-hide glue and ginger decoction).

【英译】

Line 22. 13

[In] a woman, [there are symptoms and signs of] lower abdominal fullness like protrusion, slight difficulty in urination and thirst after occurrence [of the disease] due to water and blood binding in the blood chamber. Dahuang Gansui Decoction (大黄甘遂汤, rhubarb and kansui decoction) [can be used] to treat it.

Dahuang Gansui Decoction (大黄甘遂汤, rhubarb and kansui decoction) [is composed of] 4 *liang* of Dahuang (大黄, rhubarb, Radix et Rhizoma Rhei), 2 *liang* of Gansui (甘遂, kansui, Radix Kansui) and 2 *liang* of Ejiao (阿胶, ass-hide glue, Colla Corii Asini).

These three ingredients are decocted in 3 *sheng* of water to get 1 *sheng* [after] boiling. [The decoction is] taken once the whole. And blood [stasis] should be discharged.

【原文】

（十四）

妇人经水不利下，抵当汤主之。

抵当汤方

水蛭（三十个，熬）　虻虫（三十枚，熬，去翅足）　桃仁（二十个，去皮尖）　大黄（三两，酒浸）

右四味，为末，以水五升，煮取三升，去滓，温服一升。

【今译】

妇女月经不利，用抵当汤主治。

【原文】

（十五）

妇人经水闭不利，脏坚癖不止，中有干血，下白物，矾石丸主之。

矾石丸方

矾石（三分，烧）　杏仁（一分）

右二味，末之，炼蜜和丸枣核大，内脏中，剧者再内之。

【今译】

妇女经水闭塞不利，因为胞宫内瘀血停滞不止，因灼热而有干血，又有白带时下，宜用矾石丸主治。

Volume 3

【英译】

Line 22. 14

[In] a woman，inhibited menstruation [can be] treated by Didang Decoction (抵当汤，decoction for prevention).

Didang Decoction (抵当汤，decoction for prevention) [is composed of] 30 Shuizhi (水蛭，leech，Hirudo)(simmer)，30 Mengchong (虻虫，tabanus，Tabanus)(simmer and remove the wings and legs)，20 Taoren (桃仁，peach kernel，Semen Persicae)(remove the bark and tips) and 3 *liang* of Dahuang (大黄，rhubarb，Radix et Rhizoma Rhei)(soak in wine).

These four ingredients are ground into powder and decocted in 5 *sheng* of water to get 3 *sheng* [after] boiling. The dregs are removed and [the decoction is] taken warm 1 *sheng* [each time].

【英译】

Line 22. 15

[In] a woman，menstruation is inhibited [because of] incessant hardness (blood stasis) and stagnation in the uterus [in which] there is dry blood and leukorrhea. Fanshi Pill (矾石丸，alum pill) [can be used] to treat it.

Fanshi Pill (矾石丸，alum pill) [is composed of] 3 *fen* of Fanshi (矾石，alum，Alumen)(burn) and 1 *fen* of Xingren (杏仁，apricot kernel，Semen Armeniacae Amarum).

These two ingredients are ground into powder and blended with Lianmi (炼蜜，processed honey，Mel Praeparatum) to form pills the size of jujube kernels. One pill is inserted into the uterus. [If] severe，one more pill is inserted.

【原文】

（十六）

妇人六十二种风，及腹中血气刺痛，红蓝花酒主之。

红蓝花酒方

红蓝花（一两）

右一味，以酒一大升，煎减半。顿服一半，未止，再服。

【今译】

妇女一般遭受六十二种风的侵袭，引起腹中血气刺痛，用红蓝花酒主治。

【原文】

（十七）

妇人腹中诸疾痛，当归芍药散主之。

当归芍药散方：见前妊娠中。

【今译】

妇女腹中的多种疾痛，用归芍药散主治。

【英译】

Line 22. 16

Women ［are usually attacked by］ sixty-two kinds of wind，causing stabbing pain of qi and blood in the abdomen. Honglanhua Jiu Formula（红蓝花酒方，carthamus and wine formula）［can be used］ to treat it.

Honglanhua Jiu Formula（红蓝花酒方，carthamus and wine formula）［is composed of］ 1 *liang* of Honglanhua（红蓝花，carthamus，Flos Carthami）.

This ingredient is decocted in 1 big *sheng* of wine to reduce half of it ［after］ boiling. ［The decoction is］ taken half for the first time. ［If pain is］ not eliminated，the other half is taken.

【英译】

Line 22. 17

Various pains in the abdomen of women should be treated by Danggui Shaoyao Powder（当归芍药散，Chinese angelica and poria powder）.

【原文】

(十八)

妇人腹中痛,小建中汤主之。

小建中汤方:见前虚劳中。

【今译】

妇女腹中疼痛,宜用小建中汤主治。

【原文】

(十九)

问曰:妇人病,饮食如故,烦热不得卧,而反倚息者,何也? 师曰:此名转胞,不得溺也。以胞系了戾,故致此病。但利小便则愈,宜肾气丸主之。

肾气丸方:方见虚劳中。

干地黄(八两) 薯蓣(四两) 山茱萸(四两) 泽泻(三两) 茯苓(三两) 牡丹皮(三两) 桂枝 附子(炮,各一两)

右八味,末之,炼蜜和丸梧子大。酒下十五丸,加至二十五丸,日再服。

【今译】

问:妇女患病,饮食如常,但却烦热而不能躺卧,反而倚床呼吸,这是什么原因呢?

老师:此病名为转胞,患者不能小便。因为膀胱缭绕不畅,导致此病的发生。一旦小便通利,病就痊愈,用肾气丸主治。

【英译】

Line 22.18

Abdominal pain in women [should be] treated by Xiao Jianzhong Decoction（小建中汤，minor decoction for strengthening the middle）.

【英译】

Line 22.19

Question：[When] a woman suffers from a disease，taking food is normal，[but there is] vexation and inability to lie down. [Hence the patient] leans against the bed to breathe. What is the reason?

The master said：This [disease] is called turned bladder [because the patient is] unable to urinate. Such a disease is caused by twisted bladder. [When] urination is normalized，[it can be] cured. The appropriate [formula for] treating it is Shenqi Pill（肾气丸，kidney qi pill）.

Shenqi Pill（肾气丸，kidney qi pill）[is composed of] 8 *liang* of Gandihuang（干地黄，dried rehmannia，Radix Rehmanniae），4 *liang* of Shuyu（薯蓣，dioscorea，Rhizoma Dioscoreae），4 *liang* of Shanzhuyu（山茱萸，cornus，Fructus Corni），3 *liang* of Zexie（泽泻，alisma，Rhizoma Alismatis），3 *liang* of Fuling（茯苓，poria，Poria），3 *liang* of Mudanpi（牡丹皮，moutan，Cortex Moutan Radicis），1 *liang* of Guizhi（桂枝，cinnamon twig，Ramulus Cinnamomi）and 1 *liang* of Fuzi（附子，aconite，Radix Aconiti Lateralis Preparata）(fry heavily).

These eight ingredients are ground into powder and blended with Lianmi（炼蜜，processed honey，Mel Praeparatum）to form pills the size of firmiana seeds. [Each time] 15 pills are taken with wine and twice a day. [The dosage can] increase to 25 pills.

【原文】

(二十)

蛇床子散方温阴中坐药。

蛇床子仁

右一味,末之,以白粉少许,和令相得,如枣大,绵裹内之,自然温。

【今译】

妇女阴中寒冷,用温阴中坐药蛇床子散方主治。

【原文】

(二十一)

少阴脉滑而数者,阴中即生疮,阴中蚀疮烂者,狼牙汤洗之。

狼牙汤方

狼牙(三两)

右一味,以水四升,煮取半升,以绵缠筋如茧,浸汤沥阴中,日四遍。

【今译】

少阴脉滑而数的,为阴中生疮,阴中生疮而糜烂的,宜用狼牙汤洗涤治疗。

【英译】

Line 22.20

Shechuangzi Powder（蛇床子散，cnidium seed powder）: For warming the genitals to treat [cold in the genitals in women].

Shechuangzi Powder（蛇床子散，cnidium seed powder）[is composed of] only Shechuangzi（蛇床子，cnidium seed，Fructus Cnidii）.

This ingredient is ground into powder and blended with a little white powder (processed galenite) the size of a jujube. [The powder is] wrapped in gauze and inserted into the internal (vagina) to warm [it] spontaneously.

【英译】

Line 22.21

Slippery and rapid shaoyin pulse [indicates] sores in the vagina. [When] sores in the vagina are putrefying and eroding，Langya Formula（狼牙汤，langya herb formula）[can be used] to treat it.

Langya Formula（狼牙汤，langya herb formula）[is composed of] 3 *liang* of Langya（狼牙，this ingredient is difficult to identify now）.

This ingredient is decocted in 4 *sheng* of water to get 0.5 *sheng* [after] boiling. [It is] wrapped in gauze to thicken like a cocoon. The decoction is trickled into the vagina，four times a day.

【原文】

(二十二)

胃气下泄，阴吹而正喧，此谷气之实也，膏发煎导之。

膏发煎方：见黄疸中。

【今译】

胃气下泄，前阴排气有声，连续不断，这是大便不通所致，用膏发煎导而治之。

【原文】

(二十三)

小儿疳虫蚀齿方：疑非仲景方

雄黄　葶苈

右二味，末之，取腊月猪脂熔，以槐枝绵裹头四五枚，点药烙之。

【今译】

小儿疳虫蚀齿方：这可能不是张仲景的药方。

【英译】

Line 22.22

Stomach qi is drained downward with flatulence from the vagina caused by constipation. [It should be treated by] Zhugao Fajian Formula (猪膏发煎方, pork lard and human hair Formula) to abduct it.

Zhugao Fajian Formula (猪膏发煎方, pork lard and human hair Formula) is already mentioned in treatment of jaundice.

【英译】

Line 22.23

Xiao'er Ganchong Shichi Formula (小儿疳虫蚀齿方, formula for treating infantile malnutrition and injury of teeth by worms): This formula perhaps was not made by Zhang Zhongjing.

Xiao'er Ganchong Shichi Formula (小儿疳虫蚀齿方, formula for treating infantile malnutrition and injury of teeth by worms) [is composed of] Xionghuang (雄黄, realgar, Realgar) and Tingli (葶苈, lepidium/descurainiae, Semen Lepidii seu Descurainiae).

These two ingredients are ground into powder. The pork lard, collected in November (in traditional Chinese calendar), is dipped into four or five pieces of Huaizhi (槐枝, pagoda tree twigs, Ramulus Pagodae) wrapped in gauze. [After] ignition, [it is applied to the affected region].

杂疗方第二十三

【原文】

(一)

退五脏虚热,四时加减柴胡饮子方

(冬三月加)柴胡(八分)　白术(八分)　大腹槟榔(四枚,并皮子用)　陈皮(五分)　生姜(五分)　桔梗(七分)

(春三月加)枳实　(减)白术(共六味)

(夏三月加)生姜(三分)　枳实(五分)　甘草(三分,共八味)

(秋三月加)陈皮(三分,共六味)

右各㕮咀,分为三贴。一贴以水三升,煮取二升。分温三服,如人行四五里进一服,如四体壅,添甘草少许,每贴分作三小贴,每小贴以水一升,煮取七合,温服,再合滓为一服,重煮,都成四服。

【今译】

退除五脏虚热,应当随一年四季加减柴胡饮子方治疗。

Chapter 23
Formulas for Treating Miscellaneous Diseases

【英译】

Line 23. 1

To eliminate deficiency-heat from the five zang-organs, Chaihu Decoction (柴胡饮, bupleurum decoction) should be modified in the four seasons.

In the three months in winter, add 8 *fen* of Chaihu (柴胡, bupleurum, Radix Bupleuri), 8 *fen* of Baizhu (白术, rhizome of largehead atractylodes, Rhizoma Atractylodis Macrocephalae), 4 big pieces of Binglang (槟榔, areca, Semen Arecae)(the bark is also used), 5 *fen* of Chenpi (陈皮, tangerine peel, Pericarpium Citri Reticulatae), 5 *fen* of Shengjiang (生姜, fresh ginger, Rhizoma Zingiberis Recens) and 7 *fen* of Jiegeng (桔梗, platycodon grandiflorum, Radix Platycodi).

In the three months in spring, add Zhishi (枳实, processed unripe bitter orange, Fructus Aurantii Immaturus) and remove Baizhu (白术, rhizome of largehead atractylodes, Rhizoma Atractylodis Macrocephalae)(altogether six ingredients).

In the three months in summer, add 3 *fen* of Shengjiang (生姜, fresh ginger, Rhizoma Zingiberis Recens), 5 *fen* of Zhishi (枳实, processed unripe bitter orange, Fructus Aurantii Immaturus) and 3 *fen* of Gancao (甘草, licorice, Radix Glycyrrhizae Praeparata)(altogether eight ingredients).

In the three months in autumn, add 3 *fen* of Chenpi (陈皮, tangerine peel, Pericarpium Citri Reticulatae)(altogether six ingredients).

These ingredients are chewed and divided into three packets, each of which is decocted in 3 *sheng* of water to get 2 *sheng* [after] boiling. [The decoction is] divided into three [doses] and taken warm. One [dose] is taken after the time it takes for a person to walk for four or five *li* (2 or 2. 5 miles). If the four limbs are congested, slightly increase Gancao (甘草, licorice, Radix Glycyrrhizae Praeparata). Each packet is divided into three small packets. Each small packet is decocted in 1 *sheng* of water to get 7 *ge* [after] boiling. [The decoction should be] taken warm. The dregs are put together to make another packet and boiled again to produce doses.

【原文】

(二)

长服诃黎勒丸方

诃黎勒(煨)、陈皮、厚朴(各三两)

右三味,末之,炼蜜丸如梧子大,酒饮服二十丸,加至三十丸。

【今译】

因饮食不节的长服方为诃黎勒丸方。

【英译】

Line 23.2

The formula often used [for resolving improper appetite] is Helile Pill (河黎勒丸, chebule pill).

Helile Pill (河黎勒丸, chebule pill) [is composed of] 3 *liang* of Helile (河黎勒, chebule, Fructus Chebulae) (simmer), 3 *liang* of Chenpi (陈皮, tangerine peel, Pericarpium Citri Reticulatae) and 3 *liang* of Houpo (厚朴, magnolia bark, Cortex Magnoliae Officinalis).

These three ingredients are ground into powder and blended with Lianmi (炼蜜, processed honey, Mel Praeparatum) to form pills the size of firmiana seeds. [Each time] 20 pills are taken with wine. [The dosage can be] increased to 30 pills.

【原文】

（三）

三物备急丸方

大黄（一两） 干姜（一两） 巴豆（一两，去皮心，熬，外研如脂）

右药各须精新，先捣大黄、干姜为末，研巴豆内中，合治一千杵，用为散，蜜和丸亦佳，密器中贮之，莫令歇。主心腹诸卒暴百病，若中恶客忤，心腹胀满，卒痛如锥刺，气急口噤，停尸卒死者，以暖水若酒服大豆许三四丸，或不下，捧头起，灌令下咽，须臾当差。如未差，更与三丸，当腹中鸣，即吐下，便差。若口噤，亦须折齿灌之。

【今译】

以三种药物为主治疗各种暴病的备急丸方。

【英译】

Line 23.3

［The formula used to treat fulminant diseases with three important medicinals is］Sanwu Beiji Pill（三物备急丸，pills made of three medicinals for emergency）.

Sanwu Beiji Pill（三物备急丸，pills made of three medicinals for emergency）［is composed of］1 *liang* of Dahuang（大黄，rhubarb，Radix et Rhizoma Rhei），1 *liang* of Ganjiang（干姜，dried ginger，Rhizoma Zingiberis）and 1 *liang* of Badou（巴豆，croton，Fructus Crotonis）（remove the bark and center，simmer and grind like lard）.

These ingredients should be pure and new. Dahuang（大黄，rhubarb，Radix et Rhizoma Rhei）and Ganjiang（干姜，dried ginger，Rhizoma Zingiberis）are ground into powder，Badou（巴豆，croton，Fructus Crotonis）is grated［and mixed］into it. Altogether it is grated for one thousand times to make into powder and blended with honey to form into pills. ［These pills］are stored in a sealed container to avoid leakage［of the content］. ［This formula is able］to treat various fulminant diseases in the abdomen. If［there are symptoms and signs of］malignant stroke，［invasion of］pathogenic factors，distension and fullness in the heart and abdomen，malignant pain like being needled，rapid breath，lockjaw and sudden cessation of breath［as if being］dead，three or four pills the size of soybeans should be taken with warm water or wine. If［it is］not swallowed，the head［of the patient］is raised up to pour［the pills］into the throat［so as to get them down］. After a while［the patient will］recover. If［the patient fails］to recover，3 more pills should be taken. When［there is］borborygmus，there will be vomiting and diarrhea，［and then the patient］will recover. If there is lockjaw，the teeth should be knocked out to pour［the pills into the throat］.

【原文】

(四)

治伤寒令愈不复,紫石寒食散方。

紫石英　白石英　赤石脂　钟乳(碓炼)　栝蒌根　防风　桔梗

文蛤　鬼臼(各十分)　太乙余粮(十分,烧)　干姜、附子(炮,去皮)、桂

枝(去皮,各四分)。

右十三味,杵为散,酒服方寸匕。

【今译】

治疗伤寒,使其不能复发的,是紫石寒食散方。

【原文】

(五)

救卒死方。

薤捣汁,灌鼻中。

【今译】

猝死救治方,为薤捣汁,灌入鼻中治疗。

【英译】

Line 23.4

To treat cold damage and to prevent [it] from recurring [after recovery], Zishi Hanshi Powder（紫石寒食散，fluorite and cold food powder）[is the appropriate formula].

Zishi Hanshi Powder（紫石寒食散，fluorite and cold food powder）[is composed of] 10 *fen* of Zishiying（紫石英，fluorite，Fluoritum），10 *fen* of Baishiying（白石英，white quartz，Album Quartz），10 *fen* of Chishizhi（赤石脂，halloysite，Halloysitum Rubrum），10 *fen* of Zhongrushi（钟乳石，stalactite，Statactitum）（refine and pound），10 *fen* of Gualougen（栝蒌根，trichosanthes root，Radix Trichosanthis），10 *fen* of Fangfeng（防风，saposhnikovia，Radix Saposhnikoviae），10 *fen* of Jiegeng（桔梗，platycodon grandiflorum，Radix Platycodi），10 *fen* of Wenge（文蛤，meretrix clam shell，Concha Meretricis），10 *fen* of Guijiu（鬼臼，common dysosma，Rhizoma Dysosmae Versipellis），10 *fen* of Taiyiyuliang（太乙余粮，limonite，Limonitum）（burn），4 *fen* of Ganjiang（干姜，dried ginger，Rhizoma Zingiberis），4 *fen* of Fuzi（附子，aconite，Radix Aconiti Lateralis Preparata）（fry heavily，remove the bark）and 4 *fen* of Guizhi（桂枝，cinnamon twig，Ramulus Cinnamomi）（remove the bark）.

These thirteen ingredients are ground into powder and [each time] 1 *fangcunbi* is taken with wine.

【英译】

Line 23.5

[To rescue a person who is] suddenly dead，Jiuzusi Formula（救卒死方，formula for saving sudden death）[is the appropriate formula]. [The ingredients in this formula are] crushed with Xie（薤，long-stamen onion，Bulbus Allii Macrostemonis）into juice to pour into the nose [to treat the patient].

【原文】

又方

雄鸡冠割取血,管吹内鼻中。

【今译】

另外一个药方,是从雄鸡冠中割取血,用苇管或笔管吹入鼻中。

【原文】

猪脂如鸡子大,苦酒一升,煮沸,灌喉中。

【今译】

鸡蛋大的一块猪脂,用苦酒一升煮沸,灌入喉中。

【原文】

鸡肝及血涂面上,以灰围四旁,立起。

【今译】

把鸡肝及血涂在脸面上,用灰围在四周,必站立而起。

【原文】

大豆二七粒,以鸡子白并酒和,尽以吞之。

【今译】

大豆二十七颗,与鸡蛋清和酒融合一起,全部通食。

【英译】

Another formula: To take blood by cutting off the comb of a rooster and blow it into the nose [of the patient] with a tube.

【英译】

A piece of pork lard, the size of a chicken's egg, is boiled in 1 *sheng* of vinegar and poured in the throat [of the patient for treatment].

【英译】

The liver and blood taken from a chicken are smeared over [the patient's] face with ash surrounding along all sides [of the face]. [The patient] will immediately stand up.

【英译】

Twenty-seven soybeans are mixed in wine with the white part of chicken's egg and swallowed all.

【原文】

（六）

救卒死而壮热者方。

矾石半斤，以水一斗半，煮消，以渍脚，令没踝。

【今译】

救卒死并能壮热的处方。

【原文】

（七）

救卒死而目闭者方。

骑牛临面，捣薤汁灌耳中，吹皂荚末鼻中，立效。

【今译】

救卒死而目闭的处方。

【原文】

（八）

救卒死而张口反折者方。

灸手足两爪后十四壮了，饮以五毒诸膏散。

【今译】

救卒死而角弓反张的处方。

Volume 3

【英译】

Line 23.6

The formula for rescuing [those who are] suddenly dead and strengthening heat: [This formula is composed of] 0.5 *jin* of Fanshi (矾石, alum, Alumen). [This ingredient is] melted in 1.5 *dou* of water through boiling and [used to] soak the feet and submerge the ankles.

【英译】

Line 23.7

The formula for rescuing [those who are] suddenly dead with eyes closed: To ride an ox close to the face [of the patient], to crush Xie (薤, long-stamen onion, Bulbus Allii Macrostemonis) into juice and pour [it] into the ears [of the patient], to blow powder of Zaojia (皂荚, gleditsia, Radix Gleditsiae) into the nose [of the patient]. [The treatment is] immediately effective.

【英译】

Line 23.8

The formula for rescuing [those who are] suddenly dead with opisthotonus: To burn 14 cones of moxa over the fingers of both hands and toes of both feet [of the patient] first. [Then] paste and powder made of five toxic medicinals are taken.

【原文】

(九)

救卒死而四肢不收失便者方。

马屎一升,水三斗,煮取二斗以洗之,又取牛洞一升,温酒灌口中,灸心下一寸,脐上三寸,脐下四寸,各一百壮,差。

【今译】

救卒死而四肢不收、大小便失禁的处方。

【原文】

(十)

救小儿卒死而吐利,不知是何病方。

狗屎一丸,绞取汁,以灌之。无湿者,水煮干者,取汁。

【今译】

救小儿卒死、呕吐、腹泻,致病原因不明的处方。

【原文】

(十一)

尸蹶,脉动而无气,气闭不通,故静而死也治方。

菖蒲屑,内鼻两孔中吹之,令人以桂屑着舌下。

【今译】

突然晕倒,脉动而无气,气息闭塞而不通,静而不动若尸体,以此方治疗。

【英译】

Line 23.9

The formula for rescuing [a person who is] suddenly dead with flaccidity of the four limbs: [This formula is composed of] 1 *sheng* of horse dung. [It is decocted in] 3 *dou* of water to get 2 *dou* [after] boiling to wash [the patient]. [Then] 1 *sheng* of sloppy excrement of cow is collected and poured into the mouth [of the patient] with wine. [Finally] moxibustion [is applied to the regions] 1 *cun* below the heart, 3 *cun* above the umbilicus and 4 *cun* below the umbilicus with one hundred cones. [The patient will be] recovered [after such a treatment].

【英译】

Line 23.10

To rescue infants [who are] suddenly dead or [suffer from] vomiting and diarrhea, what is the formula?

[This is the formula:] To wring one piece of dog's dung to get liquid. [This liquid is] poured [into the throat of the patient]. [If dog's dung is] not damp, [it should be] boiled in water to get liquid.

【英译】

Line 23.11

[The patient is] suddenly faint, the pulse is moving but there is no breath [because] qi is blocked. That is why this formula can treat [the patient who is] quiet but dead.

Changpu（菖蒲, acorus, Acorus Calamus）is ground into powder and blown into the nostrils [of the patient]. The patient is asked to hold cinnamon powder under the tongue.

Another formula: To scrape off hair in an area from the left corner [of the head], burn [it] into ash, mix with wine and pour into the throat. [The patient] will immediately stand up.

【原文】

又方

剔取左角发方寸,烧末,酒和,灌令入喉,立起。

【今译】

另外一个处方:从左角取一方寸的头发,烧成灰,与酒融合在一起,灌入喉咙,患者就会站立起来。

【原文】

(十二)

救卒死、客忤死,还魂汤主之方。

麻黄(三两,去节)　杏仁(去皮尖,七十个)　甘草(一两,炙)

右三味,以水八升,煮取三升,去滓。分令咽之,通治诸感忤。

【今译】

救卒死、客忤死等病患,宜用还魂汤主治。

【原文】

又方

韭根(一把)　乌梅(二七个)　吴茱萸(半升,炒)。

右三味,以水一斗煮之,以病人栉内中,三沸,栉浮者生,沉者死。煮取三升,去滓,分饮之。

【今译】

另外一个处方。

【英译】

Line 23. 12

Huanhun Decoction（还魂汤，decoction for restoring ethereal soul）：For rescuing ［a person who is］ suddenly dead and death ［caused by attack of］ pathogenic factors.

Huanhun Decoction（还魂汤，decoction for restoring ethereal soul）［is composed of］3 *liang* of Mahuang（麻黄，ephedra，Herba Ephedrae）(remove the twigs)，70 pieces of Xingren（杏仁，apricot kernel，Semen Armeniacae Amarum)(remove the peel and tip)and 1 *liang* of Gancao（甘草，licorice，Radix Glycyrrhizae Praeparata）（broil）.

These three ingredients are decocted in 8 *sheng* of water to get 3 *sheng* ［after］ boiling. The dregs are removed and divided ［into doses］ for swallowing. ［It can］ treat all ［types of cases］.

【英译】

Another formula

［This formula is composed of］1 handful of Jiugen（韭根，garlic chive root，Radix Allii Tuberosi），14 pieces of Wumei（乌梅，mume，Fructus Mume）and 0.5 *sheng* of Wuzhuyu（吴茱萸，evodia，Fructus Evodiae）（fry）.

These three ingredients are decocted in 1 *dou* of water. ［Then］ the comb of the patient is put into it to boil for three times to get 3 *sheng*. ［If］ the comb floats，［the patient］ will recover；［if］ the comb sinks，［the patient］ will die. The dregs are removed and ［the decoction is］ divided ［into doses］ for taking.

【原文】

(十三)

救自缢死方

救自缢死，旦至暮，虽已冷，必可治。暮至旦，小难也，恐此当言阴气盛故也。然夏时夜短于昼，又热，犹应可治。又云：心下若微温者，一日以上，犹可治之方。

徐徐抱解，不得截绳，上下安被卧之。一人以脚踏其两肩，手少挽其发，常弦弦勿纵之；一人以手按据胸上，数动之；一人摩捋臂胫，屈伸之。若已殭，但渐渐强屈之，并按其腹。如此一炊顷，气从口出，呼吸眼开，而犹引按莫置，亦勿苦劳之。须臾可少与桂汤及粥清，含与之，令濡喉，渐渐能咽，及稍止。若向令两人以管吹其两耳，深好。此法最善，无不活也。

【今译】

救自缢死亡的药方

救自缢死亡，如果其人上吊从早上到夜晚，虽然尸体已经变冷，但仍然可治。如果其人上吊从夜晚到早上，救治就比较难，恐怕与阴气盛有关。但夏时夜短昼长，天气又热，更应当可治。又有一个说法：心下如果有微温的，虽然发生了一日以上，但依然可治。

解救时应徐徐抱住解开绳子，不要骤然截绳，使其仰卧被上。让一人用脚踏主死者的两肩，用手挽住其头发，把头向上拉紧，使脖子平直；另一人用手按压死者的胸部，持续揉按；再一人按摩并屈伸其臂腿。如果自缢者身体已经僵硬，但要渐渐强使其身体弯曲，并按揉其腹部。这

Volume 3

【英译】

Line 23. 13

The formula for rescuing suicide from hanging

[In] rescuing suicide [from hanging], [if hanging continues from] dawn to dusk, though the body is already cold, [the person] still can be rescued. [If hanging continues from] dusk to dawn, [it is] a little bit difficult to rescue because yin qi is exuberant. But in summer, night is short and daytime is long, and it is hot. [That is why it is] still treatable. It is also said that if there is slight warmth below the heart and [although it has existed for] over one day, it is still treatable.

To rescue [the person], gently embrace [him] and relieve [the rope], do not cut the rope, and lay [him] on a mattress in a supine way. One person steps on both shoulders [of the patient] with his feet and mildly pulls the hair with his hands, keeping tight, not loosening. The second person presses the chest [of the patient] with his hands with rapid movement. The third person scrapes and rubs the arms and shins [of the patient], bending and stretching them. If [the body is] already stiff, gradually force it to bend and together press the abdomen. [Such a way of rescuing continues for a period of] time it takes for cooking a meal, [the patient will] begin to breathe and open the eyes. [The way to] stretch and press [the patient] should continue, but do not exhaust [the patient]. After a while [the patient is] given a little Guizhi Decoction (桂枝汤, cinnamon twig decoction) and clear porridge, keeping it in the mouth, moistening the throat, slowly swallowing and gradually stopping. If another two persons blow air into both ears [of the

样经过一顿饭的时间,就会使自缢者气从口出,呼吸恢复,眼睛睁开,此时还应继续按摩,但不宜太过。过一会可取少量桂枝汤及清粥,令其含在口中,濡润喉咙,渐渐就能吞咽了,稍止一会。再令两人用笔管吹其两耳,以通气。这是最好的方法,没有救不活的自缢者。

【原文】

(十四)

凡中暍死,不可使得冷,得冷便死,疗之方:

屈草带,绕暍人脐,使三两人溺其中,令温。亦可用热泥和屈草,亦可扣瓦椀底,按及车缸,以着暍人,取令溺须得流去。此谓道路穷,卒无汤,当令溺其中,欲使多人溺,取令温。若有汤便可与之,不可泥及车缸,恐此物冷。暍既在夏月,得热泥土、暖车缸,亦可用也。

【今译】

夏季中暑晕倒而死的,不能用冷敷法治疗,用冷敷法就会导致死亡。治疗方法如下:

将草绳屈作圆圈,绕在患者脐中,让三两个人尿在其中,使其有温暖之感。也可用热泥和圈起来的草,或用车缸放置在患者的肚脐周围,也让人尿在其中,但也要将其流去。这是在贫穷之地使用的救治办法,因为当地没有药物应急。所以就更应让多人撒尿其中,以便取暖。如果有汤药可供使用,就不宜再使用热泥和车缸,担心这些东西会变冷。因为中暑是在夏天,有热泥土和热车缸,也是可以用的。

patient] with tubes, it is quite ideal. This is the best [way to rescue suicide] and no one cannot be rescued.

【英译】

Line 23. 14

Death [caused by] heatstroke [in summer] cannot [be treated by] cold [compress because] cold [compress] will cause death. [The following is] the formula for treating it.

A piece of grass rope is used to encircle the umbilicus and three or two persons are asked to urinate into the encircled umbilicus to warm [this region]. Hot mud with furled grasses can also be used. [The umbilicus] can also be covered with the bottom of a ceramic bowl and pressed with the linchpin of a cart to touch [the umbilicus of] the patient. A person is asked to urinate into it till the urine flows away. Such a way [of treatment is used] in a poor place [where there is] no hot water. [That is why some people are] asked to urinate in it to warm [this region]. If there is hot water to use, mud and linchpin cannot be used [because they] may be cold. [If] heatstroke occurs in summer, [it is easy] to get hot mud and warm linchpin, and [they] can also be used [to warm the patient].

【原文】

(十五)

救溺死方。

取灶中灰两石余以埋人，从头至足。水出七孔，即活。

右疗自缢、溺、暍之法，并出自张仲景为之。其意殊绝，殆非常情所及，本草所能关，实救人之大术矣。伤寒家数有暍病，非此遇热之暍。

【今译】

救溺死者的药方。

从灶中取两石多的灰，从头到足将其掩埋。如果水从七大孔窍出，患者就会复活。

以上所谈到的自缢、溺水和中暑的治疗之法，均系张仲景所创建。意义非凡，并非一般性的治疗方法，与本草也有关系，是救人活命的大法。伤寒病患者都有发热之症，但并非中暑。

【原文】

(十六)

治马坠及一切筋骨损方。

大黄（一两，切，浸，汤成下）　绯帛（如手大，烧灰）　乱发（如鸡子大，烧灰用）　久用炊单布（一尺，烧灰）　败蒲（一握，三寸）　桃仁（四十九个，去皮尖，熬）　甘草（如中指节，炙，锉）

右七味，以童子小便量多少煎汤成，内酒一大盏，次下大黄，去滓，分温三服。先锉败蒲席半领，煎汤浴，衣被盖覆，斯须通利数行，痛楚立差，利及浴水赤，勿怪，即瘀血也。

【今译】

从马上坠落摔伤筋骨的治疗处方。

【英译】

Line 23. 15

The formula for rescuing death from drowning

To collect two *dan* or more ashes from a stove to cover the person from the head to the feet. [When] water flows out from seven orifices, [the person] will be rescued.

[The formula for] treating suicide, drowning and summer-heat mentioned above were all developed by Zhang Zhongjing, significantly unique, not just ordinary treatments or related to materia medica. [It is] in fact a great formula for rescuing people. People with cold damage often suffer from heat disease, but not just [caused by] exposure to heat.

【英译】

Line 23. 16

The formula for treating injury of sinews and bones due to falling from a horse

[This formula is composed of] 1 *liang* of Dahuang (大黄, rhubarb, Radix et Rhizoma Rhei) (cut, soak till decoction is finished), a hand-sized piece of Feibo (绯帛, crimson silk) (burn into ash), a chicken's egg-size of Luanfa (乱发, human hair, Crinis Carbonisatus) (burn into ash), 1 *chi* of Jiuyong Chuidanbu (久用炊单布, a piece of cloth used for cooking for a long time) (burn into ash), 3 *cun* of Baipu (败蒲, rotten typha, Pollen Typhae), 49 pieces of Taoren (桃仁, peach kernel, Semen Persicae) (remove the bark and tip, simmer) and a middle finger-sized piece of Gancao (甘草, licorice, Radix Glycyrrhizae Praeparata) (broil and grate).

These seven ingredients are decocted in infantile urine and a large cup of wine. Then Dahuang (大黄, rhubarb, Radix et Rhizoma Rhei) is added. The dregs are removed and [the decoction is] divided into three [doses] and taken warm. Half of Baipu (败蒲, rotten typha, Pollen Typhae) mat is grated and decocted. [The patient is] bathing [in it]. [Then the patient is] covered with clothes or quilt. [After] several times of diarrhea, pain will be relieved. [If] diarrhea and bath water turn red, do not feel strange. It is blood stasis.

禽兽鱼虫禁忌并治第二十四

【原文】

（一）

凡饮食滋味，以养于生，食之有妨，反能为害。自非服药炼液，焉能不饮食乎？切见时人，不闲调摄，疾疢竞起，若不因食而生，苟全其生，须知切忌者矣。所食之味，有与病相宜，有与身相害，若得宜则益体，害则成疾，以此致危，例皆难疗。凡煮药饮汁以解毒者，虽云救急，不可热饮，诸毒病得热更甚，宜冷饮之。

【今译】

凡是饮食的精华，均可以养生，但若不知禁忌，食之不但无益，而且会危害健康。除了服药炼丹的道家不饮食而外，任何人怎么会不靠饮食来生存呢？常见当时的人，不懂得自我调摄，疾病因此而起，人人都是靠饮食而生，而要保全人生，就必须懂得所有禁忌。所食用的食物，有的适宜于治疗疾病，有的则会伤害身体。如果食用了有益健康的食物，就会保健身体，如果食用了有害健康的食物，就会生病。由此而导致的疾病，均难治疗。凡是煎煮药的饮汁是用以解毒病的，虽然说是救急，但不可热饮，凡是致病的毒邪必热，热饮会使其更加严重，宜用冷饮主治。

Volume 3

Chapter 24
[Diseases Caused by] Fowls, Beasts, Fish and Insects:
Contraindications and Treatment

【英译】

Line 24. 1

All flavors (essence) of food and drink can nourish the body. [However there are] foods unable [to nourish] but to harm [the body]. Except [Daoists who practice] alchemy [and do not eat foods like five grains and meat, but take solomon's seal and lily etc.], who do not depend on food to live? Look at people around now, [they] do not know how to regulate and cultivate [their health] and therefore give rise to [various] diseases. [All the people] depend on food to live. In order to protect health, [one] must know the contraindications [in taking food]. Among the food to be taken, some are appropriate for [treating] disease, some are harmful to health. If [one takes] the appropriate, [it] replenishes the body; [if one takes] the harmful, [it will] cause disease. All the diseases caused by [inappropriate foods] are difficult to cure. The decoctions and juices for resolving toxins, though quite effective for emergency, cannot be taken hot [because] all the pathogenic factors [that have caused the diseases] will be worsened by heat. [Thus it is] appropriate to drink them cold.

【原文】

(二)

肝病禁辛,心病禁咸,脾病禁酸,肺病禁苦,肾病禁甘。春不食肝,夏不食心,秋不食肺,冬不食肾,四季不食脾。辨曰:春不食肝者,为肝气王,脾气败,若食肝,则又补肝,脾气败尤甚,不可救。又肝王之时,不可以死气入肝,恐伤魂也。若非王时,即虚,以肝补之佳,余脏准此。

【今译】

肝病禁用辛味食物,心病禁用咸味食物,脾病禁用酸味食物,肺病禁用苦味食物,肾病禁用甘味食物。春季肝旺,不能食用肝;夏季心旺,不能食用心;秋季肺旺,不能食用肺;冬季肾旺,不能食用肾;同时,一年四季都不能食用脾。原因是:春天之所以不食用肝,是因为肝气旺盛,脾气虚弱,如果食用肝,则肝得以补,而脾气更弱,不可救治。另外,肝旺盛的时候,死气不能入肝,入肝就会伤魂。如果非肝旺盛时,肝就会虚,食用肝以补肝效果更佳,其他脏器的情况也可以此类推。

【原文】

(三)

凡肝脏,自不可轻噉,自死者弥甚。

【今译】

凡是肝脏,自然不可轻易食用,自死动物的肝脏毒性更多,更不可食用。

【英译】

Line 24.2

[In] liver disease, pungent [food is] forbidden; [in] heart disease, salty [food is] forbidden; [in] spleen disease, sour [food is] forbidden; [in] lung disease, bitter [food is] forbidden; [in] kidney disease, sweet [food is] forbidden. [In] the spring, [animal's] liver is forbidden to eat; [in] the summer, [animal's] heart is forbidden to eat; [in] the autumn, [animal's] lung is forbidden to eat; [in] the winter, [animal's] kidney is forbidden to eat. [In] the four seasons, [animal's] spleen is forbidden to eat. This is the explanation: [The reason why animal's] liver is forbidden to eat [in] the spring [is that in this time] liver qi is exuberant but spleen qi is weak. If [animal's] liver is eaten, the liver will be supplemented, but spleen qi is further weakened and cannot be rescued. Furthermore, [when] the liver is exuberant, dead qi cannot enter the liver, otherwise the ethereal soul will be damaged. If the liver is not exuberant, it is of deficiency and will be well nourished by [eating animal's] liver. The other viscera [can be cultivated] in the same way.

【英译】

Line 24.3

[In] all [animals], the liver cannot be casually eaten, especially when [they have] died naturally.

【原文】

（四）

凡心皆为神识所舍，勿食之，使人来生复其报对矣。

【今译】

凡是心都是神识所舍之处，不能食用，食用了会使人的来生遭受报应。

【原文】

（五）

凡肉及肝，落地不着尘土者，不可食之。猪肉落水浮者，不可食。

【今译】

凡是肉和肝，落到地上不沾尘土的，就不可食用。猪肉落水后浮起的，也不可食用。

【原文】

（六）

诸肉及鱼，若狗不食，鸟不啄者，不可食。

【今译】

凡是肉及鱼类，如果狗都不食，鸟也不啄的，人也不可食用。

Volume 3

【英译】

Line 24.4

[In] all [animals], the heart is the chamber of mind and cannot be eaten [because it will] cause retribution in the next life of a person.

【英译】

Line 24.5

Any meat and liver [of animals] are inedible [if they are] not stained with dust when dropping on the ground. [If] pork floats when dropping in water, [it is] inedible.

【英译】

Line 24.6

Any meat and fish are inedible if dogs do not eat and birds do not peck.

【原文】

（七）

诸肉不干，火炙不动，见水自动者，不可食之。

【今译】

凡是久放而不干的肉类，用火烤而不动的，见水能自动的，不可食用。

【原文】

（八）

肉中有米点者，不可食之。

【今译】

肉中有米粒一样的红点，不可食用。

【原文】

（九）

六畜肉，热血不断者，不可食之。父母及身本命肉，食之令人神魂不安。

【今译】

宰杀的牲畜，热血之气没有消散的，不可食用。父母及自己生辰时所属之肉，食用了会使人神魂不安。

Volume 3

【英译】

Line 24.7

Any meat that does not move when roasted in fire and moves when put in water is inedible.

【英译】

Line 24.8

[If] there are red spots like grains in meat, it is inedible.

【英译】

Line 24.9

The meat of six domestic animals, [when] the blood [in it] is still warm, cannot be eaten. [If] the meat [related to] parents' and one's own life (birthday), [it cannot be eaten,] otherwise [it will] disquiet one's spirit and ethereal soul.

【原文】

（十）

食肥肉及热羹，不得饮冷水。

【今译】

吃肥肉，喝热羹，不能同时饮冷水。

【原文】

（十一）

诸五脏及鱼，投地尘土不污者，不可食之。

【今译】

凡动物的五脏和鱼，掉到地上而没有沾上尘土的，不可食用。

【原文】

（十二）

秽饭，馁鱼，臭肉，食之皆伤人。

【今译】

凡是污染的饭食、馁烂的鱼和发臭的肉，吃了都会伤人。

【英译】

Line 24. 10

Cold water cannot be drunken [when] eating fatty meat and hot soup.

【英译】

Line 24. 11

Any internal organs [of animals] and fish may be inedible [if they] are not stained with dust when dropping on the ground.

【英译】

Line 24. 12

Any dirty food, spoiled fish and malodorous meat will damage people if eaten.

【原文】

（十三）

自死肉，口闭者，不可食之。

【今译】

凡自行死亡的动物，口闭与否，其肉均不可食用。

【原文】

（十四）

六畜自死，皆疫死，则有毒，不可食之。

【今译】

自行死亡的六畜（马、牛、羊、鸡、犬、猪），都是因病死亡，肉中一定有毒，不可食用。

【原文】

（十五）

兽自死，北首及伏地者，食之杀人。

【今译】

动物自行死亡，头朝北倒伏在地，其肉吃了就会致人死亡。

Volume 3

【英译】

Line 24. 13

[In any] dead [animals], no matter the mouth is open [or not], the meat is inedible.

【英译】

Line 24. 14

[Among any of] the six animals, [including horse, cow, sheep, chicken, dog and pig], [death is] all caused by disease. [Therefore the meat is] inedible [because] there is toxin [in it].

【英译】

Line 24. 15

[When] an animal died on the ground with the head facing the north, [its meat cannot be eaten, otherwise] it will kill the person [who has eaten the meat].

【原文】

(十六)

食生肉,饱饮乳,变成白虫。

【今译】

吃生肉,喝饱饮乳酪,在体内就会变成寸白虫。

【原文】

(十七)

疫死牛肉,食之令病洞下,亦致坚积,宜利药下之。

【今译】

因患疫病而死亡的牛,肉中有毒,食后则导致洞泻,亦可致坚癖积聚,宜用利药攻下治疗。

【原文】

(十八)

脯脏米瓮中,有毒,及经夏食之,发肾病。

【今译】

干肉储藏在米瓮中,都会有毒,夏季食用后,就会引发肾病。

【英译】

Line 24. 16

[If one] eats raw meat and drinks much milk, [it will] transform into taenia [in his body].

【英译】

Line 24. 17

[When] a cow died due to epidemics, [there is toxin in the meat]. To eat [its meat] will cause profuse diarrhea or accumulation of hardness. Medicinals for purgation is appropriate [for treating it].

【英译】

Line 24. 18

Dried meat stored in a rice jar is inevitably toxic. [If kept in the rice jar] for the whole summer, [it] will cause kidney disease [if] eaten.

【原文】

(十九)

治自死六畜肉中毒方。

黄柏屑,捣服方寸匕。

【今译】

治疗因食用自行死亡的六畜之肉而中毒的药方为黄柏屑,捣碎后每次服用一方寸匕。

【原文】

(二十)

治食郁肉漏脯中毒方。

烧犬屎,酒服方寸匕,每服人乳汁亦良。饮生韭汁三升,亦得。

【今译】

治疗食用遭受污染或潮湿的肉脯而中毒的药方:

烧犬屎,每次用酒服用一方寸匕,用人乳服用也可以。饮用生韭菜汁三升,也行。

Volume 3

【英译】

Line 24. 19

To treat poisoning due to [eating] the meat of six domestic animals that died on their own, the formula is Huangbo Powder（黄柏屑, phellodendron powder）. [This ingredient is] grated [into powder] and taken 1 *fangcunbi* [each time].

【英译】

Line 24. 20

To treat poisoning due to eating contaminated or dampened dried meat, the formula is to burn dog dung. [Each time] 1 *fangcunbi* is taken with wine. Each time [it can also be] taken with human milk. [Besides, it is] also possible to drink 3 *sheng* of garlic chive juice.

【原文】

（二十一）

治黍米中藏干脯食之中毒方

大豆浓煮汁，饮数升即解。亦治诸肉漏脯等毒。

【今译】

治疗因食用黍米中储藏的干肉而中毒的药方

将大豆煮成浓汁，饮用数升后就能解毒。这个方子也可用以治疗因食用各种干肉受潮而中毒的疾病。

【原文】

（二十二）

治疗吃生肉中毒的处方

掘地深三尺，取其下土三升，以水五升，煮数沸，澄清汁，饮一升即愈。

【今译】

治食生肉中毒方

挖地深三尺，取地下土三升，用五升水煮数次，澄清后饮一升就能治愈。

Volume 3

【英译】

Line 24.21

To treat poisoning due to eating dried meat stored in millet, the formula is to boil Dadou (大豆, yellow soybean, Semen Sojae) into liquid. [After] taking several *sheng* [of the liquid], [the toxin will be] resolved. [Such a formula can] also treat poisoning due to eating dampened dried meat.

【英译】

Line 24.22

To treat poisoning due to eating raw meat, the formula is to dig [a hole] 3 *cun* deep into the earth and take out 3 *sheng* of soil from the bottom [of the hole]. [The soil is] boiled in 5 *sheng* of water for several times. To take 1 *sheng* of the settled liquid will cure [the patient].

【原文】

(二十三)

治六畜鸟兽肝中毒方

水浸豆豉,绞取汁,服数升愈。

【今译】

治疗食用六畜鸟兽肝而中毒的处方

用水浸泡豆豉,绞取其汁,服用数升就能治愈。

【原文】

(二十四)

马脚无夜眼者,不可食之。

【今译】

马的前两足膝上没有夜眼,其肉是不可食用的。

【原文】

(二十五)

食骏马肉,不饮酒,则杀人。

【今译】

食用骏马肉时,若不饮酒,则会致命。

Volume 3

【英译】

Line 24. 23

To treat poisoning due to eating the liver of six domestic animals, birds and beasts, the formula is to soak fermented soybeans in water and get juice through squeezing. [After] taking several *sheng* [of the juice], [the patient will be] cured.

【英译】

Line 24. 24

[If] a horse has no night eyes [on the front knees], [its meat is] inedible.

【英译】

Line 24. 25

[If a person] eats the meat of a galloping horse without drinking wine, [it] will kill him.

【原文】

(二十六)

马肉不可热食,伤人心。

【今译】

马肉不可趁热而食,这样会伤害人心。

【原文】

(二十七)

马鞍下肉,食之杀人。

【今译】

马鞍下的肉,吃了就会致人死亡。

【原文】

(二十八)

白马黑头者,不可食之。

【今译】

身白而黑头的马,其肉不可食用。

【英译】

Line 24. 26

Horse meat cannot be eaten hot，[otherwise it will] damage the heart of the person.

【英译】

Line 24. 27

The meat under a horse's hoof [is inedible]. Eating it will kill the person.

【英译】

Line 24. 28

White horse with black head is inedible.

【原文】

(二十九)

白马青蹄者,不可食之。

【今译】

身白而蹄青的马,其肉不可食用。

【原文】

(三十)

马肉狁肉共食,饱醉卧,大忌。

【今译】

马肉和猪肉一同食用,大饱大醉而入睡,则是大忌。

【原文】

(三十一)

驴马肉合猪肉食之,成霍乱。

【今译】

驴肉、马肉和猪肉一起食用,会造成霍乱。

Volume 3

【英译】

Line 24.29

White horse with blue hooves is inedible.

【英译】

Line 24.30

Eating the meat of horse and pig together [will not necessarily cause disease]. [But] sleeping [right after] overeating and overdrinking is a great contraindication.

【英译】

Line 24.31

Eating the meat of donkey, horse and pig together will cause huoluan (simultaneous vomiting and diarrhea).

【原文】

(三十二)

马肝及毛不可妄食,中毒害人。

【今译】

马肝上有毛的不可随意食用,不然就会中毒害人。

【原文】

(三十三)

食马肝毒中人未死方

雄鼠屎二七粒,末之,水和服,日再服。

【今译】

食用马肝中毒没有导致人死亡的治疗处方

用雄鼠屎十四粒,捻成末,融入水中服用,一天服用两次。

【原文】

又方

人垢取方寸匕,服之佳。

【今译】

另外一个处方

取一方寸匕的人头发垢,服用了效果也不错。

Volume 3

【英译】

Line 24.32

The liver of a horse with hair is inedible. Poisoning [from it] will damage the person [eating it].

【英译】

Line 24.33

To treat poisoning from eating horse liver without killing the person, the formula is to collect 14 droppings of a male mouse, grate into powder and mix with water for taking. [It is] taken twice a day.

【英译】

Another formula

Collect 1 *fangcunbi* of filth from the head of a person. Taking it is effective [in resolving toxin].

【原文】

(三十四)

治食马肉中毒欲死方

香豉(二两)　杏仁(三两)

右二味,蒸一食顷,熟,杵之服,日再服。

【今译】

治疗食用马肉中毒欲死的处方。

【原文】

又方

煮芦根汁,饮之良。

【今译】

另一处方

将芦根煮成汁,饮用之后效果良好。

【原文】

(三十五)

疫死牛,或目赤,或黄,食之大忌。

【今译】

牛染疫而死,两目或赤或黄,尤当忌食。

【英译】

Line 24.34

To treat poisoning from eating horse meat 〔that causes the person〕 on verge of death, the formula 〔is composed of〕 2 *liang* of Xiangchi（香豉, fermented soybean, Sojae Semen Fermentatum）and 3 *liang* of Xingren（杏仁, apricot kernel, Semen Armeniacae Amarum）.

These two ingredients are steamed as long as it takes for eating a meal. 〔When well〕 boiled, 〔it is〕 grated for taking. 〔It is〕 taken twice a day.

【英译】

Another formula

Lugen（芦根, phragmites, Rhizoma Phragmitis）is boiled into juice. Taking it is effective 〔in resolving toxin〕.

【英译】

Line 24.35

Cow that died from epidemics with red or yellow eyes is absolutely forbidden to eat.

【原文】

（三十六）

牛肉共猪肉食之，必作寸白虫。

【今译】

牛肉与猪肉一同食用，必然导致体内出现寸白虫。

【原文】

（三十七）

青牛肠，不可合犬肉食之。

【今译】

青牛肠是不可以与犬肉同食的。

【原文】

（三十八）

牛肺，从三月至五月，其中有虫如马尾，割去勿食，食则损人。

【今译】

从三月到五月，牛肺中有马尾一样的吸虫或蛔虫，应当将肺割去，如果食用了就会损伤人。

【英译】

Line 24.36

Eating the meat of cow and pig together will inevitably cause taenia [inside the body].

【英译】

Line 24.37

The intestines of a blue cow cannot be eaten together with dog meat.

【英译】

Line 24.38

From March to May, there are worms in the lung of a cow like the hair on a horse's tail. [To eat the meat of the cow, its lung should be] cut off, avoiding eating. [It] will damage the person eating it.

【原文】

(三十九)

牛羊猪肉,皆不得以楮木、桑木蒸炙。食之,令人腹内生虫。

【今译】

使用牛肉、羊肉、猪肉,不能用楮木和桑木蒸煮。不然的话食用后会令人腹内生虫。

【原文】

(四十)

噉蛇牛肉杀人,何以知之?噉蛇者,毛发向后顺者是也。

【今译】

牛吃了蛇而被毒死,人吃了死牛肉后也会毒死,怎么才能知道牛是吃蛇中毒而死的呢?吃了蛇而被毒死的牛,全身的毛则向后而顺。

【原文】

(四十一)

治噉蛇牛肉食之欲死方

饮人乳汁一升,立愈。

【今译】

牛因吃蛇而中毒死亡,人因吃此死牛肉而中毒欲死,其治疗处方是饮人乳汁一升,就能立刻治愈。

【英译】

Line 24.39

The meat of cows, sheep and pigs cannot be steamed and roasted by burning mulberry wood. Otherwise it will cause worms in the abdomen.

【英译】

Line 24.40

A cow died from poisoning of a snake it has eaten. [If a person has eaten the beef from this cow, he will be] killed. How [can one] know [it]? [If this cow died from poisoning by] eating a snake, the hair over its body turns backwards.

【英译】

Line 24.41

To treat [a person] about to die after eating the meat of a cow killed by a snake, the formula is to drink 1 *sheng* of human milk [that will] immediately cure [the patient].

【原文】

又方

以泔洗头,饮一升,愈。

牛肚细切,以水一斗,煮取一升,暖饮之,大汗出者愈。

【今译】

另外一个处方

用泔水洗头,洗后饮一升去垢水,就能治愈。

将牛胃细切,用水一斗煮,煮后取一升,暖而饮之,大汗出后就能痊愈。

【原文】

(四十二)

治食牛肉中毒方

甘草煮汁,饮之即解。

【今译】

治疗食用牛肉中毒的处方

甘草煮成汁,饮用后就能解毒。

【英译】

Another formula：

Wash the head with water that has rinsed rice and drink 1 *sheng* [of the water that is used to wash the head]. [The patient will be] cured.

The stomach of a cow is finely chopped and boiled in 1 *dou* of water to get 1 *sheng* which should be taken warm. [When] great sweating [is induced], [the patient will be] cured.

【英译】

Line 24.42

To treat poisoning from eating meat of a cow, the formula is to boil Gancao（甘草，licorice，Radix Glycyrrhizae Praeparata）into juice. Drinking the juice will immediately resolve [the toxin].

【原文】

(四十三)

羊肉其有宿热者,不可食之。

【今译】

羊肉中其有宿热的,不可食用。

【原文】

(四十四)

羊肉不可共生鱼、酪食之,害人。

【今译】

羊肉不可与生鱼和酪食一起吃,这样吃对人有危害。

【原文】

(四十五)

羊蹄甲中有珠子白者,名羊悬筋,食之令人癫。

【今译】

羊蹄甲里如果有珠子似的白色斑点,叫作羊悬筋,食了会令人发癫。

Volume 3

【英译】

Line 24.43

Mutton is hot [in nature]. [People with heat disease] cannot eat it.

【英译】

Line 24.44

Sheep meat cannot be eaten together with raw fish and fermented milk. [Otherwise it will] harm the person.

【英译】

Line 24.45

[If] there are white spots like pearl in the hooves of sheep, it is called suspended sinews of sheep. Eating it will cause epilepsy.

【原文】

(四十六)

白羊黑头,食其脑,作肠痈。

【今译】

体白头黑的羊,吃了其脑,就会引发肠痈。

【原文】

(四十七)

羊肝共生椒食之,破人五脏。

【今译】

羊肝与生椒一起食用,就会破坏人体的五脏。

【原文】

(四十八)

猪肉共羊肝和食之,令人心闷。

【今译】

猪肉与羊肝一起食用,会令人心中郁闷。

【英译】

Line 24.46

Eating the brain of a white sheep with black head will cause intestinal abscess.

【英译】

Line 24.47

Eating sheep liver with raw pepper will break the five zang-organs of a person.

【英译】

Line 24.48

Eating pork together with sheep liver will cause depression.

【原文】

(四十九)

猪肉以生胡荽同食,烂人脐。

【今译】

猪肉与生胡荽一同食用,会使人的肚脐溃烂。

【原文】

(五十)

猪脂不可合梅子食之。

【今译】

猪脂不可与梅子一同食用。

【原文】

(五十一)

猪肉和葵食之,少气。

【今译】

猪肉和葵菜一同食用,可导致少气。

【英译】

Line 24.49

Eating pork together with raw Husui（胡荽，coriander, Coriandrum Sativum）will putrefy the umbilicus of the person.

【英译】

Line 24.50

Pork lard cannot be eaten together with Meizi（梅子，mume, Fructus Mume）.

【英译】

Line 24.51

Eating pork together with Jinkui（锦葵，mallow，Malva Sinensis Cavan）causes insufficiency of qi [in the chest].

【原文】

(五十二)

鹿肉不可和蒲白作羹,食之发恶疮。

【今译】

鹿肉不可与蒲白一同作成羹,食用后会引发恶疮。

【原文】

(五十三)

麇脂及梅李子,若妊娠食之,令子青盲,男子伤精。

【今译】

如果妇女妊娠后食用麇脂及梅李子,会使胎儿色盲。男子食用则会损伤肾精。

【原文】

(五十四)

獐肉不可合虾及生菜、梅李果食之,皆病人。

【今译】

獐子肉不可与虾及生菜、梅李果等一同食用,都会引发疾病。

【英译】

Line 24.52

Venison cannot be made into soup together with Pubai （蒲白，typha rhizome，Rhizoma Typhae）. Eating it will cause malignant sores.

【英译】

Line 24.53

If a pregnant woman eats elk's fat together with Meilizi （梅李子，plum，Prunus Salicina），[it will] cause blindness of the fetus. [If] a man eats，[it will] damage [kidney] essence.

【英译】

Line 24.54

Meat of river deer cannot be eaten together with shrimp，raw vegetables and mume fruit. [Eating] any of them will cause disease.

【原文】

(五十五)

痼疾人不可食熊肉,令终身不愈。

【今译】

患痼疾的人不可吃熊肉,不然将终身不愈。

【原文】

(五十六)

白犬自死,不出舌者,食之害人。

【今译】

白狗自行死亡后舌头没有露出,食用后会危害人体。

【原文】

(五十七)

食狗鼠余,令人发瘘疮。

【今译】

吃了狗或老鼠吃剩下的食物,会引发瘰疬。

Volume 3

【英译】

Line 24.55

A patient with obstinate disease cannot eat bear meat，[otherwise the disease] cannot be cured all his life.

【英译】

Line 24.56

[If one eats] a white dog that has died without sticking out the tongue，[it] will harm him.

【英译】

Line 24.57

Eating a dog's or a rat's leftover will cause scrofula.

【原文】

(五十八)

治食犬肉不消,心下坚或腹胀,口干大渴,心急发热,妄语如狂,或洞下方:

杏仁(一升,合皮,熟,研用)

右一味,以沸汤三升和,取汁,分三服,利下肉片,大验。

【今译】

治疗食用狗肉后不能消化,心下坚硬或腹部胀满,口干大渴,心急发热,妄语如狂,或洞泻不止。其治疗之方如下:

杏仁一升,与其皮一起煮熟,研成末使用。然后用三升水煮沸成汤,取用其汁,分为三剂服用。服用后可排泄所停滞的肉片,很有疗效。

【原文】

(五十九)

妇人妊娠,不可食兔肉、山羊肉及鳖、鸡、鸭,令子无声音。

【今译】

妇女妊娠后,不可食用兔肉、山羊肉及鳖、鸡、鸭等肉,如果食用了就会使胎儿失去声音。

【英译】

Line 24.58

To treat indigestion [after] eating dog meat [marked by] hardness below the heart, or abdominal distension, dryness of the mouth, great thirst, manic talk, or incessant diarrhea, the formula is to decoct 1 *sheng* of Xingren（杏仁, apricot kernel, Semen Armeniacae Amarum）(cook with the peel and grind thoroughly).

This ingredient is decocted in 3 *sheng* of water to get juice. [The juice is] divided into three [doses] for taking. [After taking the juice, stagnated dog] meat will be discharged, quite effective.

【英译】

Line 24.59

[After] pregnancy, women cannot eat meat of rabbit, goat, turtle, chicken and duck, [otherwise] the fetus will become mute.

【原文】

（六十）

兔肉不可合白鸡肉食之，令人面发黄。

【今译】

兔肉不可与白鸡肉一同食用，否则会使人面色发黄。

【原文】

（六十一）

兔肉着干姜食之，成霍乱。

【今译】

兔肉如果与干姜一同食用，就会导致霍乱。

【原文】

（六十二）

凡鸟自死，口不闭，翅不合者，不可食之。

【今译】

凡是鸟自行死亡的，口就不闭，翅膀也不收，不可食用。

Volume 3

【英译】

Line 24.60

Rabbit meat cannot be eaten together with white chicken, [otherwise it will] make the person's face yellow.

【英译】

Line 24.61

Rabbit meat cannot be eaten together with dried ginger, [because it can] cause huoluan (霍乱, simultaneous vomiting and diarrhea).

【英译】

Line 24.62

The birds that died on their own without closing the beaks and folding the wings are inedible.

【原文】

（六十三）

诸禽肉肝青者，食之杀人。

【今译】

凡是禽兽的肉及肝出现青黑色的，食用后就会中毒死亡。

【原文】

（六十四）

鸡有六翮四距者，不可食之。

【今译】

鸡有六个翅膀和四只爪的，不可食用。

【原文】

（六十五）

乌鸡白首者，不可食之。

【今译】

乌鸡头是白的，不可食用。

Volume 3

【英译】

Line 24.63

[If] the meat and liver of any poultry are blue, eating it will kill the person.

【英译】

Line 24.64

The chickens with six wings and four claws are inedible.

【英译】

Line 24.65

The black chickens with white heads are inedible.

【原文】

(六十六)

鸡不可共葫蒜食之,滞气。

【今译】

鸡肉不可与大蒜一同食用,否则就会引起滞气。

【原文】

(六十七)

山鸡不可合鸟兽肉食之。

【今译】

山鸡不可与鸟兽肉一同食用。

【原文】

(六十八)

雉肉久食之,令人瘦。

【今译】

雉肉吃的时间长了,就会令人消瘦。

Volume 3

【英译】

Line 24.66

Chickens cannot be eaten together with garlic [for it can cause] stagnation of qi.

【英译】

Line 24.67

Red junglefowl cannot be eaten together with [the meat of] birds and beasts.

【英译】

Line 24.68

Pheasant cannot be eaten over time, [otherwise it will] make the person emaciated.

【原文】

（六十九）

鸭卵不可合鳖肉食之。

【今译】

鸭蛋不可与鳖肉一同食用。

【原文】

（七十）

妇人妊娠，食雀肉，令子淫乱无耻。

【今译】

妇女妊娠后，如果食用雀肉，就会使胎儿以后淫乱无耻。

【原文】

（七十一）

雀肉不可合李子食之。

【今译】

雀肉不可与合李子一同食用。

【英译】

Line 24.69

Duck eggs cannot be eaten together with turtle meat.

【英译】

Line 24.70

[If] a woman eats sparrow [after] pregnancy, [it will] make the fetus promiscuous and shameless [in the future].

【英译】

Line 24.71

Sparrow meat cannot be eaten together with Lizi (李子, plum, Prunus Salicina).

【原文】

(七十二)

燕肉勿食,入水为蛟龙所嗷。

【今译】

燕子肉不可食用,不然入水后就会为蛟龙吞噬。

【原文】

(七十三)

鸟兽有中毒箭死者,其肉有毒,解之方:

大豆煮汁及蓝汁,服之解。

【今译】

鸟兽被有毒的箭射死了,其肉就有毒,可解其毒的处方是,大豆煮汁及蓝汁,服用之后就解毒了。

【原文】

(七十四)

鱼头正白,如连珠至脊上,食之杀人。

【今译】

鱼头上有白色斑点,像珠子一样连续到脊背上,食用了就会危害生命。

Volume 3

【英译】

Line 24.72

Swallow meat cannot be eaten. [The person who has eaten swallow meat will be] eaten by loong [when he has] entered water.

【英译】

Line 24.73

The meat of birds and beasts killed by poisoned arrow contains toxin [which can be] resolved by juice of Dadou (大豆, yellow soybean, Semen Flavum Sojae) and juice of Liaolan (蓼蓝, indigo plant, Herba Indigo).

【英译】

Line 24.74

Eating fish with white spots on the head and stretching to the spine will kill the person.

【原文】

(七十五)

鱼头中无鳃者,不可食之,杀人。

【今译】

鱼头中没有鳃的,不可食用,使用了就会致命。

【原文】

(七十六)

鱼无肠胆者,不可食之,三年阴不起,女子绝生。

【今译】

鱼无肠胆的,不可食用,食用后,会导致男子三年阳痿,女子会导致绝生。

【原文】

(七十七)

鱼头似有角者,不可食之。

鱼目合者,不可食之。

【今译】

鱼头上好像长有角的,不可食用。

鱼的眼睛闭合的,不可食用。

Volume 3

【英译】

Line 24.75

Fish without gills is inedible, [eating it will] kill the person.

【英译】

Line 24.76

Fish without intestines and gallbladder is inedible. [Eating it will cause] impotence in men in three years and infertility in women.

【英译】

Line 24.77

Fish seeming to have horns on the head is inedible.

Fish with closed eyes is inedible.

【原文】

(七十八)

六甲日,勿食鳞甲之物。

【今译】

六甲之日是六甲之神日,所以不可食用鳞甲之物。

【原文】

(七十九)

鱼不可合鸡肉食之。

【今译】

鱼不可与鸡肉一同食用。

【原文】

(八十)

鱼不得和鸬鹚肉食之。

【今译】

鱼不得和鸬鹚肉一同食用。

【英译】

Line 24.78

On the six jiazi days, [animals, beasts or birds with] scales or shells cannot be eaten [because these six days are the days when the concerned gods are on duty].

【英译】

Line 24.79

Fish cannot be eaten together with chickens.

【英译】

Line 24.80

Fish cannot be eaten together with cormorant.

【原文】

(八十一)

鲤鱼鲊不可合小豆藿食之,其子不可合猪肝食之,害人。

【今译】

鲤鱼鲊不可与小豆藿一同食用,鲤鱼子也不可与猪肝一同食用,如果食用了就会伤害人。

【原文】

(八十二)

鲤鱼不可合犬肉食之。

【今译】

鲤鱼不可与狗肉一同食用。

【原文】

(八十三)

鲫鱼不可合猴雉肉食之。一云不可合猪肝食。

【今译】

鲫鱼不可与猴子和野鸡肉一同食用。还有一种说法,也不可与猪肝一同食用。

Volume 3

【英译】

Line 24. 81

Salted carp cannot be eaten together with the leaves of red beans. Its roes cannot be eaten with pork. [Eating it will] damage the person.

【英译】

Line 24. 82

Carp cannot be eaten together with dog meat.

【英译】

Line 24. 83

Carp cannot be eaten together with the meat of monkey or pheasant. Another saying is that it cannot be eaten together with pig liver.

【原文】

(八十四)

鳀鱼合鹿肉生食,令人筋甲缩。

【今译】

鳀鱼与鹿肉一起生吃,会使人筋脉爪甲痉挛萎缩。

【原文】

(八十五)

青鱼鲊不可合生葫荽及生葵,并麦中食之。

【今译】

青鱼鲊不可与生葫荽、生葵及麦酱一同食用。

【原文】

(八十六)

鳅、鳝不可合白犬血食之。

【今译】

泥鳅和鳝鱼不可与白色狗的血一同食用。

【英译】

Line 24.84

Eating raw Chinese catfish together with venison will cause shrinkage of sinews and nails.

【英译】

Line 24.85

Salted blue fish cannot be eaten together with raw coriander, raw mallow and wheat.

【英译】

Line 24.86

Loach and eel cannot be eaten together with blood from a white dog.

【原文】

(八十七)

龟肉不可合酒、果子食之。

【今译】

龟肉不可与酒及果子一同食用。

【原文】

(八十八)

鳖目凹陷者,及厌下有王字形者,不可食之。

【今译】

鳖的眼睛凹陷,鳖甲上有王字形的,不可食用。

【原文】

(八十九)

其肉不得合鸡鸭子食之。

【今译】

其肉不可与鸡子和鸭子一同食用。

【英译】

Line 24.87

Tortoise meat cannot be eaten together with wine and fruit.

【英译】

Line 24.88

Turtles with sunken eyes and lines below the abdomen like the structure of the Chinese character king (the structure 王 is composed of three transverse lines with one vertical line in the middle) is inedible.

【英译】

Line 24.89

The meat [mentioned above] cannot be eaten together with chicken and duck eggs.

【原文】

（九十）

龟鳖肉不可合苋菜食之。

【今译】

龟和鳖肉不可与苋菜一同食用。

【原文】

（九十一）

虾无须，及腹下通黑，煮之反白者，不可食之。

【今译】

虾没有须，腹下呈黑色，煎煮之后反而发白的，不可食用。

【原文】

（九十二）

食脍，饮奶酪，令人腹中生虫，为瘕。

【今译】

吃切细的肉，喝奶酪，会令人腹中生虫，变成瘕聚。

Volume 3

【英译】

Line 24. 90

Tortoise and turtle meat cannot be eaten together with amaranth.

【英译】

Line 24. 91

Shrimp without palpus [but] with black abdomen that turns white [after] boiling is inedible.

【英译】

Line 24. 92

Eating minced meat and drinking koumiss will cause worms in the abdomen and [form] mass.

【原文】

（九十三）

鲙食之，在心胸间不化，吐复不出，速下除之，久成症病，治之方：

橘皮（一两）　大黄（二两）　朴硝（二两）

右三味，以水一大升，煮至小升，顿服即消。

【今译】

　　吃鲙过多，停滞在心胸间不能消化，怎么也吐不出，应采取措施快速下除。如果拖延久了就会引发症病，应以此方治疗。

【原文】

（九十四）

食鲙多不消，结为症病，治之方：

马鞭草

右一味，捣汁饮之，或以姜叶汁，饮之一升，亦消。又可服吐药吐之。

【今译】

　　食用细切的鱼肉多不消，就会结聚成为病症，马鞭草是其治疗处方。

Volume 3

【英译】

Line 24. 93

[The following is] the formula for treating the disease [marked by], [after] eating minced fish, no transformation in the heart and chest and failure to vomit [it out]. [It must be] immediately resolved, endurance will result in disease.

This formula [is composed of] 1 *liang* of Jupi (橘皮, tangerine peel, Pericarpium Citri Reticulatae), 2 *liang* of Dahuang (大黄, rhubarb, Radix et Rhizoma Rhei) and 2 *liang* of Poxiao (朴硝, impure mirabilite, Sodium Sulphatae).

These three ingredients are decocted in 1 big *sheng* of water to get 1 small *sheng* [after] boiling. [This decoction is] taken once the whole and [it will be] resolved.

【英译】

Line 24. 94

[If] minced fish is taken but not digested, [it will] bind into disease. The formula for treating it is Mabiancao (马鞭草, verbena, Herba Verbenae).

This ingredient is grated into juice for drinking. Or [it is mixed with] the juice of ginger leaves. [After] taking 1 *sheng*, [it will be] resolved. [It can also be treated by] taking medicinals for inducing vomiting to vomit it.

【原文】

(九十五)

食鱼后中毒,面肿烦乱,治之方:

橘皮

浓煎汁,服之即解。

【今译】

吃鱼之后中毒,面部肿胀,烦躁慌乱,治疗的处方是橘皮。浓浓地煎煮后取其汁,服后就能解毒。

【原文】

(九十六)

食鯸鮧鱼中毒方

芦根

煮汁,服之即解。

【今译】

吃了河豚鱼中毒,解毒的处方是芦根。煎煮后取其汁,服用之后就能解毒。

【英译】

Line 24. 95

Poisoning from eating fish [causes] facial swelling, vexation and derangement. The formula for treating [it is] Jupi (橘皮, orange peel, Pericarpium Reticulatae).

This ingredient is boiled to get juice. Taking it will resolve [toxin].

【英译】

Line 24. 96

[To resolve] poisoning from eating globefish, the formula is Lugen (芦根, phragmites, Rhizoma Phragmitis).

This ingredient is boiled to get juice. Taking it will resolve [toxin].

【原文】

（九十七）

蟹目相向，足斑目赤者，不可食之。

【今译】

螃蟹两眼对视，足上有斑纹，两目发赤，不可食用。

【原文】

（九十八）

食蟹中毒治之方

紫苏

煮汁，饮之三升。紫苏子捣汁饮之，亦良。

【今译】

吃螃蟹中毒的治疗处方是紫苏。煮煎后取汁，每次服饮三升。用紫苏子捣其汁后饮之，效果亦好。

【原文】

又方

冬瓜汁，饮二升。食冬瓜亦可。

【今译】

另外一个处方是取冬瓜汁，饮用二升就可解毒。直接吃冬瓜效果也很好。

【英译】

Line 24. 97

Crabs with eyes facing each other, spots over the feet and red eyes are inedible.

【英译】

Line 24. 98

The formula for treating posioning from eating crabs is Zisu (紫苏, perilla, Folium Perillae).

This ingredient is boiled to get juice. [The juice is] taken 3 *sheng* [each time]. To pound this ingredient and drink the juice, [the effect is] also excellent.

【英译】

Another formula is to drink juice of Donggua (冬瓜, wax gourd, Benincasa Hispida). To eat it also quite effective.

【原文】

(九十九)

凡蟹未遇霜,多毒。其熟者,乃可食之。

【今译】

凡是没有遇到霜的螃蟹,多有毒素。但煮熟以后,还是可以食用的。

【原文】

(一百)

蜘蛛落食中,有毒,勿食之。

【今译】

蜘蛛掉落到了食物中,食物中就会有毒素,不能吃。

【原文】

(一百零一)

凡蜂蝇虫蚁等,多集食上,食之致瘘。

【今译】

凡是蜂、蝇、虫、蚁等均有毒,经常飞落在食物上,吃了这样的食物就会导致瘘疮。

【英译】

Line 24. 99

[When] a crab has not encountered frost, [there must be] much toxin in it. [But when] well cooked, [it is] still edible.

【英译】

Line 24. 100

[When] a spider has dropped on food, [there must be] toxin [in the food]. Do not eat it.

【英译】

Line 24. 101

Bees, flies, worms and ants [are all toxic]. [Whenever they have flown over and] dropped on the food, [the food is toxic]. Eating it will cause fistula.

果实菜谷禁忌并治第二十五

【原文】

(一)

果子生食,生疮。

【今译】

吃生果子,会生疮。

【原文】

(二)

果子落地经宿,虫蚁食之者,人大忌食之。

【今译】

果子落地,经过一夜就会腐烂,如果虫蚁吃过,就会有毒,人应禁忌食用。

Chapter 25
[Diseases Caused by] Fruits, Vegetables and Grains:
Contraindications and Treatment

【英译】

Line 25. 1

Eating raw fruit may cause sores.

【英译】

Line 25. 2

[When] a fruit has dropped on the ground, [it will be rotted].
[If] worms and ants have eaten [some of] it, eating [the rest of] it
is absolutely forbidden.

【原文】

(三)

生米停留多日,有损处,食之伤人。

【今译】

生米放置了好几天,被虫鼠损处,食用后就会伤人。

【原文】

(四)

桃子多食令人热,仍不得入水浴,令人病淋沥寒热病。

【今译】

桃子吃多了,会令人心里烦热,但仍不能入冷水沐浴,这样会令人恶寒发热,或患淋沥病。

【原文】

(五)

杏酪不熟,伤人。

【今译】

杏酪没有酿造成熟,吃了会伤人。

【英译】

Line 25.3

[When] uncooked rice has been kept for several days, [it] may be damaged [by worms or mice]. Eating it will harm the person.

【英译】

Line 25.4

Eating too many peaches will make the person hot. [If he] enters [cold] water to bathe, [it will] cause [aversion to cold and fever or] strangury.

【英译】

Line 25.5

[If] paste [made of] apricot [kernel] is not well cooked, [eating it will] damage the person.

【原文】

（六）

梅多食，坏人齿。

【今译】

梅子吃多了，会损坏牙齿。

【原文】

（七）

李不可多食，令人胪胀。

【今译】

李子不可多吃，吃多了令人腹胀。

【原文】

（八）

林檎不可多食，令人百脉弱。

【今译】

林檎不可多吃，吃多了令人百脉虚弱。

【英译】

Line 25.6

Eating too many mumes will ruin the teeth.

【英译】

Line 25.7

Plum cannot be eaten too many. [It will] cause abdominal distension.

【英译】

Line 25.8

Chinese crabapple cannot be eaten too much. [It will] weaken all the vessels [in the body].

【原文】

(九)

橘柚多食,令人口爽,不知五味。

【今译】

橘子和柚子吃多了,令人感到口淡,不能辨别其他滋味。

【原文】

(十)

梨不可多食,令人寒中。金疮、产妇,亦不宜食。

【今译】

梨不可多吃,吃多了令人脾胃虚寒。有创伤的人和产妇,也不宜食用。

【原文】

(十一)

樱桃、杏多食,伤筋骨。

【今译】

樱桃和杏子吃多了,就会损伤筋骨。

【英译】

Line 25.9

Eating too much tangerine or pomelo makes the mouth uncomfortable and unable to differentiate the five flavors.

【英译】

Line 25.10

Pears cannot be eaten too much. [Eating much of it will] make the middle (spleen and stomach) cold. People with traumatic injury and women with pregnancy should not eat it.

【英译】

Line 25.11

Eating too many cherries and apricots will injure the sinews and bones.

【原文】

（十二）

安石榴不可多食，损人肺。

【今译】

安石榴不能多吃，吃多了会损伤肺脏。

【原文】

（十三）

胡桃不可多食，令人动痰饮。

【今译】

胡桃不能多吃，吃多了令人呕吐痰饮。

【原文】

（十四）

生枣多食，令人热渴、气胀。寒热羸瘦者，弥不可食，伤人。

【今译】

生枣吃多了，令人发热、口渴、气胀。恶寒、发热、羸瘦的人，尤其不能吃，吃了就会伤人。

Volume 3

【英译】

Line 25. 12

Pomegranates cannot be eaten too many. [It will] injure the lung.

【英译】

Line 25. 13

Walnuts cannot be eaten too many. [It will] cause vomiting of phlegm and retained fluid.

【英译】

Line 25. 14

Raw jujubes cannot be eaten too many. [It will] cause fever, thirst and qi distension. Those with aversion to cold, fever and emaciation are absolutely forbidden to eat [because it] damages health.

【原文】

（十五）

食诸果中毒治之方

猪骨（烧灰）

右一味，末之，水服方寸匕。亦治马肝、漏脯等毒。

【今译】

治疗因食各种果实而中毒的处方是猪骨（烧灰）。压成粉末，每次用水服用一方寸匕。也可用以治疗因食马肝和漏脯而中毒的患者。

【原文】

（十六）

木耳赤色及仰生者，勿食。菌仰卷及赤色者不可食。

【今译】

木耳颜色变红，形式仰卷，不可以食用。仰卷及红色的菌类均不可食用。

【英译】

Line 25. 15

The formula for treating poisoning from eating various fruits is Zhugu（猪骨，pig's bone，Os Suis）（burn to ash）.

This ingredient is ground into powder and taken 1 *fangcunbi* [each time] with water. [It] can also treat poisoning from horse liver and minced meat.

【英译】

Line 25. 16

The Chinese wood fungus that becomes red and curls upward cannot be eaten. Any mushrooms appearing like that are also inedible.

【原文】

(十七)

食诸菌中毒闷乱欲死治之方

人粪汁饮一升,土浆饮一二升。大豆浓煮汁饮之。服诸吐利药,并解。

【今译】

因食用各种菌类而中毒,闷乱欲死的治疗处方如下:

饮用人粪汁一升,饮用泥水一或二升,或饮用大豆浓汁。服用一些其他引发呕吐和泄泻的药物,就能解毒。

【原文】

(十八)

食枫柱菌而哭不止,治之以前方。

【今译】

食用枫柱菌后哭啼不止的,可用前面提到的处方治疗。

Volume 3

【英译】

Line 25. 17

The formula for treating poisoning from eating various mushrooms, [marked by] depression, derangement and impending death, is the following.

To drink 1 *sheng* of juice squeezed from human stool, to drink 1 or 2 *sheng* of water from soil, or to drink some thick juice from soybeans, or to take other medicinals for inducing vomiting and diarrhea to resolve [toxin].

【英译】

Line 25. 18

Eating mushrooms from liquidambar wood causes incessant crying. [It can be] treated by the formula mentioned above.

【原文】

（十九）

误食野芋,烦毒欲死,治之以前方。

【今译】

误食野芋后,烦躁、中毒、欲死,可以前面提到的处方治疗。

【原文】

（二十）

蜀椒闭口者有毒,误食之,戟人咽喉,气病欲绝。或吐下白沫,身体痹冷,急治之方:

肉桂,煎汁饮之,多饮冷水一二升。或食蒜,或饮地浆,或浓煮豉汁饮之,并解。

【今译】

蜀椒闭口的有毒,误食之后,损伤咽喉,气机闭阻欲绝。或使人吐下白沫,身体痹冷,急治之方如下:

肉桂,煎煮后取汁服饮,多饮一二升冷水。或者吃蒜,或者饮地浆,或者饮用煮煎的豉子浓汁,合用以解其毒。

【英译】

Line 25. 19

Wrong eating of taro rhizome causes vexation, poisoning and impending death. [It can be] treated by the formula mentioned above.

【英译】

Line 25. 20

Zanthoxylum that is not split open is toxic. Wrong eating will irritate the throat and cause [disorder of] qi activity [which is] about to end, or vomiting and diarrhea of white foam, generalized impediment and cold. [Following is] the formula for treating [it] urgently.

Rougui （肉桂, cinnamon, Cinnamomi) is decocted to get juice. [The juice is] taken with more than 1 or 2 *sheng* of cold water. [Besides,] garlic can be eaten, or water from the earth can be drunken, thick boiled juice of soybeans can be taken. Combined [use of these ingredients will] resolve [toxin].

【原文】

（二十一）

正月勿食生葱，令人面生游风。

【今译】

正月不要吃生葱，吃了会令人面生游风。

【原文】

（二十二）

二月勿食蓼，伤人肾。

【今译】

二月不宜食用蓼茎，食用了会伤肾。

【原文】

（二十三）

三月勿食小蒜，伤人志性。

【今译】

三月不能吃小蒜，吃了伤人的志性。

Volume 3

【英译】

Line 25.21

[In] January [in the traditional Chinese calendar], raw scallion should not be eaten. [It will] cause wind wandering on the face (facial sores or redness and swelling of face).

【英译】

Line 25.22

[In] February [in the traditional Chinese calendar], smartweed should not be eaten. [It] damages the kidney.

【英译】

Line 25.23

[In] March [in the traditional Chinese calendar], rocambole should not be eaten. [It] damages the will [controlled by the kidney] and nature [controlled by the heart].

【原文】

(二十四)

四月、八月勿食胡荽,伤人神。

【今译】

四月和八月不能吃胡荽,吃了会伤人的神。

【原文】

(二十五)

五月勿食韭,令人乏气力。

【今译】

五月不能吃韭菜,吃了会令人缺乏气力。

【原文】

(二十六)

五月五日勿食生菜,发百病。

【今译】

五月五日不能吃生菜,吃了易发百病。

【英译】

Line 25.24

[In] April and August [in the traditional Chinese calendar], coriander cannot be eaten. [It] damages the spirit of a person.

【英译】

Line 25.25

[In] May [in the traditional Chinese calendar], garlic chive should not be eaten. [It] causes deficiency of qi and energy.

【英译】

Line 25.26

[On] May fifth [in the traditional Chinese calendar], any raw vegetables should not be eaten. [Otherwise it will] cause various diseases.

【原文】

（二十七）

六月、七月勿食茱萸，伤神气。

【今译】

六月和七月不能吃茱萸，吃了会损伤神气。

【原文】

（二十八）

八月、九月勿食姜，伤人神。

【今译】

八月和九月不能吃生姜，吃了伤人的神。

【原文】

（二十九）

十月勿食椒，损人心，伤心脉。

【今译】

十月不能吃蜀椒，吃了损害心脏，伤害心脉。

【英译】

Line 25.27

[In] June and July [in the traditional Chinese calendar], cornel should not be eaten. [It] damages spirit and qi.

【英译】

Line 25.28

[In] August and September [in the traditional Chinese calendar], ginger should not be eaten. [It] damages the spirit of a person.

【英译】

Line 25.29

[In] October [in the traditional Chinese calendar], pepper [growing in Sichuan] should not be eaten. [It] ruins the heart and damages the vessels in the heart.

【原文】

（三十）

十一月、十二月勿食薤，令人多涕唾。

【今译】

十一月和十二月不能吃生薤，吃了令人多涕多唾。

【原文】

（三十一）

四季勿食生葵，令人饮食不化，发百病。非但食中，药中皆不可用，深宜慎之。

【今译】

一年四季都不能吃生葵，吃了令人饮食不消化，引发百病。不但饮食中不能吃，作为药用，也要慎重。

【原文】

（三十二）

时病差未健；食生菜，手足必肿。

【今译】

患病者尚未康健的时候，如果吃了生菜，手足必然肿胀。

【英译】

Line 25.30

[In] November and December [in the traditional Chinese calendar], [raw] onion should not be eaten. [It] causes profuse snivel and spittle.

【英译】

Line 25.31

[In] the four seasons, raw mallow should not be eaten. [It] causes indigestion of food and various diseases. [It is] not only forbidden to eat, [but also] forbidden to use as medicinal.

【英译】

Line 25.32

[When] seasonal disease is not cured, eating raw vegetables will cause swelling of hands and feet.

【原文】

(三十三)

夜食生菜,不利人。

【今译】

夜晚吃生菜,不利消化。

【原文】

(三十四)

十月勿食被霜生菜,令人面无光,目涩,心痛,腰疼,或发心疟。疟发时,手足十指爪皆青,困萎。

【今译】

十月不能吃被霜打过的生菜,吃了令人面色无光,两目干涩,心痛,腰疼,或者引发心疟。心疟发作时,手指和脚趾都变青,精神困倦萎靡。

【原文】

(三十五)

葱、韭初生芽者,食之伤人心气。

【今译】

葱和韭菜刚生芽就吃了,会伤人的心气。

【英译】

Line 25.33

Eating raw vegetables at night causes indigestion.

【英译】

Line 25.34

[In] October [in the traditional Chinese calendar], raw vegetables exposed to frost should not be eaten. [It will] cause dull facial complexion, dryness of eyes, heart pain, lumbago, or malaria in the heart. [When] malaria occurs, all the fingers and toes become blue with cachexia.

【英译】

Line 25.35

Eating scallion and garlic chive that are just sprouting damages heart qi.

【原文】

(三十六)

饮白酒,食生韭,令人病增。

【今译】

喝白酒,吃生韭菜,会令人病情加剧。

【原文】

(三十七)

生葱不可共蜜食之,杀人。独颗蒜弥忌。

【今译】

生葱不能与蜂蜜一同食用,食用了就会致命。独颗蒜更不能与蜂蜜一起吃。

【原文】

(三十八)

枣合生葱食之,令人病。

【今译】

枣与生葱一同食用,会令人生病。

Volume 3

【英译】

Line 25.36

Drinking alcohol and eating raw garlic chive will worsen disease.

【英译】

Line 25.37

Raw scallion should not be eaten together with honey. ［Eating it will］ kill the person. Garlic with single clove is especially forbidden ［to eat with honey］.

【英译】

Line 25.38

Eating jujube together with scallion will cause disease.

【原文】

（三十九）

生葱和雄鸡、雉、白犬肉食之,令人七窍经年流血。

【今译】

生葱和雄鸡、雉鸟、白狗肉一同食用,会令人七窍经常流血。

【原文】

（四十）

食糖、蜜后四日内,食生葱、韭,令人心痛。

【今译】

吃了糖喝了蜂蜜四天之内,如果又吃了生葱和韭菜,会令人心痛。

【原文】

（四十一）

夜食诸姜、蒜、葱等,伤人心。

【今译】

夜晚吃了任何姜、蒜、葱等,都会伤人心。

【英译】

Line 25.39

Eating raw scallion with the meat of roosters, pheasants and white dogs will cause frequent bleeding from the seven orifices.

【英译】

Line 25.40

Within four days after eating sugar and honey, eating raw scallion and garlic chive will cause heart pain.

【英译】

Line 25.41

Eating any ginger, garlic and scallion at night will damage the heart.

【原文】

(四十二)

芜菁根多食之,令人气胀。

【今译】

芜菁根吃多了,就会令人气胀。

【原文】

(四十三)

薤不可共牛肉作羹食之,成瘕病。韭亦然。

【今译】

薤白、韭菜和牛肉不可一起做成肉羹吃,吃了就会引起瘕积病。

【原文】

(四十四)

莼多食,动痔疾。

【今译】

莼菜吃多了,会使人气壅,导致痔疾的发生。

Volume 3

【英译】

Line 25.42

Eating too much turnip root will cause qi distension.

【英译】

Line 25.43

Meat broth made together with onion，garlic chive and beef will cause lump disease.

【英译】

Line 25.44

Eating too much water shield causes hemorrhoids.

【原文】

(四十五)

野苣不可同蜜食之,作内痔。

【今译】

野苣不能与蜂蜜一同食用,否则就会引发内痔。

【原文】

(四十六)

白苣不可共酪同食,作䘌虫。

【今译】

白苣不能与乳酪一起食用,否则就会引发䘌虫。

【原文】

(四十七)

黄瓜食之,发热病。

【今译】

黄瓜吃多了,就会引发热病。

Volume 3

【英译】

Line 25.45

Bitter sow thistle cannot be eaten together with honey. [It will] cause internal hemorrhoids.

【英译】

Line 25.46

Lettuce cannot be eaten together with koumiss. [It will cause] ground beetles.

【英译】

Line 25.47

Eating too much cucumber will cause heat disease.

【原文】

(四十八)

葵心不可食,伤人。叶尤冷,黄背赤茎者,勿食之。

【今译】

冬葵叶的嫩心不可食用,食用了将伤人。其叶子尤其冷苦,黄背叶和赤色茎,也不可食用。

【原文】

(四十九)

胡荽久食之,令人多忘。

【今译】

胡荽吃的时间久了,会令人记忆力减退。

【原文】

(五十)

病人不可食胡荽及黄花菜。

【今译】

患病之人不可食用胡荽及黄花菜。

【英译】

Line 25. 48

[The tender] center of mallow cannot be eaten. [It] damages the person [eating it]. Its leaves are especially cold. [The one with] yellow back and red stalk is also inedible.

【英译】

Line 25. 49

Eating coriander over time causes hypomnesis.

【英译】

Line 25. 50

Patients should not eat coriander and day lily.

【原文】

(五十一)

芋不可多食,动病。

【今译】

芋不能多吃,多吃了会引起肠胃病。

【原文】

妊妇食姜,令子余指。

【今译】

妇女怀孕后吃生姜,会使胎儿长出多余的手指。

【原文】

(五十三)

蓼多食,发心痛。

【今译】

蓼实吃多了,就会引发心痛。

【英译】

Line 25.51

Taro should not be eaten too much. [It will] cause [intestinal and stomach] disease.

【英译】

Line 25.52

Eating ginger [after] pregnancy will cause the fetus to have extra fingers.

【英译】

Line 25.53

Eating too much water pepper [fruit] will cause heart pain.

【原文】

(五十四)

蓼和生鱼食之,令人夺气,阴核疼痛。

【今译】

蓼实和生鱼一同食用,会使人肺气夺失,引起阴囊疼痛。

【原文】

(五十五)

芥菜不可共兔肉食之,成恶邪病。

【今译】

芥菜不能与兔肉一起食用,一起食用会引发恶邪病。

【原文】

(五十六)

小蒜多食,伤人心力。

【今译】

小蒜吃多了,就会损伤人的心力。

【英译】

Line 25.54

Eating water pepper [fruit] together with fish will exhaust qi and cause scrotum pain.

【英译】

Line 25.55

Eating mustard leaf together with rabbit meat will cause malignant disease.

【英译】

Line 25.56

Eating too much rocambole will damage heart strength.

【原文】

(五十七)

食躁或躁方

豉,浓煮汁饮之。

【今译】

因食菜中毒而烦躁或非因饮食中毒而自行烦躁的治疗处方是,将豆豉浓煮成汁,饮而治之。

【原文】

(五十八)

钩吻与芹菜相似,误食之,杀人,解之方:

荠苨(八两)

右一味,水六升,煮取二升,分温二服。钩吻生地傍无他草,其茎有毛者,以此别之。

【今译】

钩吻与芹菜相似,误食后会夺人性命,解毒之方是荠苨(八两)。

【英译】

Line 25.57

The formula [for treating] vexation [due to] food or [due to] self agitation is to boil Douchi (豆豉，fermented soybean，Semen Glycines Fermentatum) to get thick juice. Taking [it will resolve vexation].

【英译】

Line 25.58

Yellow jessamine is similar to celery. Eating it wrong will kill the person. The formula for resolving it is Qini (荠苨，apricot-leaved adenophora，Radix Adenophorae Trachelioidis).

8 *liang* of this ingredient is decocted in 6 *sheng* of water to get 2 *sheng* [after] boiling. [The decoction is] divided into two [doses] and taken warm. The place where Gouwen (钩吻，yellow jessamine，Herba Gelsemii) grows has no other grasses. Downy stalk is the only mark to differentiate it.

【原文】

(五十九)

菜中有水莨菪,叶圆而光,有毒,误食之,令人狂乱,状如中风,或吐血,治之方:

甘草煮汁,服之即解。

【今译】

菜中有水莨菪,其叶子圆而有光,但却有毒,误食之会令人狂乱,就像中风一样,或者吐血。其治疗方子为将甘草煮成汁,服用后就能解毒。

【原文】

(六十)

春秋二时,龙带精入芹菜中,人偶食之为病,发时手青腹满,痛不可忍,名蛟龙病,治之方:

硬糖(二三升)

右一味,日两度服之,吐出如蜥蜴三五枚,差。

【今译】

在春秋两个季节,像蛟龙一样的蜥蜴类虫子遗精于芹菜中,人若偶而食之就会发病,发病时手青腹满,痛不可忍,此病名叫蛟龙病,其治疗方子如下:

硬糖(二三升),每天服用两次,服用后会吐出像蜥蜴一样的虫子三五枚,病就治好了。

【英译】

Line 25.59

Among vegetables, there is water henbane with round and shiny leaves which is toxic. Eating it by mistake will cause mania like wind stroke or blood vomiting. The formula for treating [it is] juice of Gancao (甘草, licorice, Radix Glycyrrhizae) [made by] boiling. Taking it will resolve [toxin].

【英译】

Line 25.60

In spring and autumn, [there are insects like] flood loong that excretes some sperms in the celery. [If] a person has eaten it by accident, [it will cause] blueness in the hands, abdominal fullness and unbearable pain. [This is] called flood loong disease. The formula for treating it is 2 or 3 *sheng* of Yingtang (硬糖, hard malt sugar, Durum Maltosum). [It is] taken twice a day. [When] 3 or 5 [insects] like lizard are vomited out, [the disease will be] cured.

【原文】

（六十一）

食苦瓠中毒治之方

黍穰煮汁，数服之解。

【今译】

吃苦瓠（即苦壶芦）中毒，治疗的方子为黍穰煎煮的汁，服用数次就可解毒。

【原文】

（六十二）

扁豆，寒热者不可食之。

【今译】

恶寒发热的患者不可食用扁豆。

【原文】

（六十三）

久食小豆，令人枯燥。

【今译】

长时间食用小豆，会令人皮肤枯燥。

【英译】

Line 25. 61

［For］ treating poisoning from eating bitter calabash，the formula is Shurang（黍穰，broomcorn millet or grain stalk）. ［It is］ boiled to get juice. Taking ［the juice］ several times will resolve ［toxin］.

【英译】

Line 25. 62

［Patients with］ aversion to cold and fever should not eat lablab ［because it is sweet in taste，warm in property and stagnant in nature，tending to promote qi］.

【英译】

Line 25. 63

Eating rice bean for a long time causes dryness ［of the skin and emaciation］.

【原文】

(六十四)

食大豆屑,忌噉猪肉。

【今译】

吃大豆屑后,不能再吃猪肉,否则难以消化。

【原文】

(六十五)

大麦久食,令人作疥。

【今译】

大麦吃的时间久了,令人发作疥疮。

【原文】

(六十六)

白黍米不可同饴、蜜食,亦不可合葵食之。

【今译】

白黍米不能与饴糖和蜂蜜一同食用,也不可与冷滑的葵一起食用。

【英译】

Line 25.64

It is forbidden to eat pork [after] eating soybean flakes [because it will cause indigestion, especially for children].

【英译】

Line 25.65

Eating barley for a long time will cause sores.

【英译】

Line 25.66

Broomcorn millet cannot be eaten together with malt sugar and honey, or with mallow [which is cold in nature and slippery in property].

【原文】

(六十七)

蚝麦面多食,令人发落。

【今译】

荞麦面吃多了,会令人头晕目眩。

【原文】

(六十八)

盐多食,伤人肺。

【今译】

盐吃多了,会损伤肺脏。

【原文】

(六十九)

食冷物,冰人齿。食热物,勿饮冷水。

【今译】

吃了过冷的食物,会使牙齿冰冷。吃热烫的食物时,不要立刻饮用冷水。

【英译】

Line 25.67

Eating too much buckwheat flour will cause dizziness and blurred vision.

【英译】

Line 25.68

Eating a great deal of salt will damage the lung.

【英译】

Line 25.69

Eating cold food will freeze the teeth. [When] eating hot food, avoid drinking cold water [immediately, otherwise it will damage the spleen and stomach, resulting in vomiting or dampness syndrome/pattern].

【原文】

（七十）

饮酒食生苍耳,令人心痛。

【今译】

饮酒后吃生苍耳,会令人心痛。

【原文】

（七十一）

夏月大醉汗流,不得冷水洗着身及使扇,即成病。

【今译】

夏天醉酒后大汗淋漓,不能用冷水洗身,也不能用扇子扇风,否则就会引发疾病。

【原文】

（七十二）

饮酒大忌灸腹背,令人肠结。

【今译】

饮酒后不能灸治腹背,否则会令人肠结。

Volume 3

【英译】

Line 25. 70

Eating fresh xanthium ［after］ drinking wine will cause heart pain.

【英译】

Line 25. 71

［In］ summer，［if there is］ profuse sweating ［when a person is］ drunken，he should not wash ［the body with］ cold water or ［resolve sweating by］ using fan，［otherwise it will］ cause disease.

【英译】

Line 25. 72

［It is］ forbidden to ［treat］ the abdomen and back with moxibustion ［after］ drinking wine ［because it will］ cause binding of the intestines.

【原文】

(七十三)

醉后勿饱食,发寒热。

【今译】

醉后不能吃的太饱,否则将引发寒热之症。

【原文】

(七十四)

饮酒食猪肉,卧秫稻穰中,则发黄。

【今译】

饮酒后再吃猪肉,吃饱后躺卧在高粱和稻草中,会导致周身发黄。

【原文】

(七十五)

食饴多饮酒,大忌。

【今译】

食用饴糖后又多饮酒,应当大忌。

【英译】

Line 25.73

[It is] forbidden to overeat [when a person is] drunken, [otherwise it will] cause aversion to cold and fever.

【英译】

Line 25.74

Lying on sorghum or rice straw [after] drinking wine and eating pork will cause generalized yellowing.

【英译】

Line 25.75

[It is] absolutely forbidden to drink wine [after] eating malt sugar.

【原文】

(七十六)

凡水及酒照见人影动者,不可饮之。

【今译】

凡是水和酒能照见人影,人没有动而影子却在晃动的,不可饮用。

【原文】

(七十七)

醋合酪食之,令人血瘕。

【今译】

醋与酪一起食用,会令人产生血瘕。

【原文】

(七十八)

食白米粥,勿食生苍耳,成走疰。

【今译】

吃白米粥时,不能吃生苍耳,否则就会造成走疰。

【英译】

Line 25.76

[It is] forbidden to drink water and wine that can reflect and stir the silhouette [of a person because of profuse toxin in it].

【英译】

Line 25.77

Eating vinegar together with koumiss will cause blood stagnation.

【英译】

Line 25.78

[It is] forbidden to eat raw xanthium [when] eating white rice porridge [because it will] cause running fixation (paralysis or rheumatism).

【原文】

(七十九)

食甜粥已,食盐即吐。

【今译】

吃了甜粥后再吃盐,就会引起呕吐。

【原文】

(八十)

犀角筋搅饮食,沫出,及浇地坟起者,食之杀人。

【今译】

用犀角筷子捣搅饮食,会产生白色泡沫,如果将其倒在地上而喷起,说明食中有毒,吃了会导致死亡。

【英译】

Line 25.79

Eating salt after eating sweet porridge will cause vomiting.

【英译】

Line 25.80

[If there] appears froth in food or drink [when stirred by] rhinoceros horn or [if the food or drink] sprays [when] poured on the ground, eating it will kill the person.

【原文】

(八十一)

饮食中毒烦满治之方

苦参(三两) 苦酒(一升半)

右二味,煮三沸,三上三下。服之,吐食出,即差。或以水煮亦得。

又方

犀角汤亦佳。

【今译】

饮食中毒后引发烦躁腹满的,治疗方子为苦参(三两)和苦酒(一升半)。煎煮三次,三上三下。服用后吐出所饮用的食物,就会解毒。或者用水煎煮,效果也可以。

另外一个处方是犀角汤,效果也很好。

【原文】

(八十二)

贪食,食多不消,心腹坚满痛治之方

盐(一升) 水(三升)

右二味,煮令盐消。分三服,当吐出食,便差。

【今译】

贪食,吃多了就会不消化,导致心腹坚硬、胀满、疼痛,治疗方子为盐(一升)和水(三升),通过煎煮使盐消化。分为三剂服用,服用后吐出所饮食物,身体就会康复。

Volume 3

【英译】

Line 25.81

Vexation and abdominal fullness [caused by] poisoning from food taken [can be] treated by the formula [composed of] 3 *liang* of Kushen (苦参, flavescent sophora, Radix Sophorae Flavescentis) and 1.5 *sheng* of Kujiu (苦酒, rice vinegar, Acetum). These two ingredients are boiled for three times, rising and falling thrice respectively. [When] food taken is vomited out, [toxin will be] resolved. To boil it with water, [the effect is] the same.

Another formula is Xijiao Decoction (犀角汤, rhinoceros horn, Cornu Rhinoceri), [the effect is] also excellent.

【英译】

Line 25.82

The formula for treating hardness, fullness and pain in the heart and abdomen [caused by] indigestion [due to] lycorexia [is composed of] 1 *sheng* of salt and 3 *sheng* of water. These two ingredients are decocted till salt is melted. [The decoction is] divided into three [doses]. [When] the food is vomited out [after] taking [the decoction], [the patient will be] cured.

【原文】

(八十三)

矾石生入腹,破人心肝,亦禁水。

【今译】

生的明矾食入腹后,会破坏心肝,也不能喝水。

【原文】

(八十四)

商陆,以水服,杀人。

【今译】

用水服用商陆会导致死亡。

【原文】

(八十五)

葶苈子,傅头疮,药成入脑,杀人。

【今译】

葶苈子可以治疗头疮,但若使疮毒入脑,导致死亡。

【英译】

Line 25.83

Eating raw Fanshi（矾石，alum，Alums）will injure the heart and liver. [It is] also forbidden to drink water [because water will melt alum and damage fluid in the body].

【英译】

Line 25.84

Taking Shanglu（商陆，phytolacca，Radix Phytolaccae）with water will cause death.

【英译】

Line 25.85

Tinglizi（葶苈子，semen tingli，Semen Lepidii）can be used to treat head sore. [But if] toxin enters the brain, [it will cause] death.

【原文】

(八十六)

水银入人耳及六畜等,皆死。以金银着耳边,水银则吐。

【今译】

水银进入人耳或六畜吃了,都会引起死亡。如果及时将金银放在耳边,水银就会被吐出来。

【原文】

(八十七)

苦练无子者杀人。

【今译】

金铃子不结子,毒性大,服用了会导致死亡。

【原文】

(八十八)

凡诸毒,多是假毒以投,不知时,宜煮甘草荠苨汁饮之,通除诸毒药。

【今译】

凡是有毒的食物都是人为所致,食用者不知道有人投毒时,吃了宜用煮甘草荠苨汁治疗,可消解一切毒素。

【英译】

Line 25.86

[When] mercury enters human ears or is eaten by six domestic animals, all will be killed. [But if] ears [are immediately] touched by gold and silver [jewelry], mercury will be vomited out.

【英译】

Line 25.87

Taking Kulian（苦练）, [actually referring to Jinlingzi（金铃子, Chinaberry, Fructus Tosendan）, quite toxic], [will cause] death.

【英译】

Line 25.88

[No food is toxic.] Toxic [foods] are mostly caused [by someone secretly adding] toxin [to the food]. [If the person who has eaten poisoned food] without knowing [it], boiled Gancao Qini Juice（甘草荠苨汁, licorice and adenophora juice）is the appropriate [formula for treating it]. All the toxin can be resolved.

图书在版编目(CIP)数据

金匮要略英译：英文/(东汉)张仲景著；刘希茹今译；李照国英译.—上海：上海三联书店,2022.8
(国学经典外译丛书.第一辑)
ISBN 978 - 7 - 5426 - 7799 - 0

Ⅰ.①金⋯　Ⅱ.①张⋯②刘⋯③李⋯　Ⅲ.①《金匮要略方论》—译文—英文　Ⅳ.①R222.3

中国版本图书馆 CIP 数据核字(2022)第 142545 号

国学经典外译丛书·第一辑

金匮要略英译

著　　者 / (东汉)张仲景
今　　译 / 刘希茹
英　　译 / 李照国
责任编辑 / 杜　鹃
装帧设计 / 徐　徐
监　　制 / 姚　军
责任校对 / 王凌霄

出版发行 / 上海三联书店
　　　　　(200030)中国上海市漕溪北路 331 号 A 座 6 楼
邮　　箱 / sdxsanlian@sina.com
邮购电话 / 021 - 22895540
印　　刷 / 上海颛辉印刷厂有限公司

版　　次 / 2022 年 8 月第 1 版
印　　次 / 2022 年 8 月第 1 次印刷
开　　本 / 640mm×960mm　1/16
字　　数 / 620 千字
印　　张 / 42.75
书　　号 / ISBN 978 - 7 - 5426 - 7799 - 0/R·125
定　　价 / 130.00 元

敬启读者,如发现本书有印装质量问题,请与印刷厂联系 021 - 56152633